Simple, Fast and Easy NCLEX® REVIEW

Your Ultimate Study Guide for Passing the NCLEX-RN and PN

NOTICE

Know and consider your scope of nursing practice and roles in the management, delegation and prioritization of care as you apply the information in this book in the NCLEX-RN and PN exam.

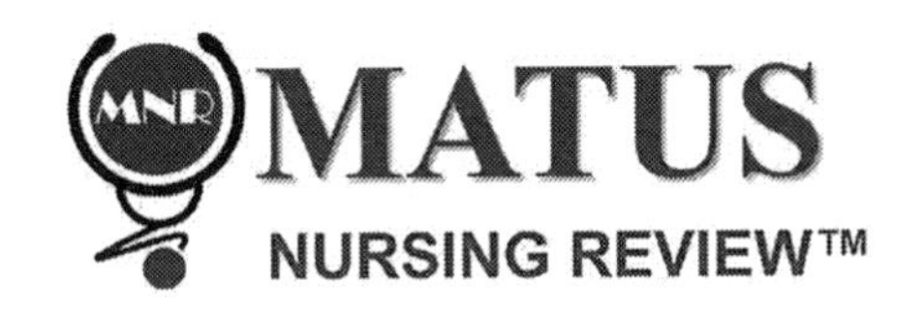

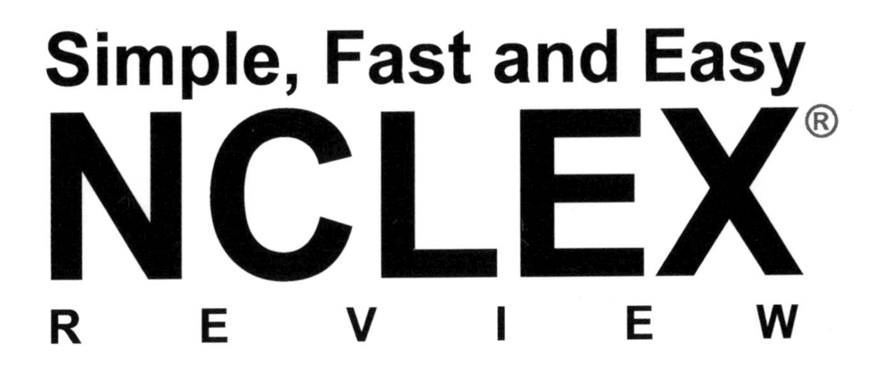

Your Ultimate Study Guide for Passing the NCLEX-RN and PN

ALAN JOHN MATUS, MSN, RN, CNE

California, USA 2018

Simple, Fast and Easy NCLEX® Review

Printed in the United States of America
First edition: March 2018
ISBN-13: 978-0-578-50890-0

Library of Congress Control Number: 2018902613

For special sales about buying this book in bulk quantities, please email: info@matusnursingreview.com

NOTICES

This book is solely intended for use in preparation for the National Council Licensure Examination. This is not a guide to the care and treatment of clients. Attention has been taken to verify the accuracy of the nursing contents and guideline practices presented. The author will not be held responsible for errors or omissions or for any consequences from the application of the information contained in this material. Application of information in clinical practice remains the sole responsibility of the licensed professional nurse. In view of continuous research, modification in public regulations and the ever-changing flow of information relating to medications and treatments, it is recommended that the reader review the latest updates in drug therapy and check the FDA status of each drug or device being intended for use in actual clinical nursing practice.

About the Author

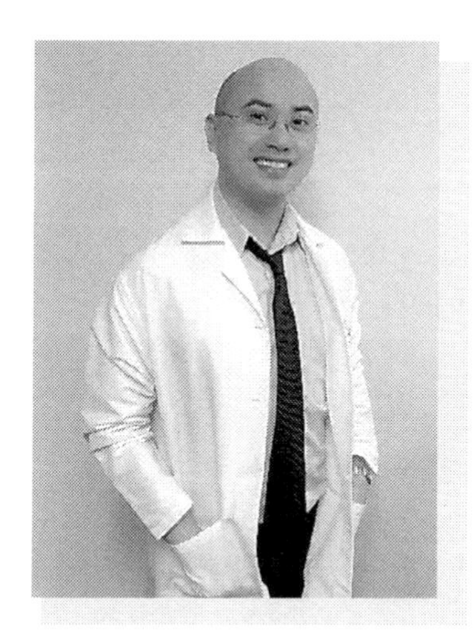

Alan John Matus is a seasoned nursing faculty and NCLEX instructor whose passion for NCLEX review spans over almost two decades. Before coming to the US, he served as a review instructor for the Nursing Board Exam and CGFNS Exam in the Philippines. He graduated Magna Cum Laude for his Bachelor of Science in Nursing Degree and was ranked as 3rd place topnotcher for the Philippines Nurse Licensure Exam. In 2011, he earned his Master of Science in Nursing - Nurse Educator Degree at California State University-Dominguez Hills. He was also inducted to the Phi Kappa Phi Honor Society and The Honor Nursing Society, Sigma Theta Tau International. In 2016, he passed the Nurse Educator Certification Exam (CNE) by the National League for Nursing. As a Certified Nurse Educator, he serves as a leader and role model demonstrating his expertise in academic nursing education. Alan has been a faculty in various nursing programs and specializes in NCLEX review, curriculum development, teaching strategies and assessment and evaluation of learning. For several years, he also served as the nurse educator for a care coordination initiative of a large health system and his collaborative work with skilled nursing facilities has been cited in several journal articles. Alan is the founder and lead instructor of Matus Nursing Review which provides live and online NCLEX review classes to nursing graduates. Currently, he is also the Director of Nursing Program of a nursing school in Los Angeles and oversees the overall supervision and implementation of the program curriculum. With his professional and leadership experience, Alan brings a wealth of knowledge that will greatly benefit many future nurses.

"As the US health care system undergoes a dramatic transformation, NCLEX remains inseparable from current nursing practice. My goal is to fill the knowledge gaps, inspire and enhance critical-thinking skills through innovative and engaging educational approaches in order for nursing graduates to pass the NCLEX, make a difference and thrive in the real world of health care."

Preface

Welcome to the first edition of Simple, Fast and Easy NCLEX Review! I hope that this book will help you pass your NCLEX exam by learning core nursing content in a concise, easy-to-read format.

As a nurse educator for many years, I understand that preparing for the NCLEX exam can be overwhelming especially if you do not have a clear grasp of topics or have been out of school for a long time. With so much information to learn, it is easy to get distracted and lose interest. You may also be taking the NCLEX for the first or second time but often find it challenging to open your books due to the excessive information that you have to read. This book is an essential study resource and has been designed for you to easily learn nursing concepts in the NCLEX. As you read this book, please take note of the following:

✓ Capitalized or bold texts that emphasize key concepts to remember
✓ NCLEX Alert! boxes that highlight care priority
✓ Fun acronyms that make recall of information much easier
✓ Tables that compare and contrast various similar disease conditions

I encourage you to read every chapter in this book, page by page, at least multiple times so you can connect the dots and understand the concepts. You may also cover the other half of the page to test your ability to recall information. My experience as a nursing faculty has greatly helped me create this material to facilitate your study preparation for the NCLEX exam. Thank you very much for allowing me to be a part of your journey to become a successful licensed professional nurse.

Alan John Matus

Are you ready? Know your ABC's to conquer the NCLEX!

Passing the NCLEX requires an organized, systematic plan to achieve your goal. As you prepare for your NCLEX exam, remember this "ABC Roadmap to NCLEX Success"!

A – Attitude and Determination
This is the most crucial factor as you prepare for the NCLEX. Without the burning fire to achieve your goal, you will easily give up when you encounter frustrations. You must stay inspired to wake up each morning excited to open your books. Remember, it is easy to get bored, tired and distracted when studying, so make sure that you always think of your purpose why you want to pass the NCLEX!

B – Basic Core Content Mastery
Some students think that answering thousands of NCLEX-style questions will make them pass. However, unless you have the mastery of basic nursing concepts, you will have a hard time passing the NCLEX. You should know core nursing content in order to enhance your critical thinking skills.

C – Critical Thinking and Test-Taking Skills
Once you have mastered core concepts in nursing, you will be ready to tackle critical-thinking questions. The magic of learning occurs when you answer NCLEX-style questions and read the rationales of answers. Make sure that the questions you answer are mostly on the application and analysis levels as these are the common types of questions in the NCLEX. What matters is not just the quantity but the quality of questions that you answer!

Now you know what the "ABC Roadmap to NCLEX Success" is all about. If you achieve all of these elements, then you will surely make it. Again, remember that it all starts with the right attitude so that you can put the time and effort to prepare and pass the NCLEX!

The ABC Roadmap To NCLEX Success

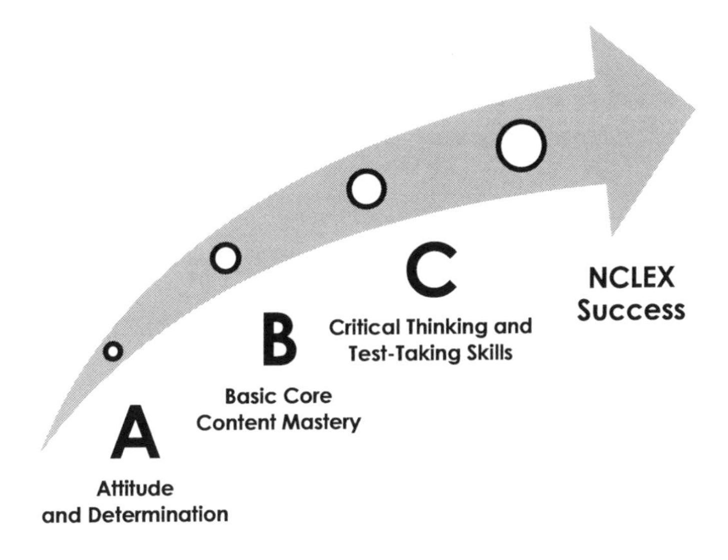

NCLEX Preparation Tips

As the days draw near towards your NCLEX exam, please note these important tips as you embark on your roadmap to NCLEX success!

Weeks Before the Exam

- Set a regular study schedule and adhere to it. Make a calendar of topics to study outlining your weak and strong areas. Make sure that you balance study hours with time for relaxation. Your brain needs to rest too!
- Explore study techniques that help you learn best. Remember, each person learns differently. Know your core content and practice lots of NCLEX questions!
- Surround yourself with people that will motivate you to reach your goal. Always remind yourself by asking, *"What is the best reason why I need to pass the NCLEX?"*.
- Be mindful when scheduling your NCLEX date. If you are not a morning person, it is better not to schedule the exam very early in the morning. Schedule your exam on the time you feel you will perform best!

The Day Before the Exam

- Relax and feel confident. Do something fun – watch a movie, have a laugh with friends or walk in the beach. You have prepared well-enough for the NCLEX, so take a deep breath and BELIEVE in yourself!
- Visit the testing venue if possible. Consider the travel time, traffic and weather on the day and time of your exam. If necessary, you may book a hotel near the testing venue.
- Call a supportive friend or relative to get one last encouragement and positive reinforcement.
- Have a good night rest. Sleep is very important so that you can concentrate well in answering questions. Never take any new medication that may affect your performance during the test!
- Prepare necessary items the night before the exam such as ID, eyeglasses and other important documents.
- Set an alarm clock. In fact, you can use more than one alarm clock if you want to make sure you wake up on time!

On the Day of Exam

- Have a healthy, nourishing and balanced breakfast. Do not drink anything that will make you feel anxious during the test.
- Bring some snacks that you can eat during the test break. Remember, you cannot think right when you are hungry!
- Wear clothing preferably in layers to make you comfortable in the testing room.
- Arrive at the testing venue early! You don't want severe anxiety to affect your concentration. Remember, you spent so much effort to prepare for this big day!
- Make sure that you follow instructions by the proctor especially items pertaining to exam integrity, breaks and use of computer. Do not bring items that are not allowed during the test.

During the Exam

- A little anxiety is helpful but when you start to feel more anxious, take several deep breaths, concentrate and tell yourself, *"I am ready and I can do this!".* Use the power of positive thinking!
- Read the question carefully.
- Understand what is being asked.
- Re-read the stem if necessary.
- Look for critical words - *most appropriate, early, late, best, first, initial, immediate, most likely.*
- Read the choices and use the process of elimination.
- Eliminate obviously wrong distractors immediately!
- Check what nursing action should be done before reporting the situation.
- If a client is in severe distress, intervene immediately.
- Remember your principles of prioritization and delegation of care.
- Assume that all clients are being cared for in an ideal hospital environment. Everything is ready and available!
- Do your best on every test item but do not take too much time on any question.
- Do not overthink! Remember, NCLEX is only testing you on core competencies expected from a BRAND NEW NURSE. The questions are not meant to trick you!

After Taking the Exam

- Finally, you made it through the big day! Take a deep breath and wait for the result of your exam patiently. Always remember, you are on your way to fulfilling your one ultimate dream – to become a licensed professional nurse!

Table of Contents

The National Council Licensure Examination (NCLEX®)

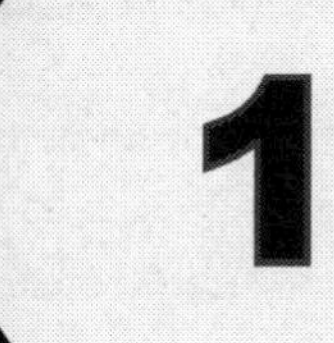

A. The NCLEX Process

❑ The __________ is the organization that develops and administers the NCLEX-PN and NCLEX-RN.	National Council of State Boards Nursing (NCSBN)
❑ What will the examinee receive once declared eligible to take the NCLEX by the State Board of Nursing?	Authorization to Test (ATT)
❑ Each ATT validity period is determined by the ________.	State Board of Nursing
❑ The average length of an ATT is ________.	90 days
❑ Examinee should schedule an NCLEX appointment to test through ______________________.	Pearson VUE
❑ What material provides the test blueprint for the NCLEX?	NCLEX Test Plan
❑ The ________________ estimates the ability of the examinee based on all the previous answers and difficulty of question items.	Computerized Adaptive Test (CAT)
❑ In addition to multiple-choice items, examinees will answer _________________________ that include Multiple-response items (Select all that apply), Hot spot items, Fill-in-the-blank items, Exhibit format, Ordered Response items and Audio and Graphic formats.	Alternate-Style Questions
❑ Minimum and maximum number of questions for NCLEX-PN	85 and 205
❑ Minimum and maximum number of questions for NCLEX-RN	75 and 265
❑ Maximum exam length for NCLEX-PN and NCLEX-RN	5 and 6 hours
❑ In Quick Results Service, the "unofficial" results are available how many hours after the exam?	48 hours, only in selected states*

B. Client Needs Categories in the NCLEX Exam

SAFE AND EFFECTIVE ENVIRONMENT	PHYSIOLOGICAL INTEGRITY	PSYCHOSOCIAL INTEGRITY	HEALTH PROMOTION AND MAINTENANCE
Protects clients from hazards.	Provision of comfort and assistance with ADL's and prevention of complications.	Promotion and maintenance of health and prevention and early identification of mental health problems.	Promotion and maintenance of health and prevention and early identification of health problems.

C. NCLEX Facts - *True or False?*

- ❑ I need to be well-prepared so I should wait longer after graduation before taking the NCLEX.

FALSE – After graduation, your nursing knowledge is still fresh especially after taking the exit exam. Prepare for your NCLEX wisely but do not wait for many months before taking the exam.

- ❑ As long as I answer thousands of NCLEX-style questions, I will surely pass the NCLEX.

FALSE – There's no shortcut to NCLEX success! Mastery of nursing core content is an essential prerequisite to enhance your critical thinking skills in answering NCLEX questions.

- ❑ I should not take the NCLEX if I am experiencing severe personal life stress.

TRUE - Psychological preparation is important to concentrate and answer NCLEX questions correctly.

- ❑ I should not touch the white board until the tutorial is over.

TRUE - When a white board is provided during the exam, the examinee should avoid writing anything until the exam starts to prevent suspicions of cheating.

- ❑ I should not bring in writing instruments for the NCLEX.

TRUE - Proctors will provide you materials during the exam. You do not need to bring your own writing materials.

- ❑ I should read the question carefully and understand what is asked before looking at the options.

TRUE - Failure to understand what is being asked in the main scenario will affect your chances of picking the right answer. So, read the stem of the question carefully!

- ❑ I will fail the NCLEX if I make mistakes in the first few number of questions.

  FALSE - The NCLEX gives examinees a chance to catch up even if answers on the first few items are wrong.

- ❑ I should answer the questions quickly so I do not run out of time.

  FALSE - Although spending too much time on any question is discouraged, answering in a hasty manner will result into poor analysis of question items.

- ❑ The computer will give questions based on my weak areas.

  FALSE - The computer chooses questions based on the examinee's performance on each question and picks an easier or harder question based on answers to prior questions. This is how the Computerized Adaptive Testing (CAT) operates.

- ❑ I can't skip questions.

  TRUE – The NCLEX does not allow examinees to skip or return to previous items.

- ❑ Most questions will be on the application and analysis levels.

  TRUE – Most of the questions will be on the application and analysis level. The NCLEX is an exam that evaluates critical thinking in clinical nursing practice.

- ❑ There are pilot questions and I will notice them for sure.

  FALSE – The 15 pilot questions are not recognizable during the exam and do not count towards exam performance.

- ❑ The NCLEX exam will usually include generic drug names only.

  TRUE – In most occasions, NCLEX will provide the generic names of medications as they tend to be more consistent.

- ❑ If I failed answering the "Select All That Apply (SATA)" questions, I will fail the NCLEX.

  FALSE – Every question in the NCLEX will affect overall test performance and scoring except the pilot questions.

- ❑ SATA questions may have one possible answer only, more than one answer, or all choices are correct.

  TRUE – Previously, SATA questions have a minimum of 2 correct answers, however this has changed. When answering SATA questions, treat each option as a true or false statement and eliminate those you think are wrong!

- ❑ Calculation items should be rounded at the end of the calculation.

  TRUE – Numbers should only be rounded when writing the final answer.

- ❑ Words such as "identify all except," "Which of the following is not," and "Choose the one that is not" are not found in the NCLEX exam.

  TRUE – These words or phrases are not found in the NCLEX.

- ❑ If the questions become more difficult, it means that I am doing a great job.

  TRUE – Yes, you will receive more difficult questions when your answers are correct!

- ❑ NCLEX will always include items reflecting the latest research findings.

  FALSE – NCLEX Test Plans are updated every 3 years to reflect current practice. Question items are not updated as soon as the latest clinical updates occur.

- ❑ The NCLEX exam is more difficult in other states.

  FALSE – The NCLEX is a national exam and the test difficulty does not vary in every state.

- ❑ The first optional break will be offered after 2 hours of testing and the next optional break is offered after 3 ½ hours during the test.

  TRUE - The breaks are optional. Remember, the breaks count against the testing time!

- ❑ If the computer does not stop at 75 or 85, I still have a chance to pass.

  TRUE – Yes, you still have a chance! The computer will only stop giving items when it is 95% certain that your ability is clearly above or clearly below passing standard.

- ❑ I will surely fail if I run out of time.

  FALSE – If you have answered the minimum number of items, the computer examines your last 60 ability estimates. You will pass if your last 60 ability estimates are above the passing standard.

- ❑ I should **NEVER** divulge any information about the questions I answered in the NCLEX exam.

  TRUE – The NCLEX has strict guidelines on protecting the integrity of the test questions. Examinees are expected to follow these policies to avoid suspension or revocation of the nursing license.

> ***NCLEX Alert!*** *Please visit www.ncsbn.org for updates about the NCLEX process.*

Test-Taking Strategies 2

A. Taking the NCLEX

How does the NCLEX setting look like?

- All clients receive care in an ideal, complete clinical setting
- Everything is ready, available and accessible for client care
- NCLEX questions are based on textbook concepts and not the real clinical world

Why do you pick the wrong answers?

- You did not understand what's being asked
- You overanalyze the case scenario
- You read very fast or very slow
- You simply are not familiar with the concept
- You had a mental block due to anxiety

What are Positive and Negative Questions?

- **Positive**
  You must select a choice that is correct
- **Negative**
  You must select a choice that is wrong

> ***NCLEX Alert!*** *Key words for negative questions include "needs further teaching" or "requires further intervention". Negative questions are usually harder to answer than positive questions.*

B. Conquer the NCLEX: Test-Taking Strategies

- ❑ Take your time and read the question carefully.
- ❑ Make sure that you understand what is being asked in the stem of the question. If you did not understand the stem, re-read if necessary.
- ❑ Read the choices and eliminate wrong distractors immediately! You want to focus on choices that will help you arrive at the right answer.
- ❑ A distractor should be completely accurate. If a distractor contains wrong information, do not choose that option.
- ❑ Avoid choices that include absolute words such as: *always, none, must, never, only, all and every.*
- ❑ Client refers to an adult person age 18-65 years-old. If the client is a child, it will be specifically stated.
- ❑ If the stem of the question includes descriptions about cultural and religious beliefs, they will usually be relevant in selecting the right answers.
- ❑ In most cases, do not answer restrain the client or give antipsychotic drugs. NCLEX wants a nurse who will apply alternative or least invasive interventions for a client.
- ❑ Check what nursing action may be done before reporting. NCLEX will usually test your ability to assess or intervene before calling the health care provider. Remember, most of the questions in the NCLEX will be in the application or higher level of learning, which means you have to use your critical-thinking skills and promote client safety first!

> ***NCLEX Alert!*** *If a client is in severe distress, intervene immediately! There is no need to perform additional assessment if the stem contains enough information about the client's condition.*

Bloom's Taxonomy of Learning

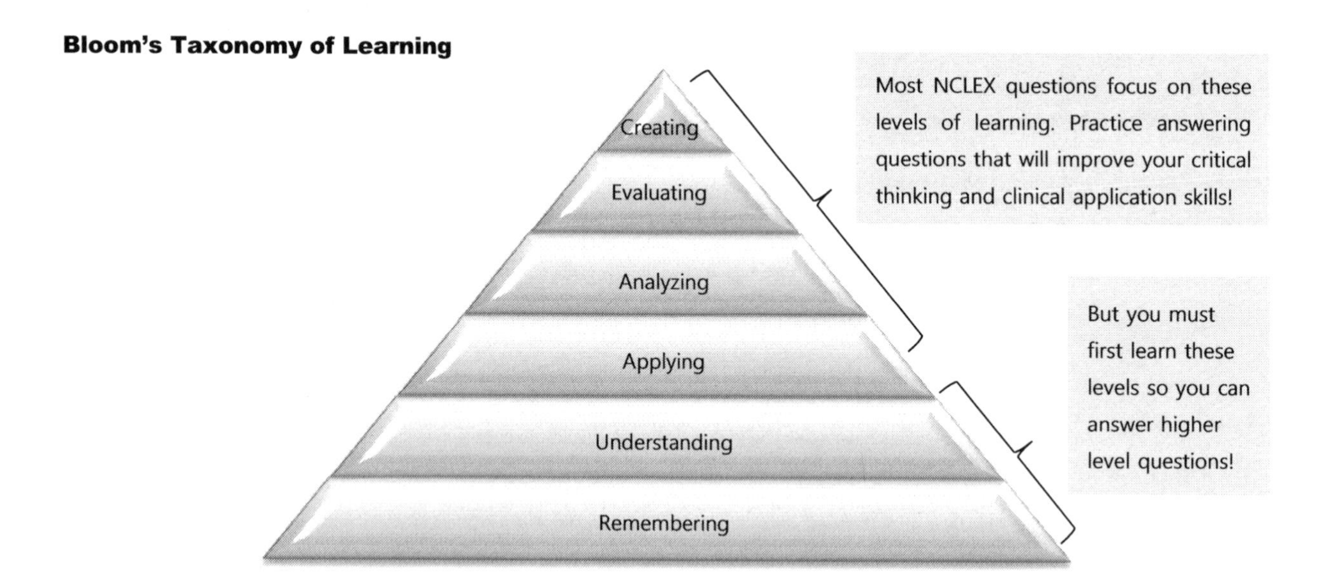

> ***NCLEX Alert!*** *Don't overanalyze every question. Just read the question for what it is and don't apply any extra information that are not there. Remember, NCLEX is just trying to see if you have the minimum competency required to safely practice as a new nurse - and that's it! NCLEX is all about safety!*

C. Prioritization of Client Care

High-Priority Conditions – *These should be on top of your list to learn before taking the NCLEX!*

- ❑ Burns of the face and neck
- ❑ Hip displacement
- ❑ Compartment syndrome
- ❑ Fat embolism
- ❑ Rhabdomyolosis
- ❑ Dumping syndrome
- ❑ Hepatic encephalopathy
- ❑ Acute pancreatitis
- ❑ Acute cholecystitis
- ❑ Acute intestinal obstruction
- ❑ Status asthmaticus
- ❑ Pulmonary embolism
- ❑ Severe pneumothorax
- ❑ Mediastinal shifting
- ❑ Acute asthmatic attack
- ❑ Ventricular fibrillation
- ❑ Pacemaker malfunction
- ❑ Cardiac arrest
- ❑ Hypertensive crisis
- ❑ Myocardial infarction
- ❑ Cardiac tamponade
- ❑ Acute pulmonary edema
- ❑ Ruptured aneurysm
- ❑ Severe hypoglycemia
- ❑ Diabetic ketoacidosis
- ❑ Hyperglycemic, Hyperosmolar, Non-Ketotic Coma
- ❑ Thyroid storm
- ❑ Myxedema coma
- ❑ Adrenal/Addisonian Crisis
- ❑ Anaphylaxis
- ❑ Sepsis
- ❑ Increased intracranial pressure
- ❑ Spinal and neurogenic shock
- ❑ Autonomic dysreflexia
- ❑ Myasthenic and cholinergic crisis
- ❑ Status epilepticus
- ❑ Stroke
- ❑ Meningitis
- ❑ Head injury
- ❑ Agranulocytosis/Neutropenia
- ❑ Thrombocytopenia
- ❑ Wound dehiscence and evisceration
- ❑ Retinal detachment
- ❑ Acute renal failure
- ❑ Acute larygospasm/Croup
- ❑ Sickle cell crisis
- ❑ Disseminated intravascular coagulation
- ❑ Pathologic jaundice in newborns
- ❑ Prolapsed umbilical cord
- ❑ Acute suicidal ideation
- ❑ Tardive dyskinesia
- ❑ Neuroleptic malignant syndrome
- ❑ Hypertensive crisis
- ❑ Severe hypo/hyperkalemia
- ❑ Severe hypo/hypercalcemia
- ❑ Severe hypo/hypernatremia
- ❑ Severe hypo/hypermagnesemia
- ❑ Severe hypo/hyperphosphatenemia
- ❑ Blood transfusion reactions
- ❑ Post-partum bleeding
- ❑ Amniotic fluid embolism
- ❑ Toxic shock syndrome
- ❑ Eclampsia
- ❑ HELLP syndrome
- ❑ Abruptio placenta
- ❑ Placenta previa

NCLEX Alert! *IMPORTANT CONCEPTS YOU SHOULD ALWAYS KEEP IN MIND!*

Presenting signs and symptoms, Priority actions, Diet, Labs, Emergency equipment, Positions, Complications

How Do You Prioritize Client Care? *Know these rules!*

Rule 1. Use the ABC principle, Maslow's Hierarchy of Needs and the Nursing Process. Always remember that physiologic needs (airway, breathing, circulation,) are more important than psychological needs.

Rule 2. Check the stem of the question for essential key words such as: *immediate, initial, most important, next, primary, first, highest priority, best.*

Rule 3. Several or all of the choices may be correct but you have to choose the best answer. So, it is always important to read all the distractors being provided!

Rule 4. Airway is a priority but not in all situations. For example, if the client has hypoglycemia, airway is not the priority unless the situation states that the client has an airway problem.

Rule 5. Prioritize **UNSTABLE** or **CRITICAL** client conditions. Clues or examples may include the following: *"marked change in symptoms, acute symptoms, sudden occurrence, symptoms unrelieved by interventions, immediate post-op, newly admitted, critical lab results, altered mental status, breathing problem, immediate danger or safety issues, low pulse oximetry reading, chest pain, low blood sugar"*

Rule 6. Prioritize **ACUTE** symptoms over expected symptoms of **CHRONIC** conditions. For example, a client who is having severe respiratory distress due to an allergy is more serious than a COPD client with dyspnea.

D. Delegation of Client Care

How Do You Delegate Client Care? *Know these rules!*

Rule 1. Remember the 5 R's of delegation: (1) The right task, (2) the right circumstance, (3) the right person, (4) the right direction or communication, and (5) the right supervision. (*American Nurses Association*)

Rule 2. Always delegate tasks based on the staff member's experience, training, skills, competence, scope of practice, job description and provisions in the State Nurse Practice Act. Care should not be delegated if there is no evidence that the staff has the competence to perform the task without supervision.

Rule 3. RN's do not delegate clients who: *are critical, unstable, newly-admitted, newly diagnosed, immediate post-operative, require continuous vital signs monitoring, need initial or complete assessment, need complete and complex teaching and have intravenous fluids and antibiotics.*

Rule 4. RN's should not assign unstable clients to the following nurses: *LPN, recent graduate nurses, unit floaters and registry, temporary or per diem nurses.*

Rule 5. Nursing assistants or unlicensed assistive personnel (UAP) may perform simple, non-complex tasks such as: *assisting with ADL's, hygiene care, positioning, ambulation, bathing, feeding, changing Foley bag, skin care, range-of-motion exercises and obtaining of vital signs of stable clients.*

NCLEX Alert! *Unlicensed assistive personnel (UAP) refers to unlicensed health care providers acting as support care team members in the provision of client care. It includes nursing assistants, nurse aides, orderlies, attendants or technicians. The UAP scope of function is determined by each State Nurse Practice Act. (National Council of State Boards of Nursing)*

RN	LPN	NURSING ASSISTANT/UAP
❑ Management of care	❑ Monitoring of stable clients	❑ Hygiene care
❑ Performing initial assessments	❑ Taking routine vital signs	❑ Positioning
❑ Assessment of unstable clients	❑ Administration of drugs except intravenous infusions	❑ Feeding
❑ Complex teaching	❑ Simple sterile procedures	❑ Bathing
❑ IV drug administration	❑ Reinforcement of teaching	❑ Ambulation
❑ Administering blood transfusion	❑ Simple teaching such as dressing change	❑ Skin care
❑ Managing invasive lines such as Swan Ganz catheter		❑ Range-of-motion exercises
		❑ Taking routine vital signs

NCLEX Alert! *RN's do not delegate what they can EAT - Evaluate, Assess, Teach. Tasks that require critical nursing judgment are not delegated. In the hospital, the LPN functions under the supervision of the RN. In the long-term care setting, the LPN is sometimes the charge nurse and is responsible for the care of clients.*

Delegation of Nursing Care - *RN, LPN OR UAP?*

1.	Assessing a newly-admitted client's pain	RN
2.	Developing the initial plan of care	RN
3.	Feeding a newly admitted stroke client with dysphagia	RN
4.	Positioning a client immediately after a hip joint surgery	RN
5.	Inserting a Foley catheter	LPN
6.	Caring for a client with newly-inserted cardiac stent	RN
7.	Changing bedsheets, bathing and collecting stool specimen	UAP
8.	Swan-Ganz catheter measurement and monitoring	RN
9.	Administering oral antihypertensive medications	LPN
10.	Administering Total Parenteral Nutrition (TPN)	RN

E. Tips on Answering Pharmacology Questions

- ❑ If you know the drug's classification, action and side effects, you will also know the interventions!
- ❑ Make sure you are familiar with the similarities in drug names: *e.g. zole, lol, mycin, zem, mycin, xaban.*
- ❑ Always assume a medication order is present.
- ❑ Note that some drugs have multiple actions and uses: *e.g. atropine sulfate, beta-blockers, benzodiazepines*
- ❑ You can't memorize everything about drugs but make sure, you know what most new nurses should know!

Do you know your drug prefixes or suffixes? How many more of these do you know?

NAMES	DRUG	NAMES	DRUG
- prazole	Proton Pump Inhibitor	**- mab**	Immunomodulators
- dipine, -pamil, -zem	Calcium-Channel Blocker	**- lukast**	Leukotriene Inhibitors
- olol	Beta-Blocker	**- profen**	NSAIDs
- statin	Lipid-Lowering Drugs	**- salazine**	Aminosalicylates
- epam	Benzodiazepines	**- cillin**	Penicillins
- pril	ACE Inhibitors	**- sterone**	Androgens
- floxacin	Fluoroquinolones	**- xaban**	Anticoagulants
- plase	Thrombolytics	**- conazole/azole**	Antifungal
- tidine	H_2 Blockers	**- phylline**	Xanthine Derivatives
- mycin	Aminoglycosides	**- barbital**	Barbiturates
- sone	Corticosteroids	**- antidine**	Antivirals
- kinase	Thrombolytics	**- caine**	Anesthetic
- lone	Corticosteroids	**cef -**	Cephalosporins
- olam	Benzodiazepines	**- cycline**	Tetracyclines
- zosin	Alpha-Blockers	**- nitro**	Nitrates
- thiazide	Thiazide diuretics	**- semide**	Loop Diuretics
- darone	Antiarrhythmic	**- quine**	Antimalarial
- sartan	Angiotensin Receptor Blocker (ARB)	**- dronate**	Biphosphonates
- thromycin	Macrolides	**- triptan**	Anti-migraine

Do you know your drug side effects?

EXAMPLES OF DRUG ACTION	SIDE EFFECTS
Decreases blood pressure	*Orthostatic hypotension*
Diuresis	*Hypotension, dehydration, hypokalemia, hyponatremia*
Vasodilation	*Orthostatic hypotension*
Blocks $beta_1$ and $beta_2$ cell receptors	*Hypotension, heart block, bronchoconstriction*
Depresses pain perception	*Respiratory depression*
Replaces thyroid hormones	*Hyperthyroidism (tachycardia, irritability, sweating)*
Replaces antidiuretic hormone (ADH)	*Water retention, edema*
Blocks dopamine	*Extrapyramidal symptoms/Parkinsonism*
Prolongs the clotting process	*Bleeding (hematuria, ecchymosis, hematoma)*
Stimulates release of insulin	*Hypoglycemia*
Stimulates uterine contraction	*Uterine tetany*
Suppresses the immune system	*Infection*
Inhibits the breakdown of acetylcholine	*Cholinergic effects (salivation, bradycardia, wheezing)*
Stimulates peristalsis	*Abdominal cramps, diarrhea*
Increases strength of cardiac contraction	*Polyuria*
Constricts the pupils	*Poor vision in darkness*

NCLEX Alert!

ANTICHOLINERGICS *(sympathetic) are not the same as* ***ANTICHOLINESTERASE*** *(parasympathetic) drugs. Many drugs have anticholinergic effects such as antihistamines, antidepressants, antipsychotics, bronchodilators, anti-Parkinsonians, atropine and antispasmodics.*

Anticholinergic side effects include ***dry mouth, constipation, urinary retention, blurred vision, mydriasis, bronchodilation, hypertension*** *and* ***tachycardia****. Be alert for these effects when studying your drugs because they will surely be in the NCLEX!*

F. Stick to Your Game Plan: Study Techniques

- ❑ Assess your readiness by making a list of your strong and weak areas. Remember, the first step in NCLEX preparation is to identify nursing content that you need to focus on!
- ❑ Create a "things to do" list and study calendar. This is important so you can get organized and study regularly until your NCLEX exam day. Take note, learning is more effective if studying takes place in smaller chunks over time.
- ❑ The morning hours are the best times to study as you are more alert and well-rested.
- ❑ Explore your preferred location to study such as the library, home or coffee shops. Avoid places that will distract you from concentrating and learning.
- ❑ Explore different study methods such as group, individual or online study sessions.
- ❑ Understand the pathophysiology of disease conditions as this will help you identify the signs and symptoms and rationale for nursing and medical interventions.
- ❑ Use study techniques to improve retention such as mnemonics, tables, flash cards, notes, concept mapping or even teaching the topics to your own self or others!
- ❑ Write and note rationales of NCLEX practice questions – even if you get the right answers! Remember, what works in the NCLEX is understanding the why's and how's and not the memorization of answers.
- ❑ Look up terms that you are not familiar with. Keep your resources handy such as your books or the internet.
- ❑ Avoid using too many NCLEX books that will take too much of your time for preparation. You should have an NCLEX review book as your main reference and several others as additional resources.
- ❑ Answer NCLEX-style questions as many as you can and do it every day! However, make sure that you do this while mastering your core content so you can effectively practice your critical-thinking skills.

G. Wrapping it up: Strategies for Preparation

- ❑ Stay motivated and focused on your goal – that is, to be a professional nurse!
- ❑ Be careful with social affairs and distractions especially during holiday season. Discipline is key to sticking with your game plan!
- ❑ Obtain enough rest and sleep. Your body also needs to recover from the hard work of studying.
- ❑ Practice a healthy lifestyle. Exercise regularly and enjoy recreational activities.
- ❑ Eat a nutritious diet and hydrate sufficiently. Avoid using alcohol or any recreational drugs.
- ❑ Practice relaxation techniques such as deep breathing, listening to music and meditation. Take note, your ability to manage stress is crucial to your NCLEX performance!

> ***NCLEX Alert!*** *Remember, you have to keep your focus until the day of exam. A motivated attitude coupled with persistence and hard work will help you in achieving your goal – that is, to pass the NCLEX and become a professional nurse!*

Principles of Nursing Practice

3

A. Ethical Concepts

❑ Distinguishes right and wrong actions or values	Ethics
❑ Personal beliefs about right or wrong behaviors	Morality
❑ To tell the truth	Veracity
❑ To serve equal benefits	Justice
❑ To perform what is promised	Fidelity
❑ To uphold right to self-determination	Autonomy
❑ To do good to others	Beneficence
❑ To cause no harm	Nonmaleficence
❑ Conflict between ethical principles that affects ability to make decisions and perform duties	Ethical dilemma
❑ A committee that aims to resolve and create solutions to ethical issues	Ethics Committee
❑ Standing up to ensure the client's best interest and welfare	Advocate
❑ A state act that regulates the practice of nursing and provides guidelines for professional violations	Nurse Practice Act
❑ Is the Nurse Practice Act the same for all states?	No, every state has its Nurse Practice Act
❑ Principle where employer is accountable for any negligence performed by an employee	Respondeat Superior
❑ Protocols of the organization that nursing staff should follow in the performance of duties	Institutional policies and procedures

B. Legal Concepts

Legal Terms and Definitions

❑ Threat of bodily harm with an apparent ability to cause injury	Assault
❑ Unlawful physical contact upon a threat	Battery
❑ Restraint of a person without legal justification	False Imprisonment
❑ Intentional deception to gain illegal benefits	Fraud
❑ Damaging the reputation of a person such as slander or libel	Defamation

❑ Nursing actions that fail to meet standards of care such as medication errors, preventable falls and failure to perform end-of-shift hand-off	Negligence
❑ Negligence of a licensed professional nurse	Malpractice
❑ An illegal action or an infringement of a right resulting to civil liability (e.g. false imprisonment, battery, assault, fraud, defamation, invasion of privacy)	Tort
❑ A minor wrongdoing considered to be less serious than a felony (e.g. drunk driving without injury, vandalism)	Misdemeanor
❑ Serious crime that includes physical harm to victims	Felony
❑ A law that encourages a health professional to help during emergency and provides basic protection from unintended consequences	Good Samaritan Law

Informed Consent

❑ What are important items to explain to a client before any major or invasive procedure?	Risk and benefits
❑ Who can sign a consent if the client is mentally incompetent?	Guardian, next of kin or the Durable Power of Attorney (DPOA) agent
❑ Is the nurse responsible for explaining the nature of a medical procedure or surgery?	No, the nurse only serves as a witness and the surgeon should explain the nature of treatment
❑ What drugs should not be given before the client signs a consent?	Mind-altering drugs such as sedatives
❑ Who cannot give consents?	Clients who are unconscious, sedated, have dementia or minors (unless emancipated)
❑ In what situations can consents be waived?	During emergency, mental therapy and status as emancipated minor
❑ What is an emancipated minor?	Emancipated minors achieved freedom from parental control and supervision through marriage, enlistment in the Armed Forces or by a court order. They are self-responsible before the age of majority.

Patient Health Information (PHI)

❑ What law provides data privacy and security provisions for protecting medical information?	HIPAA or Health Insurance Portability and Accountability Act of 1996
❑ When can PHI be disclosed legally?	To report a reportable disease or stop a dangerous threat to client and public safety (e.g. terrorism or suicide)
❑ What are the client rights regarding medical records?	Right to review a copy, change or apply restrictions to access
❑ Examples of invasion of privacy	Sharing client information to unauthorized personnel, accessing health information, posting photos of a client in social media and publication of client medical information
❑ What is Risk Management?	The process of identification, assessment, and analysis of risks to promote patient safety and control legal accountabilities
❑ Examples of reportable incidents	Falls, skin tears, client-to-client altercation
❑ Does an incident report replace nursing documentation?	No
❑ Are incident reports noted in nursing documentation or filed in the client's chart?	No, it is an internal document

Advance Health Care Directive

❑ What is an advance health care directive?	A client appoints a health care agent who will make healthcare decisions when unable to speak for self
❑ What are examples of client wishes in advance health care directives?	Life-sustaining treatments Physician preference Organ donation wishes Palliative care Comfort measures
❑ Who cannot serve as witnesses?	Health care agent, Health care provider
❑ Can the client make changes to the advance health care directive anytime?	Yes

❑ What makes an advance health care directive valid?

Client's signature; 2 witnesses/notarized; If the client is in a skilled nursing facility, the State of California requires the signature of the ombudsman or patient advocate as witness; State laws may vary

❑ What does a "Do Not Resuscitate" (DNR) order mean?

DNR does **NOT** mean "do not treat" the client. It only means that lifesaving measures will not be done when the client goes into cardiopulmonary arrest. The client may still be treated for ongoing health issues such as pneumonia, dehydration or urinary infection.

❑ What is a Physician Orders for Life-Sustaining Treatment (POLST) form?

POLST is a form that gives seriously ill clients more control over their end-of-life care, including medical treatment, lifesaving measures (such as a feeding tube or ventilator) and CPR. This form follows the client wherever he goes. (*www.capolst.org*)

Palliative Care versus Hospice Care

PALLIATIVE CARE	HOSPICE CARE
❑ Begins early in client care ❑ Client has chronic, life-threatening illness that causes stressful symptoms ❑ Goal is management of symptoms to improve quality of life	❑ Client has terminal illness ❑ Time frame is life expectancy < 6 months ❑ Goal is management of symptoms with emphasis on pain control for a dignified, pain-free death

Client Teaching

❑ What is *teach-back* method?

Asking the client to restate what has been taught using his or her own words

❑ What is the other name of teach-back method?

"Closing the loop" or "show me method"

❑ What kind of language should be used?

Plain language in a caring way

❑ Which question should be avoided?

"Do you understand?", as this does not ensure understanding of instructions

❑ What is the best method to teach and ensure understanding of a procedure (e.g. insulin injection)?

Demonstration-Return demonstration

C. Leadership and Management

Health Care Delivery System

Description	Term
❑ System of healthcare delivery that focuses on managing use, access, cost, quality and effectiveness of healthcare services	Managed Care
❑ Interdisciplinary process involving collaboration and coordination of client care	Case Management
❑ Evaluation of the appropriateness and necessity of health care services, equipment or procedures	Utilization Review

Nursing Care Delivery Systems

Description	Term
❑ Leader assigns tasks to staff responsible for providing care to the client	Team nursing
❑ Nurse provides care from admission to discharge	Primary nursing
❑ Divides nursing care into tasks such as medication administration or wound treatments	Functional nursing

Leadership Styles

Description	Term
❑ Provides incentives or punishments to members based on performance outcomes	Transactional
❑ Visionary leader inspires and motivates employees through passion and clear goals that lead to positive changes	Transformational
❑ Lacks direct supervision of employees and is effective only for highly trained or competent employees	Laissez-Faire
❑ Managers make decisions alone without the feedback or participation of employees	Autocratic
❑ Employees share ideas to the decision-making process	Democratic

Professional Nursing

Description	Term
❑ Has passionate, magnetic personality and influences others	Leader
❑ Task-oriented, controls others and ensures compliance with policies	Manager
❑ Types of Advanced Practice Nurses	Nurse Practitioner, Nurse Anesthetist, Clinical Nurse Specialist, Nurse Midwife
❑ An approach to care that utilizes the best research evidence or findings to promote quality nursing care	Evidence-Based Practice

Question	Answer
❑ A process that focuses on enhancing workflows and actions in the delivery of health care services	Quality/Performance Improvement
❑ Standardized and evidence-based care management plans that provide a sequence of interventions and outcomes in order to achieve quality care at a lower cost	Clinical, care or critical pathways (care map)
❑ A situation arising from disagreement in beliefs and values	Conflict
❑ Three types of conflict	Organizational, Interpersonal, Intrapersonal

Modes of Conflict Resolution

Question	Answer
❑ Assertive and very uncooperative *"We are short of staff so I cannot approve your vacation request."*	Competing
❑ Middle of assertiveness and cooperativeness *"You can take a vacation but you should work extra hours this week."*	Compromising
❑ Assertive and cooperative *"You can take a vacation. Let us see if you have vacation hours yet."*	Collaboration
❑ Unassertive and highly cooperative *"You can take a vacation even though we have problems with coverage."*	Accommodating
❑ Unassertive and uncooperative *"I have no time to look at your vacation request."*	Avoiding

Discharge Planning Process

Question	Answer
❑ When does discharge planning begin?	Upon admission in facility
❑ Items to teach the client before discharge	Medication instructions, diet, emergency contacts, reporting complications, use of durable medical equipment (DME), home health care services, follow-up care and appointments
❑ A process of comparing a client's medication orders to all of the medications that the client has been taking to avoid medication errors such as omissions, duplications or dose errors	Medication reconciliation
❑ What is a discharge summary?	Document prepared by the HCP at the end of hospitalization and contains the client's chief complaint, diagnosis, treatments, progress and recommendations

Fire Extinguishers

❑ Wood, cloth, upholstery, paper, rubbish and plastic	Type A
❑ Flammable liquids	Type B
❑ Electrical equipment	Type C
❑ What does RACE stand for?	Rescue, Alert others, Confine, Extinguish
❑ What does PASS stand for?	Pull, Aim, Squeeze, Sweep

Restraints

❑ What is important to document when carrying out an order for a restraint?	Specific behavior of the client
❑ Release restraint device every 2 hours	To perform exercises, promote circulation and provide nutrition
❑ What should be tried initially before applying restraints?	Alternative interventions
❑ What are examples of alternative interventions?	Reorientation, family visit, placing client near the nursing station, toileting program, reminiscence and music therapy

Levels of Prevention

PRIMARY	SECONDARY	TERTIARY
Aims to prevent disease or injury	Aims to decrease the impact of a disease or injury	Aims to minimize the impact of an ongoing illness
❑ Education about healthy lifestyles and avoidance of risk factors (e.g. exercise) ❑ Immunization	❑ Detecting and treating disease (e.g. TB skin test) ❑ Screening test (e.g. colonoscopy)	❑ Exercise programs to prevent further heart attacks ❑ Disease management programs (e.g. diabetes, heart failure)

Biological Terrorism

❑ Caused by Clostridium botulinum bacteria found in the soil and can spread through the air, **canned food** or wound	Botulism
❑ Causes nervous paralysis and symptoms such as dysphagia, slurred speech and muscle weakness	Botulism
❑ Severely toxic and deadly nerve gas that results to paralysis	Sarin
❑ Causes painful blistering of the skin and mucous membranes and swelling of the throat when inhaled	Mustard gas
❑ Caused by spore-forming bacterium transmitted through direct contact through the GI, skin or inhalation route	Anthrax
❑ Inhalation results to flu symptoms, dyspnea and shock	Anthrax

❑ Causes papules that change to pustules on the face and extremities	Smallpox

Prioritization and Triage in the Emergency Room

EMERGENT (RED) PRIORITY 1	URGENT (YELLOW) PRIORITY 2	NON-URGENT (GREEN) PRIORITY 3
Fatal injuries	Non-life-threatening injuries	No immediate, fatal injuries
❑ Immediate attention needed ❑ Examples: *accident victims, chest pain, anaphylaxis, stroke*	❑ Needs treatment in 1-2 hours ❑ Examples: *fever, hypertension, vomiting, abdominal pain*	❑ Can wait several hours ❑ Examples: *minor wound, sprain, mild flu, colds, cough*

Phases of Disaster Management

❑ The agency of the United States Department of Homeland Security that is responsible for coordinating the federal government's response to natural and manmade disasters	Federal Emergency Management Agency (FEMA)
❑ Involves steps to decrease the impact and vulnerability to disasters such as injuries and deaths	Mitigation
❑ Focuses on training implementation to enhance capability to respond and recover from a disaster	Preparedness
❑ Focuses on savings lives and responding to the immediate dangers presented by the disaster	Response
❑ Restoration of all aspects of the disaster's impact on a community	Recovery

D. Cultural Diversity and Health Practices

❑ Eye contact may be considered rude or disrespectful	African Americans, Asian Americans, Native Americans
❑ Eye contact is a sign of trustworthiness and attentiveness	White Americans
❑ Avoiding eye contact is a sign of respect	Hispanic Americans
❑ Avoid close physical distance	White Americans
❑ Comfortable with close physical contact	Hispanic Americans
❑ Touching should be limited especially during conversations; May also apply to opposite sex	Asian Americans
❑ Touching the head is a sign of disrespect	Asian Americans
❑ Silence is valued and a form of respect	Asian Americans

❑ Disharmony between yin and yang is the cause of diseases	Asian Americans
❑ Mythologies and legends are common	Native Americans
❑ Practices Blessingway ceremony to remove ill health	Native Americans
❑ Practices simple lifestyle and separation from modern world	Amish
❑ Practices Rumspringa as a rite of passage during adolescence; Decision is made whether to leave or embrace the community	Amish
❑ Practices **shunning** (social exclusion) due to disobedience	Amish
❑ Time is important	White Americans
❑ Lactose intolerance is common	Asian Americans, Hispanic Americans African Americans, Native Americans

E. Religion and Dietary Preferences

❑ Should not eat foods in which blood has been added	Jehovah's Witnesses
❑ Only eats animal meat that has been drained or bled properly	Jehovah's Witnesses
❑ Prohibits consumption of birds of prey, pork and any meat not ritually slaughtered (halal)	Islam
❑ All vegetarian cuisines are halal and allowed	Islam
❑ During the month of Ramadan, fasting is obligated starting from dawn until sunset	Islam
❑ Lacto-Vegetarians	Hinduism, Buddhism
❑ Meats are prohibited on Ash Wednesday and Fridays during Lent	Roman Catholics
❑ Eats legumes, whole grains, nuts, fruits, and vegetables	Seventh-day Adventist
❑ Alcohol, tea and coffee are prohibited	Latter-Day Saints (Mormon), Seventh-Day Adventist
❑ Adheres to the laws of **Kosher**	Judaism
❑ Only allows meats coming from animals that are cloven-hoofed (sheep, deer, goat), vegetable eaters and chew their cud	Judaism
❑ Milk and meat products are **not** combined in a meal	Judaism
❑ 24-hour fasting is observed during Day of Atonement (Yom Kippur); exempts pregnant women and ill persons	Judaism
❑ No leavened bread is eaten during the 8-day Passover celebration in spring	Judaism
❑ Should refrain from operating electricity, setting a fire, baking and cooking during Sabbath	Judaism

F. Religion and End-of-Life Care Beliefs and Practices

❑ A rabbi may be called during the dying process	Judaism
❑ Burial takes place as soon as possible	Judaism, Islam
❑ Forbids autopsy and cremation	Judaism
❑ Believes that at death the body and the spirit separate	Latter-Day Saints (Mormons)
❑ Practices the Sacrament of the Anointing of the Sick	Roman Catholic
❑ Believes that when a person dies, he goes into sleep until God resurrects the person from the dead	Jehovah's Witness
❑ Forbids blood transfusion as a life-saving treatment	Jehovah's Witness
❑ Body is wrapped in a white shroud	Islam
❑ Daily prayers are important to prepare for death any time	Islam
❑ Bodies are buried **facing the Mecca**, the Muslim holy city	Islam
❑ Family members of the same gender as the deceased will bathe and shroud the body for burial	Islam
❑ Body will be buried within 24 hours as the soul leaves the body at the time of death	Islam
❑ A coffin is usually not used but a chamber is dug into the grave and sealed with wooden boards	Islam
❑ Believes that when they die they will be reborn again	Buddhism
❑ Practices meditation when approaching death	Buddhism
❑ Believes in reincarnation	Hinduism
❑ The dead body will be bathed by family then clothed in white traditional clothing	Hinduism
❑ Thread is applied around the neck or wrist of the dying person and a sacred basil leaf is placed on the client's tongue or a few drops of water as a purifying practice	Hinduism
❑ Practices cremation as they believe burning the body releases the spirit; Ritual includes casting the ashes in the river to send the dead person to afterlife	Hinduism

NCLEX Alert! *Make sure that you are familiar with the common cultural and religious beliefs and practices for they will most likely be in the NCLEX!*

Fundamentals of Nursing 4

A. SBAR Technique of Communication

❑ What is SBAR?	Framework and guide for communication
❑ When do you use SBAR?	Calling a physician, Handing off clients, Discharging clients, Documentation, Change of condition

SITUATION	BACKGROUND	ASSESSMENT	RECOMMENDATIONS
"What is the issue?"	*"What is the background?"*	*"What is the problem?"*	*"What will be done?"*
❑ Date the condition started ❑ What makes the symptoms worse or better?	❑ Primary diagnoses ❑ Code status ❑ Focused systems assessment ❑ Vital signs, Pain level ❑ Lab results, Drugs ❑ Effect of interventions	❑ *"I think the problem may be .....* ❑ *"I am not sure what the problem is, but the client is not getting better."*	❑ Nursing interventions ❑ Monitor vital signs ❑ New orders ❑ Laboratory tests ❑ Diagnostic tests ❑ Medication order ❑ HCP visit ❑ Transfer to ER

B. Infection Control and Infectious Diseases

Terminologies

❑ An infection that is acquired in a health care facility	Nosocomial infection
❑ The period between exposure to an infection and the appearance of the first symptoms	Incubation period
❑ Infection occurs due to a weakened immune system	Opportunistic infection
❑ Onset of disease with non-specific or general symptoms	Prodromal period
❑ Client has the organisms but has no signs or symptoms of disease (ex. + MRSA swab)	Colonization
❑ Materials that carry infection such as clothes and utensils	Fomites
❑ Reduces the number of pathogens (e.g. enemas, tube feedings)	Medical asepsis
❑ Eliminates all pathogens (e.g. Foley catheterization)	Surgical asepsis

Standard versus Transmission-Based Precautions

- Precautions used to prevent transmission of diseases that can be acquired by contact with blood, body fluids, non-intact skin and mucous membranes. These measures are used when providing care to all individuals, whether or not they appear **infected** or **symptomatic**.
  STANDARD PRECAUTIONS

- Additional precautions applied for clients who are **suspected** or **known** to be infected or colonized with infectious agents. Combined with "Standard Precautions" as needed.
  TRANSMISSION-BASED PRECAUTIONS

Means of Transmission

TRANSMISSION	DEFINITION	EXAMPLE
Airborne	Particles are suspended on air beyond 3 feet	Inhalation of measles virus
Droplet	Infection is spread within 3 feet	Sneezing, coughing
Direct contact	Host spreads the infection to another person	Sexual intercourse
Indirect contact	Contaminated material to another person	Holding a cellphone

Disease Transmissions

PRECAUTIONS	DISEASES	PPE	ROOM	OTHERS
AIRBORNE	Measles Tuberculosis Chicken pox Herpes zoster *(if immunocompromised or disseminated type)*	N-95 Mask	Private Room **Negative airflow pressure** Door is closed	Client wears mask outside of room; should only leave the room if needed
DROPLET	Respiratory Syncytial Virus (RSV) Influenza, Meningitis, Rubella, Streptococcal pneumonia, Pertussis, Mumps, SARS	Surgical Mask	Private or shared room (3 feet away) May open the door	Client wears mask outside of room

PRECAUTIONS	DISEASES	PPE	ROOM	OTHERS
CONTACT	Multidrug Resistant Organisms (MDRO's) such as MRSA and VRE RSV Scabies Impetigo Rotavirus Enterovirus Ebola Chicken pox Wounds Herpes zoster Carbapenem-resistant enterobacteriaceae (CRE)	Gown, Gloves	Private room or in a room with similarly infected client; no other infections	Dedicated equipment Supervise client during ambulation Must be continent
CONTACT PLUS	C. Difficile Norovirus	Gown, Gloves	Private room or in a room with similarly infected client; no other infections	Dedicated equipment Supervise client during ambulation Must be continent Hand washing with **soap and water** is required for all those who have had contact with the client or the client's environment

Reference: Centers for Disease Control and Prevention

Which PPE will you use?

1. Client suspected of active tuberculosis who needs a diaper change due to incontinence and severe diarrhea

   Gown and gloves for diaper change; N-95 mask for TB

2. Client with psoriasis who needs wound irrigation

   Gown, gloves, mask/goggle or a face shield for wound irrigation; no PPE needed for psoriasis as it is non-infectious

3. Client with HIV who needs a bed bath

   No PPE needed; HIV is not transmitted through body contact with intact skin

4. Client with Legionnaire's disease who needs a blood draw — Gloves for blood draw; no PPE needed for Legionnaire's disease as it is not transmissible from human to human

5. Client with "disseminated" herpes zoster who needs repositioning — Gown, gloves and N-95 mask as disseminated herpes zoster is transmitted through contact and airborne route

Personal Protective Equipment (PPE)

- ❑ Sequence for donning PPE — (1) Gown (2) Mask (3) Goggle (4) Gloves
- ❑ Sequence for removing PPE — (1) Gloves (2) Google (3) Gown (4) Mask

Multi-Drug Resistant Organisms (MDRO)

CLOSTRIDIUM DIFFICILE (C. DIFFICILE)	METHICILLIN-RESISTANT STAPHYLOCOCCUS AUREUS (MRSA)	VANCOMYCIN-RESISTANT ENTEROCOCCI (VRE)	NOROVIRUS
Transmission ❑ Contact; related to **overuse** of ATBs	Transmission ❑ Contact	Transmission ❑ Contact	Transmission ❑ Contact; **fecal-oral;** contaminated food or water or by touching surfaces; aerosolized vomit
Assessment ❑ Severe diarrhea, fever, abdominal pain, bloody stool	Assessment ❑ Boils, sepsis, pneumonia, urinary tract infection (depending on site of invasion)	Assessment ❑ UTI ❑ Wound infection ❑ Diarrhea ❑ Fever ❑ Chills	Assessment ❑ Vomiting, watery, non-bloody diarrhea with abdominal cramps
Interventions ❑ **metronidazole** (Flagyl), Vancomycin	Interventions ❑ **Vancomycin** ❑ Incision and drainage	Interventions ❑ ATBs other than Vancomycin	Interventions ❑ IVF, Oral rehydration ❑ Antiemetics

Duration of Isolation (DI)

- ❑ Measles — 4 days after rash appears
- ❑ Mumps — 9 days
- ❑ Rubella — 7 days after rash appears
- ❑ Herpes, Varicella — Until lesions are dry and crusted
- ❑ Meningitis, Scabies — Up to 24 hours after treatment

Key Points in Infection Control

- Handwashing should be done before and after client contacts.
- The name of the client and infection should **not** appear on the front door.
- Privacy curtain should be drawn between client beds in multi-bed rooms.
- Do not place clients with different types of active infections in the same room. (e.g. MRSA vs. VRE or MRSA vs. MRSA/Flu)
- Consider developmental needs when isolating children (e.g. same sex roommate for school-children).
- Assign an immune staff to clients with rubella, varicella and rubeola. The immune staff may not need to wear a mask depending on facility protocol.
- Droplet nuclei (airborne) is not the same as large droplets.
- For substantial spraying of fluids, gloves, gown and goggles (or face shield) should be worn.
- The N95 mask must be "fit tested" for each user by a trained person.
- Respirators should always be removed outside the client room, after the door is closed.
- Clients on contact precautions may be allowed to go to the activity room if the site of infection can be covered.
- Clients with active symptoms (e.g. C. difficile with diarrhea) should not join group activities.

C. Sexually Transmitted Diseases

Chlamydia

Transmission	Sexual intercourse or genital contact
Assessment	Clear urethral discharge, burning urination
Interventions	azithromycin (Zithromax) doxycycline (Vibramycin)

Gonorrhea

Transmission	Sexual intercourse
Assessment	Purulent discharge, pain on urination
Interventions	Single IM dose cephalosporin

Syphilis

Transmission	Blood, direct contact with painless chancre
Assessment	Stages: 1. PRIMARY- **painless chancre** 2. SECONDARY - rashes, fever, sore throat 3. TERTIARY - CNS damage
When is syphilis infectious?	During primary and secondary stages only
Interventions	Single IM dose penicillin G

D. Pain Management

❑ Pain for 6 months or less	Acute
❑ Pain for more than 6 months	Chronic
❑ Example: cancer pain	Chronic pain
❑ Abnormal impulses from the nervous system	Neuropathic pain
❑ Shooting, burning, stinging, electric-like pain	Neuropathic pain
❑ Example: diabetic neuropathy or phantom limb pain	Neuropathic pain
❑ Requires higher doses of the same pain drug	Pain tolerance
❑ Physical symptoms occur when stopping the drug	Dependence
❑ Temporary, severe pain even when a client is already medicated with a long-acting painkiller	Breakthrough pain
❑ What does OLDCART mean in pain assessment?	Onset, Location, Duration, Characteristics, Associated/Aggravating factors, Radiation, Treatments
❑ What is the most accurate source of pain assessment?	Verbalization of an alert client
❑ Numerical Rating Scale	Ask client to rate pain from 0 - 10
❑ Wong-Baker Faces Pain Rating Scale	Pain assessment for ages 3 and older
❑ PAINAD Scale	Pain Assessment in Clients with Advanced Dementia
❑ What is the World Health Organization (WHO) Analgesic Ladder?	A three-step process for cancer pain relief. Pain management should start with non-opioids, followed by mild opioids and finally, strong opioids until the client is free of pain

Pain Medications

❑ Why should pain medications be given before the pain gets worse?	Pain medications are more effective before the pain reaches its peak
❑ What are examples of non-narcotic drugs?	acetaminophen (Tylenol), NSAIDs such as ibuprofen (Advil, Motrin), indomethacin (Indocin) and aspirin
❑ What are the most common side effects of NSAIDs?	Gastric upset, bleeding
❑ What pain drug is considered severely hepatotoxic?	acetaminophen (Tylenol) Dose limit is 4,000 mg per day
❑ What is the antidote for acetaminophen overdose?	acetylcysteine (Mucomyst)
❑ What are examples of mild opioids?	Codeine, hydrocodone, oxycodone

❑ What opioid is available in combination products with aspirin or acetaminophen?	hydrocodone (e.g. Vicodin), oxycodone (e.g. Percocet, Oxycontin)
❑ What are examples of major opioids?	Morphine, meperidine (Demerol), hydromorphone (Dilaudid), fentanyl, methadone
❑ What opioid is similar but stronger than morphine?	Hydromorphone (Dilaudid)
❑ What opioid is also used for neuropathic pain?	Methadone
❑ What are the side effects of opioids or narcotics?	Constipation, respiratory depression, urinary retention
❑ What is the antidote for opioid overdose?	naloxone (Narcan)

E. Perioperative Nursing

❑ Who is responsible for obtaining the informed consent before any surgery?	Surgeon
❑ What interventions are included in pre-operative care?	Obtaining informed consent Explanation of risk and benefits Client should void before surgery Foley catheter inserted as ordered Ensure safety after giving pre-op drugs
❑ What items are included in preoperative instructions?	Expectations after surgery (e.g. devices) Turning and repositioning Splinting the incision site to decrease pain Deep breathing and coughing exercises Leg exercises
❑ What items are included in a preoperative checklist?	Allergies, Vital signs, Blood Type, H and P, Labs tests, ID band, Informed consent, NPO status, Last time voided, Secure valuables, Remove jewelry, hairpins, nail polish, make-up and dentures
❑ When is deep breathing and coughing highly recommended after surgery?	When surgery involves a high abdominal incision (e.g. cholecystectomy). This may cause pain and shallow breathing leading to hypoventilation and atelectasis

- ❑ What is "*The Joint Commission's Universal Protocol for Preventing Wrong Site, Wrong Procedure and Wrong Person Surgery?*"
  Requires 2 information to identify the correct client (e.g. name, date of birth)
  The surgeon marks the operative site
  "Time-out" procedure is performed to verify details of procedure

- ❑ What interventions are included in post-operative care?
  Assess airway and level of consciousness
  Provide warm blankets
  Maintain NPO until return of gag reflexes
  Promote early ambulation
  Monitor for gastric and bladder distention
  Monitor ability to void within 6 hours

> ***NCLEX Alert!*** *If the client has not voided within 6 hours after surgery, assess for bladder distention or perform a bladder scan to determine need for immediate catheterization.*

- ❑ Steps on how to perform deep-breathing and coughing exercises
  Breathe deeply through the nose
  Cough deeply splinting the operative site

- ❑ Steps on how to use an incentive spirometry
  Place mouth around mouth piece
  Inhale slowly to raise the flow indicator
  Hold breath for several seconds then exhale through pursed lips

Post-Operative Complications

❑ Tachypnea, crackles, chest pain, productive cough	Pneumonia
❑ Weak, rapid pulse, cool, clammy skin, hypotension	Hemorrhagic shock
❑ Sudden sharp chest pain, dyspnea	Pulmonary embolism
❑ Bladder sounds like a drum on percussion	Urinary retention
❑ Absent bowel sounds, failure to pass flatus	Paralytic Ileus
❑ Positive Homan's sign, warm, tender extremity	Thrombophlebitis
❑ Opening of wound edges	Dehiscence
❑ Protrusion of organs through a surgical wound	Evisceration
❑ Place client on modified Trendelenburg position	Hypovolemic shock
❑ Pour warm water over the perineum	Urinary retention
❑ Have the client hear running water	Urinary retention
❑ Place client on Low Fowler's position with knees bent	Evisceration
❑ Cover the wound with sterile normal saline	Evisceration
❑ Prevention includes early ambulation and application of sequential compression device or elastic stockings	Thrombophlebitis

F. Positioning Skills

DISEASE CONDITION OR PROCEDURE	POSITION
Abdominal aortic aneurysm surgery	❑ Semi-Fowler's position to prevent tension on surgical site
Amputation of the lower extremity	❑ Elevate foot of the bed to reduce edema ❑ Support residual limb with pillows
Autonomic dysreflexia	❑ High Fowler's position to reduce high blood pressure
Bronchoscopy	❑ Supine position with arms on side
Central line catheter insertion for TPN	❑ Trendelenburg position to prevent air embolism
Dumping syndrome	❑ Lie down after meals to slow down gastric emptying
Enema administration	❑ Left Sim's position to allow solution to flow into colon
Gastroesophageal reflux disease (GERD)	❑ Sit upright or walk around after meals to prevent reflux
Hemorrhoidectomy	❑ Side-lying position to prevent hemorrhage and pain
Increased intracranial pressure	❑ Semi-Fowler's (preferred)/Fowler's position ❑ Avoid extreme hip and knee flexion ❑ Head in midline, neutral position
Liver biopsy	During the procedure ❑ Supine with right arm above the head to expose the liver After the procedure ❑ Right side-lying position with bed flat to prevent bleeding
Mastectomy	❑ Semi-Fowler's position with the affected arm elevated ❑ Avoid abduction of arm on the operated side
Myelography/Myelogram	After the procedure ❑ Water-soluble dye (Metrizamide) - Semi-Fowler's position ❑ Oil-soluble (Pantopaque) - Flat position
Nasogastric tube insertion	❑ Sitting position with head tilted forward
Paracentesis	❑ Semi-Fowler's or sitting upright position to drain fluid
Thoracentesis	❑ Sitting on edge of bed leaning over the bedside table or side-lying position on the unaffected side
Thyroidectomy	❑ Semi-Fowler's or Fowler's position ❑ Avoid hyperextension or hyperflexion of the neck
Total hip replacement	❑ Maintain abduction of extremities ❑ Avoid internal and external rotation of hip

G. Fall Prevention

- ❑ What are the risk factors for falls? — Muscle weakness, gait problems, poor lighting, sedating drugs, Alzheimer's disease, poor vision, equipment failure
- ❑ What are examples of Fall Risk Assessment Tests? — Timed-Up and Go Test, 30-Second Chair Stand Test, Four-Stage Balance Test
- ❑ What are examples of fall prevention strategies? — Educate staff, Exercise, Review medications, Check vision, Home safety check, Check orthostatic BP, Teach client on safety

H. Management of Tubes

1. Nasogastric Tubes

- ❑ What are the purposes of NGT insertion? — For feeding, decompression and lavage
- ❑ What is the best method to verify NGT placement? — Abdominal x-ray (may use contrast media)
- ❑ When do you check NGT placement and residual volume? — Before tube feeding and giving drugs
- ❑ How do you check proper placement of the NGT? —
  1. Aspirate gastric contents and check color → should be light yellow to greenish
  2. Measure the pH → should be <4
  3. Instill 5-10 ml of air into the NG tube and listen for the whooshing sound of air
- ❑ Assess gastric residual volume (GRV) every 4 hours during the first 48 hours of feeding — >250 mL after second check→ Report
  A promotility agent may be ordered
  >500 mL → Hold feeding per facility policy
- ❑ If residual is <100 ml, is it safe to give tube feeding? — Yes (amount depends on facility policy)

2. Gastrointestinal Tube Feedings

Types of Administration

BOLUS	CONTINUOUS	INTERMITTENT	CYCLIC
❑ 300-400 mL of formula given over 20-30 minutes via an infusion pump, syringe or using gravity; Risk for aspiration	❑ Slow, continuous feeding given via an infusion pump for a longer period of time (16-24 hours)	❑ 300-400 mL given over 30-60 minutes every 4-6 hours via an infusion pump or using gravity	❑ Nocturnal tube feeding ❑ Continuous feeding over 12-16 hours

Administering Tube Feedings

❑ For continuous feeding, place the client in ___________ position at all times	Semi-Fowler's
❑ For bolus feeding, place client in _________ position for 30 minutes after feeding to prevent aspiration	High-Fowler's
❑ Change the feeding bag and tubing every ___ hours	24
❑ Do not hang formula for more than ___ hours	4
❑ Flush with ________ of water after feeding	30–50 mL
❑ How do you give medications via GT or NGT?	Verify the order Wash hands Confirm the client's identity Explain the procedure to the client Check tube placement and gastric residual amount before giving medication Aspirate drug into syringe and give drug Flush with 30-50 mL of water Clamp the tube as needed

3. Tracheostomy

❑ What are the parts of the tracheostomy tube?	Inner cannula, outer cannula, obturator
❑ What is the purpose of the inner cannula?	Collects secretions, Removed for cleaning
❑ What is the purpose of the outer cannula?	Maintains the tracheal opening
❑ What is the purpose of the obturator?	Inserted into the outer cannula to provide a smooth surface during insertion
❑ What is the purpose of a cuffed tracheostomy tube?	Seals the airway when using a ventilator
❑ Is tracheostomy suctioning done on a regular basis?	No, it is only done when necessary
❑ What is used to clean the tracheostomy site?	Hydrogen peroxide; Rinse the site with NS
❑ What safety precaution is important to remember when changing tracheostomy ties?	Ask for assistance to prevent accidental extubation and closure of the airway

4. Chest-Tube Drainage System

❑ What is the purpose of chest tubes?	Remove air and fluid the from the pleural space to restore **NEGATIVE** pressure
❑ Place the drainage system below the level of the chest at all times	To prevent backflow of drainage
❑ How do you facilitate drainage of air and fluid?	Change the client's position frequently
❑ Is stripping or milking of chest tubes allowed?	No, it will cause tension pneumothorax
❑ Is clamping of chest tubes allowed?	No, it will cause tension pneumothorax
❑ What should you do if there is a break in the system?	Submerge tube in a bottle of sterile water

- ❑ What should you do when the chest tube is pulled out from the chest accidentally? — Apply occlusive sterile dressing and report
- ❑ What device is important to prepare at the bedside? — At least two clamps or hemostats
- ❑ What procedure confirms lung re-expansion? — Chest x-ray
- ❑ What instruction is given during chest tube removal? — Take a deep breath and hold. Site is covered with sterile petroleum dressing

COLLECTION CHAMBER	WATER–SEAL CHAMBER	SUCTION CONTROL CHAMBER
❑ Drainage >70-100 mL/hour → Report to HCP ❑ Drainage suddenly changes into bright red → Report to HCP	❑ Water–seal prevents air from entering the pleural space ❑ Oscillation/Tidaling/ Fluctuation of water level → normal finding in a functioning system ❑ Fluctuation stops → indicates obstruction, kinks or defective suction → lung has re-expanded (usually 2-3 days after) ❑ Intermittent bubbling → normal finding with ongoing pneumothorax ❑ Continuous bubbling → air leak is present	❑ Suction control chamber facilitates the removal of air and fluid Wet Suction System ❑ Gentle bubbling → normal finding ❑ Vigorous bubbling → air leak is present Dry Suction System ❑ Absence of bubbling → normal finding

I. Conversions, Dosage and Intravenous Fluid Calculation

- ❑ What are the seven rights of medication administration? — Right medication, dose, client, route, time, frequency and documentation
- ❑ What are examples of household systems of measurement? — drop, teaspoon, tablespoon, ounce, pint
- ❑ What are examples of metric system of measurement? — meter, liter, gram
- ❑ What drugs are given in milliequivalent (mEq)? — potassium KCl (e.g.10 mEq)
- ❑ What drugs are given in units? — penicillin, heparin sodium, insulin
- ❑ How many mL's are in a medicine cup? — 30 mL

Household Measures

❑ 1 teaspoon = __ mL	5
❑ 1 T (tbsp) = 3 tsp = __ mL	15
❑ 1 medicine cup = __ mL	30
❑ 1 oz = __ mL	30
❑ 1 cup = __ oz	8
❑ 1 quart =__ pints	2
❑ 1 pint = __ cups	2
❑ 1 gr (grain) = __ mg	60
❑ 1 g (gram) = __ mg	1000
❑ 1 kg = __ lbs.	2.2
❑ 1 lb = __ oz	16

Converting Temperature Units

❑ How do you convert Celsius to Fahrenheit?	Multiply by 1.8 and add 32
❑ How to you convert Fahrenheit to Celsius?	Subtract 32 and divide the result by 1.8

Injection Methods

❑ 10-15 degrees	Intradermal
❑ 45-90 degrees (for normal-sized clients)	Subcutaneous
❑ 90 degrees (quick darting motion)	Intramuscular
❑ 25-27 gauge, ¼ to ⅜ inch needle	Intradermal
❑ 25-30 gauge, ⅜ to ⅝ inch needle	Subcutaneous
❑ 23 gauge, ⅝ to 1-inch needle	Intramuscular (deltoid)
❑ Uses 1 mL tuberculin syringe for skin testing	Intradermal
❑ Used for insulin and heparin injections	Subcutaneous
❑ Uses Z-track technique	Intramuscular
❑ Insert the needle in the "V" formed between the index and third fingers	Intramuscular (ventrogluteal)
❑ Risk of sciatic nerve injury	Intramuscular (dorsogluteal)
❑ Preferred site for infants	Intramuscular (vastus lateralis)
❑ Aspiration should be performed	Intramuscular (except flu vaccine)
❑ What is the purpose of the Z-track technique during IM injection?	Prevents leakage of medication and staining of the skin (e.g. iron)

Medication Calculation Formula

$$\frac{\textbf{Dose ordered} \text{ (mg, g, units, mEq)}}{\textbf{Available stock} \text{ (mg, g, units, mEq)}} \times \textbf{Quantity} \text{ (per mL, tablet)}$$

Example:

1. A client is ordered to receive Amoxicillin 0.25 g p.o. every 8 hours. The drug on hand shows Amoxicillin 125 mg per 5 mL. How many mL will you give?

   Steps: Convert 0.25 g to mg = 250 mg

   $$\frac{250 \text{ mg}}{125 \text{ mg}} \times 5 \text{ mL} = 10 \text{ mL (answer)}$$

IV Fluid Calculations

- ❑ 1 mL = _______ drops (gtts) — 10, 15, 20
- ❑ 1 mL = _______ microdrops (ugtts) — 60

IV Calculation Formulas

1. drops/minute

   $$\frac{\text{Total volume (mL)} \times \text{drop factor}}{\text{Number of hours to run} \times 60} = \text{drops per minute}$$

2. mL/hour

   $$\frac{\text{Total volume (mL)}}{\text{Number of hours to run}} = \text{number of mL/hour}$$

3. Infusion time

   $$\frac{\text{Total volume (mL) to infuse}}{\text{mL per hour being infused}} = \text{infusion time}$$

Example:

1. The physician orders 1 liter of D_5 W to infuse for 8 hours. The infusion set has a drop factor of 15 gtts/mL. What flow rate (gtts/minute) will you set on the IV infusion pump? Round off your final answer to the nearest whole number.

   Steps:

   $$\frac{1000 \text{ mL} \times 15 \text{ gtts/mL}}{8 \times 60} = 31 \text{ gtts/min (answer)}$$

J. Herbal Therapies

HERB	USES
Aloe	❑ Anti-inflammatory, Antibacterial
Angelica	❑ Muscle relaxant, Vasodilator, Decreases menopausal symptoms
Black cohosh	❑ Treats menopausal symptoms, Treats motion sickness
Bilberry	❑ Improves vision, Lowers blood glucose, Fights cancer
Cat's claw	❑ Anti-oxidant, Enhances the immune system, Antihypertensive
Chamomile	❑ Decreases muscle spasm, Anti- inflammatory, Sedative
Dehydroepiandrosterone (DHEA)	❑ Anti-aging, Treats erectile dysfunction, Prevents osteoporosis
Echinacea	❑ Enhances the immune system, Fights flu and colds
Evening primrose	❑ Treats bone loss and nerve damage, Metabolizes fatty acids
Feverfew	❑ Anti-inflammatory, Treats migraines, arthritis, vomiting and fever
Garlic	❑ Treats hypertension, Lowers cholesterol levels
Ginkgo biloba	❑ Enhances memory, Anti-oxidant
Ginseng	❑ Improves energy, Fights stress and fatigue, Lowers blood glucose
Ginger	❑ Treats nausea and vomiting, Treats motions sickness
Glucosamine	❑ Helps build cartilage to prevent arthritis
Kava	❑ Antianxiety, Muscle relaxant, Promotes sleep
Milk thistle	❑ Antioxidant, Treats liver disorders, Detoxifier
Melatonin	❑ Treats insomnia
Peppermint oil	❑ Antispasmodic, Treats irritable bowel syndrome (IBS)
Saw palmetto	❑ Antiestrogen, Treats UTI and BPH
St. John's Wort	❑ Treats depression and insomnia, Antibacterial, Antiviral
Valerian	❑ Treats insomnia, Antianxiety

NCLEX Alert! *Herbal supplements should be avoided before a major surgery as they can affect blood clotting and anesthesia.*

Drug Interactions and Effects of Herbs

HERB	DRUG OR SUBSTANCE	EFFECTS
Aloe	❑ digoxin	→ increased side effects (digoxin toxicity)
Black cohosh	❑ atorvastatin (Lipitor) ❑ acetaminophen (Tylenol) ❑ alcohol	→ hepatotoxicity
Cranberry	❑ anticoagulants	→ bleeding
Echinacea	❑ caffeine ❑ immunosuppressant	→ increased effects (jitteriness, headache, insomnia) → reduced effectiveness
Evening primrose oil	❑ anticonvulsants, phenothiazines	→ increased seizures
Feverfew	❑ anticoagulants	→ increased bleeding
Ginkgo biloba	❑ HIV drugs, alprazolam, statins, antidepressants ❑ anticoagulants, NSAIDs ❑ anticonvulsants	→ reduced effectiveness → increased bleeding → increased seizures
Ginseng	❑ warfarin, diabetes drugs	→ reduced effectiveness
Goldenseal	❑ pimozide, thioridazine ❑ antacids, H_2 antagonists, antihypertensives, anticoagulants	→ arrhythmias → reduced effectiveness
Kava	❑ alcohol ❑ CNS depressants, MAOIs, antiplatelets	→ liver toxicity → increased effects
Melatonin	❑ sedatives, benzodiazepines, hypnotics, antihistamines, narcotics, muscle relaxants ❑ diabetes drugs ❑ anticoagulants	→ increased drowsiness and dizziness → reduced effectiveness → increased bleeding
Saw palmetto	❑ finasteride (Proscar) ❑ warfarin ❑ oral contraceptives	→ increased effects → increased bleeding → reduced effectiveness

HERB	DRUG OR SUBSTANCE	EFFECTS
St. John's Wort	❑ SSRIs, tricyclics, MAOIs, nefazodone (Serzone), dextromethorphan,sedatives ❑ antihistamines, digoxin, immunosuppressants, theophylline ❑ oral contraceptives, warfarin, narcotics, omeprazole, HIV drugs	→ increased side effects → decreased levels → reduced effectiveness
Valerian	❑ skeletal muscle relaxants, sedatives, hypnotics, narcotics, antidepressants	→ increased drowsiness and dizziness
HERBS THAT INCREASE THE EFFECTS OF WARFARIN		
agrimony, ginkgo, onion, alfalfa, danshen, papain, licorice, wild carrot, red clover, cassio, aniseed, arnica flower, passion flower, horse chestnut, tonka beans, celery seed, artemesia, fenugreek, prickly ash, feverfew, fish oil, bogbean, garlic, chamomile, dihydroepiandrosterone, parsley, sweet woodruff, dandelion, bromelains, ginger, sweet clover, horseradish, turmeric, chinese wolfberry, meadowsweet, wild lettuce, clove, willow		
HERBS THAT DECREASE THE EFFECTS OF WARFARIN		
goldenseal, ginseng, St. John's Wort, yarrow, green tea		

NCLEX Alert! *DRUGS THAT INTERACT WITH GRAPEFRUIT JUICE*

Immunosuppressants, Methadone, sildenafil (Viagra), Statins, Antihistamines, Calcium channel blockers, HIV drug - saquinavir (Invirase, Fortovase), amiodarone (Cordarone), disopyramide (Norpace), carbamazepine (Tegretol), buspirone (Buspar), triazolam (Halcion), diazepam (Valium), midazolam (Versed), sertraline (Zoloft)

K. Alternative and Complementary Medicines

❑ Movement of the body part to decrease pain, promote healing and improve mobility Ex: Chiropractic therapy, massage, reflexology	Manipulative Therapy
❑ Healers can transfer healing energy into a client and cause positive results Ex. Acupuncture, qi gong, reiki and johre, magnetic therapy	Energy Medicine

❑ Health depends on a harmonious balance between the mind, body and spirit Ex: Diet, herbal therapy, detoxification, massage, meditation, yoga	Ayurveda
❑ If a substance causes a symptom in a healthy person, providing a small amount of the same substance may treat the disease Ex: Plant and mineral extracts	Homeopathy
❑ Diseases can be properly treated or prevented without the use of medications Ex: hydrotherapy, acupuncture	Naturopathy
❑ Avoids the use of highly processed or refined foods; Emphasizes consumption of organic foods and whole grains	Macrobiotic Diet
❑ Diseases are due to deficiencies in essential substances; Emphasizes nutritional supplementation	Orthomolecular Therapy
❑ Uses extracted oils from plant materials such as leaves, stems, flowers or roots to improve mental and physical state	Aromatherapy

L. Basic Life Support

Reference: Highlights of the 2015 American Heart Association (AHA) Guidelines Update for CPR and ECC
Summary of High-Quality CPR Components for BLS Providers (www.heart.org)
Note the change from A-B-C to C-A-B (Compression, Airway, Breathing) sequence

❑ What is important to check before saving a victim?	Make sure the environment is safe
❑ Recognition of cardiac arrest	Check for responsiveness No breathing or only gasping No definite pulse felt within 10 seconds
❑ Breathing and pulse check can be performed simultaneously in less than ___ seconds	10
❑ **For adults and adolescents**: If you are alone with no mobile phone, leave the victim to activate the emergency response system and get the ________ before beginning CPR. Otherwise, send someone and begin CPR immediately; use the AED as soon as available.	Automatic External Defibrillator (AED)

❑ For children (age 1 year to puberty) and infants (age <1 year, excluding newborns)	**1. Witnessed collapse** Follow steps for adults and adolescents **2. Unwitnessed collapse** Give 2 minutes of CPR Leave the victim to activate the emergency response system and get the AED Return to the child or infant and resume CPR; use the AED as soon as it is available
❑ Compression ventilation ratio without advanced airway for adults and adolescents	1 or 2 rescuers = 30:2
❑ Compression-ventilation ratio without advanced airway for children (age 1 year to puberty) and infants (age <1 year, excluding newborns)	1 rescuer = 30:2 2 or more rescuers = 15:2
❑ Compression-ventilation ratio with advanced airway; Perform continuous compressions at a rate of _____/min Give ___ breath every 6 seconds (10 breaths/min)	 100-120 1
❑ Compression depth	Adults: At least 2 inches (5 cm) Children: At least 2 inches (5 cm) Infants: About 1 ½ inches (4 cm)
❑ Hand placement for adults and adolescents	2 hands on the lower half of the breastbone (sternum)
❑ Hand placement for children (age 1 year to puberty)	2 hands or 1 hand (optional for very small child) on the lower half of the sternum
❑ Hand placement for infants (age <1 year, excluding newborns)	1 RESCUER: 2 fingers in the center of the chest, just below the nipple line 2 OR MORE RESCUERS: 2 thumb–encircling hands in the center of the chest, just below the nipple line
❑ Limit interruptions in chest compressions to less than ____ seconds	10

> ***NCLEX Alert!*** *WHAT IS HANDS-ONLY CPR?*
> *"Hands-only" CPR is CPR which does not include mouth-to-mouth resuscitation. It is an approach to save a person who suddenly collapses outside the hospital environment (e.g. workplace, gym, home). It involves two simple steps: (1) Call 911 and (2) Push hard and fast in the center of the chest.*

Advanced Nursing Concepts 5

A. Acid-Base Balance

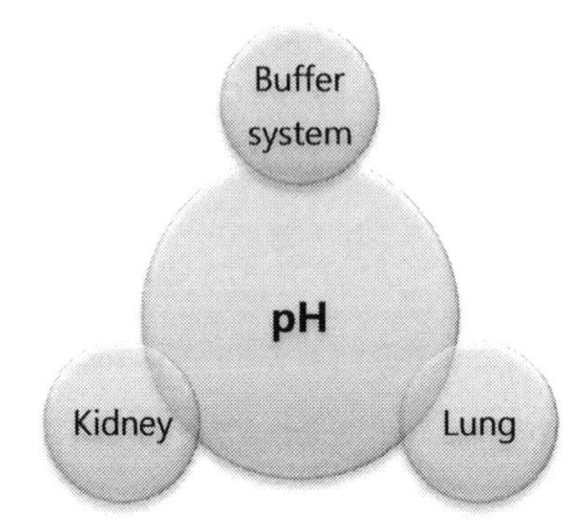

❑ What systems regulate the pH?	Buffers, Respiratory and Urinary system
❑ Which organs compensate when an acid-base imbalance occurs?	Kidneys and lungs
❑ What do the lungs regulate?	Partial pressure of CO_2 (pCO_2) level
❑ What do the kidneys regulate?	Bicarbonate (HCO_3) level
❑ Why is it important to maintain a normal pH?	A severely abnormal pH can lead to death

Normal ABG Values – *This is where you start!*

❑ Normal pH	7.35 - 7.45
❑ Normal pCO_2	35 - 45 mmHg
❑ Normal HCO_3	22 - 26 mEq/L
❑ Normal pO_2	80 - 100 mmHg
❑ Base excess	-2 to +2 mEq/L

What do these values mean? – *You must perfectly know this!*

❑ ↑ pH	alkalosis
❑ ↓ pH	acidosis
❑ ↑ pCO_2	acidosis
❑ ↓ pCO_2	alkalosis
❑ ↑ HCO_3	alkalosis
❑ ↓ HCO_3	acidosis
❑ Base excess < - 2 mEq/L	metabolic acidosis
❑ Base excess > +2 mEq/L	metabolic alkalosis

Types of Acid-Base Imbalances

	RESPIRATORY ACIDOSIS	RESPIRATORY ALKALOSIS	METABOLIC ACIDOSIS	METABOLIC ALKALOSIS
Values	↓ pH, ↑ pCO_2	↑ pH, ↓ pCO_2	↓ pH, ↓ HCO_3	↑ pH, ↑ HCO_3
Compen-Sation	Kidneys retain HCO_3	Kidneys excrete HCO_3	Lungs excrete CO_2	Lungs retain CO_2
Causes	❑ COPD ❑ Asthma ❑ Hypoventilation ❑ Sedatives	❑ Hyperventilation ❑ Anxiety ❑ Labor pain	❑ Severe diarrhea ❑ Renal failure ❑ Diabetic ketoacidosis	❑ Severe vomiting ❑ Antacids ❑ Sodium bicarbonate
Assessment	❑ Restlessness ❑ Drowsiness ❑ CNS depression	❑ **Numbness and tingling** ❑ Lightheadedness ❑ Headache ❑ Paresthesia ❑ CNS stimulation	❑ Rapid, deep respiration - Kussmaul breathing ❑ **Hyperkalemia** ❑ CNS depression	❑ Decreased respiration ❑ Twitching ❑ Dysrhythmia ❑ **Hypokalemia** ❑ CNS stimulation
Interven-tions	❑ Maintain airway ❑ Oxygen ❑ Pursed-lip breathing ❑ Semi-Fowler's position	❑ Paper bag breathing ❑ Instruct to slow down breathing	❑ Assess LOC ❑ Monitor K^+ level ❑ Sodium bicarbonate ❑ Treat the cause	❑ Assess LOC ❑ Monitor K^+ level ❑ Antiemetics ❑ Diuretics ❑ Treat the cause

NCLEX Alert!

Acidosis causes CNS depression while alkalosis causes CNS stimulation.

Acidosis also causes the potassium to leave the cells and move into the bloodstream causing hyperkalemia!

B. Arterial Blood Gas

❑ What test is done before ABG specimen withdrawal in order to determine collateral circulation by assessing the patency of the **ulnar** artery?

Allen's Test

❑ What are the steps in Allen's Test?

1. Clench the fist several times.
2. Occlude the radial and ulnar artery at the wrist.
3. Extend fingers which will show a **blanched** hand.

4. Remove pressure on the **ulnar artery** and observe for return of color of the hand. If the color of the hand does not return in 2-3 seconds, the test is positive and radial arterial puncture should not be done.

Steps in ABG Analysis – *Yes, you should know this!*

1. Analyze the pH, PCO_2 and HCO_3.
2. Identify whether the imbalance is **acidosis** or **alkalosis**. (Check the pH)
3. Identify whether the problem is **respiratory** or **metabolic**. (Check what matches the pH)
   If the pCO_2 matches the pH = respiratory; If the HCO_3 matches the pH = metabolic

Types of Compensation – *You have to learn this, in case NCLEX will ask you!*

		pH	PCO_2		HCO_3
Uncompensated	The pH is abnormal and PCO_2 or HCO_3 remains normal	abnormal	abnormal normal	NOT OPPOSITE	normal abnormal
Partially Compensated	The pH is abnormal and PCO_2 and HCO_3 are opposite	abnormal	alkalosis acidosis	OPPOSITE	acidosis alkalosis
Fully Compensated	The pH is normal and PCO_2 and HCO_3 are opposite	normal	alkalosis acidosis	OPPOSITE	acidosis alkalosis

NCLEX Alert! *FULLY COMPENSATED ACID-BASE IMBALANCE*

The pH is normal and if less than 7.40, the problem is likely acidosis.

The pH is normal and if more than 7.40, the problem is likely alkalosis.

Examples of Acid-Base Imbalances

pH (7.35-7.45)	pCO_2 (35-45 mmHg)	HCO_3 (22-26 mEq/L)	RESULT
7.31 acidosis	49 acidosis	24 normal	respiratory acidosis, uncompensated
7.31 acidosis	49 acidosis	28 alkalosis	respiratory acidosis, partially compensated
7.39 normal	49 acidosis	28 alkalosis	respiratory acidosis, fully compensated
7.49 alkalosis	37 normal	29 alkalosis	metabolic alkalosis, uncompensated
7.49 alkalosis	48 acidosis	29 alkalosis	metabolic alkalosis, partially compensated
7.45 normal	48 acidosis	29 alkalosis	metabolic alkalosis, fully compensated
7.25 acidosis	50 acidosis	18 acidosis	mixed respiratory and metabolic acidosis

C. Fluids and Electrolytes

Major Signs of Electrolyte Imbalances

	HYPO -	HYPER -
Potassium	Weakness	Weakness
Sodium	Weakness	Weakness
Calcium	Tetany	Weakness
Phosphorus	Weakness	Tetany
Magnesium	Tetany	Weakness

1. Potassium – Normal Value: 3.5 to 5.0 mEq/L

Food sources: cantaloupes, bananas, carrots, spinach, fish, tomatoes, bananas, avocados, potatoes, oranges

HYPOKALEMIA **Potassium < 3.5 mEq/L**	**HYPERKALEMIA** **Potassium > 5.0 mEq/L**
Causes ❑ Cushing's syndrome ❑ Metabolic alkalosis ❑ Vomiting, diarrhea, gastric lavage ❑ Non-potassium sparing diuretics ❑ Insulin	Causes ❑ Addison's disease ❑ Metabolic acidosis ❑ Burns (1st stage) ❑ Potassium-sparing diuretics ❑ Renal failure
Assessment ❑ **Muscle weakness** ❑ Arrhythmias ❑ Muscle cramping ❑ Hypoactive bowel sounds ❑ Shallow respiration ❑ Postural hypotension ❑ Cardiac arrest ❑ Peaked P waves; depressed ST segment and **U waves; flat T waves**	Assessment ❑ **Muscle weakness** ❑ Arrhythmias ❑ Diarrhea ❑ Bradycardia ❑ Paresthesia ❑ Cardiac arrest ❑ Wide, flat P waves; prolonged PR interval; depressed ST segment; and **tall T waves; widened QRS complex**
Interventions ❑ Monitor for dysrhythmias ❑ Encourage foods high in potassium ❑ Potassium replacement (K-dur, KCl)	Interventions ❑ Monitor for dysrhythmias ❑ Potassium-wasting diuretics ❑ IV dextrose with regular insulin to move potassium inside the cells along with glucose ❑ Sodium polysterene sulfonate (Kayexalate) ❑ $NaHCO_3$ for metabolic acidosis

NCLEX Alert! *Sodium polysterene sulfonate (Kayexalate, Kionex, Kayexate) belongs to the class of medications called cation-exchange resins. It lowers the level of potassium in the blood by binding to potassium in the intestines. It is important to monitor the bowel movements to ensure that the medication is working!*

2. Sodium - Normal Value: 135 - 145 mEq/L

Food sources: canned foods, milk, bacon, pickles, custard, processed foods, table salt, cottage cheese, hot dogs, soy sauce, ketchup, potato chips, gravy, pizza

HYPONATREMIA Sodium < 135 mEq/L	HYPERNATREMIA Sodium > 145 mEq/L
Causes ❑ Syndrome of Inappropriate Antidiuretic Hormone Secretion (SIADH) ❑ Excessive intake of water (dilutional) ❑ Diuretics ❑ Addison's disease	Causes ❑ Diabetes insipidus ❑ Dehydration ❑ Diarrhea ❑ Cushing's syndrome
Assessment ❑ **Muscle weakness** ❑ Rapid, thready pulse ❑ Postural hypotension ❑ Poor skin turgor ❑ Abdominal cramping ❑ Seizures	Assessment ❑ **Muscle weakness** ❑ Dry mucous membranes ❑ Poor skin turgor ❑ Thirst ❑ Flushed skin ❑ Fever ❑ Seizures
Interventions ❑ IV 0.9% sodium chloride ❑ Salt tablets ❑ Avoid tap water enemas	Interventions ❑ Increase water intake ❑ Diuretics ❑ Assess for heart failure

3. Calcium - Normal Value: 8.6 - 10 mg/dL (4.3 to 5.3 mEq/L)

Food sources: milk, yogurt, kale, collard, tofu, cheese, orange, spinach, sesame seeds, almonds, fish

HYPOCALCEMIA Calcium < 8.6 mg/dL	HYPERCALCEMIA Calcium > 10 mg/dL
Causes ❑ Hypoparathyroidism ❑ Renal failure ❑ Pancreatitis	Causes ❑ Hyperparathyroidism ❑ Prolonged immobilization ❑ Excessive intake of milk and vitamin D

HYPOCALCEMIA Calcium < 8.6 mg/dL	HYPERCALCEMIA Calcium > 10 mg/dL
Assessment	Assessment
❑ ↓ CALCIUM = ↑ PHOSPHORUS	❑ ↑ CA = ↓ PHOSPHORUS
❑ **Muscle tetany**	❑ **Muscle weakness**
❑ Neuromuscular irritability	❑ Abdominal distention
❑ **Numbness and tingling in extremities**	❑ Nausea and vomiting
❑ Positive Chvostek's and Trousseau's sign	❑ Decreased deep tendon reflexes
❑ Seizures	❑ Constipation
❑ Abdominal cramping	❑ Kidney stones
❑ Arrhythmias	❑ Pathologic fractures
❑ Prolongation of QT interval	❑ Shortened QT interval and widened T wave
Interventions	Interventions
❑ Seizure precautions	❑ Low calcium diet
❑ Maintain a patent airway	❑ Avoid Vitamin D and thiazide diuretics
❑ Oral/IV calcium replacement	❑ Give phosphates or calcitonin

NCLEX Alert! *Calcium and phosphorus have an inverse relationship. When calcium level in the blood increases, phosphorus decreases.*

4. Magnesium - Normal Value: 1.5 - 2.5 mEq/L

Food sources: raisins, avocados, quinoa, pork, beef, chicken, peanut butter, peas, potatoes, cauliflower, oatmeal, yogurt, milk, green, spinach, broccoli, oatmeal

HYPOMAGNESEMIA Magnesium < 1.5 mEq/L	HYPERMAGNESEMIA Magnesium > 2.5 mg/dL
Causes	Causes
❑ Diarrhea	❑ Antacids containing magnesium
❑ Alcoholism	❑ End-Stage Renal Disease (ESRD)
❑ Crohn's disease	❑ Magnesium sulfate

<table>
<tr><th>HYPOMAGNESEMIA
Magnesium < 1.5 mEq/L</th><th>HYPERMAGNESEMIA
Magnesium > 2.5 mg/dL</th></tr>
<tr><td>Assessment
❑ Muscle tetany
❑ Paresthesia
❑ Hyperactive reflexes
❑ Positive Chvostek's and Trousseau's sign
❑ Shallow respiration
❑ Seizures
❑ Muscle weakness in severe cases
❑ Tall T waves and depressed ST segment</td><td>Assessment
❑ Muscle weakness
❑ Hypotension
❑ Bradycardia
❑ Nausea and vomiting
❑ Sweating and flushing
❑ Absent deep tendon reflexes
❑ Respiratory depression
❑ Cardiac arrest
❑ Prolonged PR interval and widened QRS</td></tr>
<tr><td>Interventions
❑ Monitor for dysrhythmias
❑ Seizure precautions</td><td>Interventions
❑ Monitor for respiratory depression
❑ Loop diuretics</td></tr>
</table>

5. Phosphorus - Normal Value: 2.5 - 4.5 mEq/L

Food sources: organ meats, canned fish, soda, milk, whole-grain breads, peanuts, cereals, pork, beef, chicken, fish

<table>
<tr><th>HYPOPHOSPHATEMIA
Phosphorus < 2.5 mEq/L</th><th>HYPERPHOSPHATEMIA
Phosphorus > 4.5 mEq/L</th></tr>
<tr><td>Causes
❑ Hyperparathyroidism
❑ Renal failure</td><td>Causes
❑ Hypoparathyroidism
❑ Renal insufficiency</td></tr>
<tr><td>Assessment
❑ ↓ PHOSPHORUS = ↑ CALCIUM
❑ Muscle weakness
❑ Decreased deep tendon reflexes
❑ Shallow respiration
❑ Bone pain
❑ Confusion
❑ Seizures</td><td>Assessment
❑ ↑ PHOSPHORUS = ↓ CALCIUM
❑ Muscle tetany
❑ Hyperactive reflexes
❑ Neuromuscular irritability
❑ Muscle weakness in severe cases
❑ Positive Chvostek's or Trousseau's sign
❑ Seizures</td></tr>
<tr><td>Interventions
❑ Monitor for hypercalcemia
❑ Phosphate supplements</td><td>Interventions
❑ Monitor for hypocalcemia
❑ aluminum hydroxide gel (Amphogel)
→ lowers the phosphorus level
❑ Calcium supplements</td></tr>
</table>

D. Intravenous Therapy

❑ Preferred intravenous insertion site in adults	Upper arm, dorsum of hand
❑ Preferred intravenous insertion site in infants	Veins in the scalp and feet
❑ Sites to avoid in intravenous insertion	Swollen and paralyzed extremity, Lower extremities, Arm with dialysis shunt
❑ Use vented tubing for glass or hard bottles	To allow the fluid to flow smoothly
❑ The piggyback infusion (medication) should be hung ______________ than the primary bag to allow fluid to resume flow after piggyback administration is finished	Higher

Types of Intravenous Fluids

❑ 0.9% sodium chloride (normal saline)	Isotonic
❑ Lactated Ringer's (LR)	Isotonic
❑ 0.45% (½ normal saline)	Hypotonic
❑ 5% dextrose in water (D_5W)	Hypotonic
❑ 5% dextrose in Lactated Ringer's solution	Hypertonic
❑ 5% dextrose in 0.45% saline (D_5 ½ NS)	Hypertonic
❑ 5% dextrose in 0.9% saline (D_5 NS)	Hypertonic
❑ 10% dextrose in water ($D_{10}W$)	Hypertonic
❑ Used to increase volume, keep vein open and dilute drugs	0.9% sodium chloride (normal saline)
❑ Used for emergency fluid resuscitation; Has potassium and is not given to clients with renal failure	Lactated Ringer's
❑ Used for hyponatremia and fluid replacement	5% dextrose in 0.45% saline (D_5 ½ NS)
❑ Will cause cerebral edema in clients with head injury	5% dextrose in water (D_5W)

Complications of IV Therapy

COMPLICATIONS	ASSESSMENT
Fluid overload	Tachypnea, crackles, hypertension
Air embolism	Dyspnea, tachycardia, chest pain
Infection	Fever, chills, redness, warmth, edema, pain
Infiltration	Pain, swelling, **cold skin**
Phlebitis	**Warm skin**, redness, tenderness, slow IV infusion

Interventions for Complications of IV Therapy

❑ Phlebitis	Use a smaller gauge needle, Remove the device, Apply warm compress
❑ Infiltration (extravasation)	Remove the device, Elevate the arm

	Apply warm or cold compress
❑ Catheter embolism	Check catheter before and after insertion
❑ Fluid overload	Use an IV pump, Assess for crackles
❑ Air embolism	Prime tubing before infusion
	Replace bottle before becoming empty
	Left side in a Trendelenburg position

Central Venous Catheters

❑ Purposes	Infuse IV fluids, TPN and drugs
	Measure central venous pressure (CVP)
❑ Types	Hickman, Broviac, Groshong
❑ How do you maintain the patency of central venous catheters?	Flush with heparin
❑ What is a port-a-cath?	A specially implanted venous access device used for frequent drug administration

E. Blood Transfusion

❑ Type A blood type can receive	A, O
❑ Type B blood type can receive	B, O
❑ Type AB blood type can receive	A, B, AB, O
❑ Type O blood type can receive	O only
❑ Universal donor is Type ___; Universal recipient is Type ___	O, AB
❑ What does the positive sign mean (e.g. A^+, B^+, O^+, AB^+)?	Presence of Rh antigen
❑ Rh (+) blood can receive ________	Rh (-) or Rh (+) blood
❑ Rh (-) blood should only receive ______ blood	Rh (-)
❑ When does Rh incompatibility occur?	Rh (-) blood is exposed to Rh (+) blood

Blood Administration

❑ How long should packed RBC's be infused?	2-4 hours
❑ How long should platelets be infused?	15-30 minutes
❑ Is cross matching required for platelet transfusion?	No
❑ How long should fresh frozen plasma be infused?	15-30 minutes
❑ Does fresh frozen plasma provide platelets?	No, it provides clotting factors

Nursing Responsibilities in Blood Administration

❑ Check crossmatch record with ___ nurses	2
❑ Use only ________________ solution	Normal saline
❑ Infusions (1 unit) should not exceed _________ for packed RBCs	4 hours
❑ How often is the blood transfusion set changed?	With each unit of blood

❑ Blood should be given within ___ minutes after arrival from blood bank	30 minutes
❑ Take vital signs before transfusion and after the first _____ minutes; every hour until 1 hour after transfusion	15
❑ Administer acetaminophen or diphenhydramine	As ordered
❑ Stay with the client for the first ____ minutes	15
❑ If reaction occurs, _____________ the blood transfusion, change the IV tubing, keep the IV line open infusing with normal saline, report to HCP and return the BT bag to blood bank. Obtain urinalysis order for hemoglobinuria	Stop

Blood Transfusion Reactions

ACUTE HEMOLYTIC REACTION (ABO incompatibility)	DELAYED HEMOLYTIC REACTION	FEBRILE REACTION	ALLERGIC REACTION	TRANSFUSION-RELATED ACUTE LUNG INJURY
❑ **Low back pain** ❑ Hematuria ❑ Fever, chills ❑ Hypotension ❑ Chest pain	❑ Mild fever ❑ Jaundice ❑ Decreasing hematocrit days after BT	❑ Fever ❑ Chills ❑ Tachycardia ❑ Headache	❑ Shortness of breath ❑ Itchiness ❑ Urticaria ❑ Swelling of lips	❑ Sudden onset of pulmonary edema ❑ Rare event

F. Laboratory Values

1. Erythrocyte Tests

LAB TEST	DESCRIPTION	NORMAL VALUES
❑ RBC, Hemoglobin and Hematocrit	❑ ***Low = anemia*** ❑ ***High = polycythemia (at risk for clotting)***	Hemoglobin ❑ Male: 13-17 g/dL ❑ Female: 12-15 g/dL Hematocrit ❑ Male: 40-52% ❑ Female: 36-47% Iron ❑ Male: 65-175 mcg/dL ❑ Female: 50-170 mcg/dL Red blood cells ❑ Male: 4.7-6.1 million cells/ul ❑ Female: 4.2-5.4 million cells/ul

LAB TEST	DESCRIPTION	NORMAL VALUES
❑ Erythrocyte Sedimentation Rate (ESR)	❑ Rate at which red blood cells sediment in a period of one hour ❑ ***High = inflammation but does not identify specific disease process***	Male: 0-22 mm/hr Female: 0-29 mm/hr

2. Coagulation Tests

LAB TEST	DESCRIPTION	NORMAL VALUES
Prothrombin Time (PT) International Normalized Ratio (INR)	❑ Used to monitor warfarin therapy ❑ Therapeutic effect is achieved if PT is **1.5-2.5 times** control (normal) value ❑ ***High = at risk for bleeding***	PT: 11-14 seconds INR: 2-3 during warfarin dosing
Activated Partial Thromboplastin Time (aPTT) Partial Thromboplastin Time (PTT)	❑ Used to monitor heparin therapy ❑ aPTT is more sensitive than PTT ❑ Therapeutic effect is achieved if aPPT or PTT is **1.5-2.5 times** control (normal) value ❑ ***High = at risk for bleeding***	aPTT: 30-40 seconds PTT: 60-70 seconds
Platelet Count	❑ ***Low = at risk for bleeding (thrombocytopenia)***	150,000 – 400,000 cells/mm^3
Clotting Time	❑ ***High = at risk for bleeding***	8-15 minutes
D-dimer Test	❑ D-dimer is a protein fragment after a blood clot ❑ ***High = thrombosis, embolism***	< or =250 ng/mL DDU

3. Serum Enzyme and Protein Tests

LAB TEST	DESCRIPTION	NORMAL VALUES
Troponins	❑ Troponin I and Troponin T ❑ Proteins found in heart muscle ❑ Released in the blood when there is cardiac damage ❑ ***High = myocardial infarction***	Increases 3 hours after MI Troponin I → high for 7-10 days Troponin T → high for 10-14 days

LAB TEST	DESCRIPTION	NORMAL VALUES
Creatine kinase (CK)	❑ CK-MB (cardiac) ❑ Avoid exercise and alcohol before the test	Increases within 3-6 hours after MI, peak 18 hours, normal 2-3 days
Lactic Dehydrogenase (LDH)	❑ Enzyme found mostly in tissues	Increases 24 hours after MI, peak 48-72 hours, normal 7-14 days
Myoglobin	❑ Rises earlier than troponin, but not specific for cardiac damage	Increases 2 hours after MI
B-type natriuretic peptide (BNP)	❑ BNP is a hormone secreted by the failing heart ❑ Causes natriuresis (excretion of sodium in urine) ❑ ***High = heart failure***	<125 pg/mL

4. Gastrointestinal Tests

LAB TEST	DESCRIPTION	NORMAL VALUES
Ammonia	❑ Forms when protein is broken down and acted upon by bacteria in the intestines ❑ The liver converts ammonia to urea then eliminated in urine ❑ Place specimen on ice and send to lab within 30 minutes ❑ ***High = hepatic encephalopathy***	10 - 80 mcg/dL
Albumin	❑ Protein synthesized by the liver ❑ Maintains the osmotic pressure ❑ ***Low = malnutrition, cirrhosis***	3.5-5 g/dL
Alkaline phosphatase	❑ Increased in bone growth, liver and gallbladder disease	44-147 IU/L
Alanine aminotransferase (ALT)	❑ Formerly serum glutamate-pyruvate transaminase (SGPT) ❑ ***High = liver disease***	20-60 IU/L
Aspartate aminotransferase (AST)	❑ Formerly serum glutamic oxaloacetic transaminase (SGOT) ❑ ***High = liver disease***	Male: 6-34 IU/L Female: 8-40 IU/L.

LAB TEST	DESCRIPTION	NORMAL VALUES
Amylase	❑ Inflamed pancreas releases amylase into the blood ❑ Avoid alcohol before the test ❑ ***High = acute pancreatitis***	23-85 U/L
Lipase	❑ ***High = acute pancreatitis***	0-160 U/L
Bilirubin	❑ Produced by the liver, spleen and bone marrow; and hemolysis ❑ Fasting required ❑ ***High = liver disease, hemolysis***	Direct (GI): 0-0.3 mg/dL Indirect (Blood): 0.2-1.2 mg/dL Total: < 1.5 mg/dL
Lipids		Cholesterol: <200 mg/dL HDLs: male (40-50 mg/dL) female (50-59 mg/dL) LDLs: <100 mg/dL (optimal) Triglycerides: <150 mg/dL

5. Glucose Tests

LAB TEST	DESCRIPTION	NORMAL VALUES
2-Hour Post-Prandial Blood Glucose	❑ Measures blood glucose 2 hours after eating a meal, timed from the beginning of the meal	<140 mg/dL
Glycosylated Hemoglobin (HgbA1C)	❑ Blood glucose adhered to hemoglobin of the RBC ❑ Reflects glucose level control (average) for the past 3-4 months	Normal: <5.7% Prediabetes: 5.7% to 6.4% Diabetes: 6.5% or higher
Fasting Blood Glucose	❑ Blood sample taken after fasting ❑ Do not give morning insulin	Normal: < 100 mg/dL Prediabetes: 100 mg/dL to 125 mg/dL Diabetes: 126 mg/dL or higher
Glucose Tolerance Test	1. Avoid coffee, alcohol, and smoking before the test 2. Do not give morning insulin 3. Client fasts overnight 4. Blood sugar level is measured 5. Client drinks a glucose liquid 6. Blood sugar levels are tested at multiple time intervals	Normal: < 140 mg/dL Prediabetes: 140 mg/dL to 199 mg/dL Diabetes: 200 mg/dL or higher *Reference:* *American Diabetes Association (www.diabetes.org)*

6. Urinary Tests

LAB TEST	DESCRIPTION	NORMAL VALUES
Serum Creatinine	❑ Specific indicator of renal function ❑ Avoid exercise before the test ❑ ***High = renal disease***	0.6 - 1.3 mg/dL
Blood Urea Nitrogen	❑ ***High = renal disease***	8 - 25 mg/dL
Creatinine Clearance	❑ Accurate measurement of renal function as to how much creatinine is excreted by the kidneys ❑ Includes collecting a **24-hour urine sample** followed by drawing a blood sample to compare creatinine levels ❑ ***Low = renal disease***	Male: 97-137 mL/min Female: 88-128 mL/min
Urinalysis with reflex culture and sensitivity (C/S) test	❑ Reflex culture means that C/S test will only be done if urinalysis result is abnormal	Color: Pale yellow Odor: Aromatic Specific gravity: 1.010 - 1.030 pH: 4.5 - 7.8 Protein: none or some traces Hemoglobin: none Ketones: none Bilirubin: none Glucose: none Bacteria: <1000 colonies/mL

7. Additional Laboratory Tests

LAB TEST	DESCRIPTION	NORMAL VALUES
Thyroid Tests	❑ TSH (thyrotropin) ❑ Thyroxine (T4) ❑ Thyroxine, free (FT4) ❑ Triiodothyronine (T_3) ❑ ***High = hyperthyroidism*** ❑ ***Low = hypothyroidism***	TSH: 0.5-4.70 μg/mL T_4 : 4.5-12.5 μg/dL FT_4 : 0.7-1.9 μg /dL T_3 : 80-180 μg /dL

LAB TEST	DESCRIPTION	NORMAL VALUES
White Blood Cell Count WBC Differential Count ❑ *Lymphocytes* ❑ *Monocytes* ❑ *Basophils* ❑ *Eosinophils* ❑ *Neutrophils*	1. Shift to the left - increased immature neutrophils due to infection or inflammation 2. High WBC count with a left shift - increased neutrophils due to severe infection 3. Low WBC count with a left shift - recovery from bone marrow suppression 4. Shift to the right - more mature WBC	White Blood Cell Count (WBC) ❑ 5000-10000 cells/mm^3
HIV Testing	❑ ELISA, Western blot antibody tests ❑ NAAT (nucleic acid amplification)	
CD4 (T cell) Counts	❑ Monitors progression of HIV disease	500-1600 cells/mm^3
Viral Load Testing	❑ Monitors HIV infection status	

8. Therapeutic Drug Levels

DRUG	THERAPEUTIC VALUES
phenytoin (Dilantin), theophylline, acetaminophen	10-20 mcg/mL
gentamycin	5-10 mcg/mL
valproic acid (Depakene)	50-100 mcg/mL
digoxin (Lanoxin)	0.5-2 ng/mL
lithium (Lithobid)	0.5-1.3 mEq/L
magnesium sulfate	4-7 mg/dL
carbamazepine (Tegretol)	5-12 mcg/mL

NCLEX Alert! *PEAK and TROUGH LEVELS – WHAT ARE THEY?*

*Peak and trough specimens are serum samples collected to determine the level of an antibiotic or other drugs in the blood. The **trough level** (lowest concentration) includes a specimen being collected **30 minutes prior** to the IV administration of the drug. The **peak level** (highest concentration) includes a specimen being collected **30 minutes after** the IV infusion.*

G. Drug Antidotes

DRUG TOXICITY OR CLINICAL CONDITION	ANTIDOTE
Acetaminophen (Tylenol)	acetylcysteine (Mucomyst)
Atropine and scopolamine	pilocarpine
Benzodiazepines	flumazenil (Romazicon)
Myasthenic Crisis	edrophonium (Tensilon), neostigmine (Prostigmine)
Cholinergic Crisis (anticholinesterase overdose)	atropine sulfate
Warfarin	phytomenadione (Vitamin K)
Digoxin	digoxin immune fab (Digibind)
Extrapyramidal symptoms (EPS)	diphenhydramine (Benadryl), benztropine (Cogentin), biperiden (Akineton), trihexyphenidyl HCl (Artane)
Heparin	Protamine sulfate
Hyperkalemia	Insulin & glucose, $NaHCO_3$, Kayexalate, Kionex
Insulin reaction/shock (hypoglycemia)	Dextrose 50% IV, Glucagon injection
Iron	deferoxamine mesylate (Desferal)
Isoniazid (peripheral neuropathy)	Pyridoxine (Vitamin B_6)
Lead poisoning	Dimercaprol, edetate calcium, disodium
Magnesium sulfate	Calcium gluconate
Narcotic opioids (respiratory depression)	nalmefene (Selincro), naloxone (Narcan), nalorphine (Nalline)
Thrombolytics	aminocaproic acid (Amicar)

NCLEX Alert! *Make sure that you remember the drug antidotes as they are frequently used during emergencies to reverse the effects of the drugs!*

Integumentary System 6

A. The Integumentary System

❑ Functions	Protection Thermoregulation Vitamin synthesis (Vitamin D)
❑ Outer layer of the skin	Epidermis
❑ Cells that produce melanin and determines skin color	Melanocytes
❑ Is the skin darker due to melanin?	Yes
❑ Irregular patches of melanin	Freckles
❑ Also known as the "true skin"	Dermis Has blood vessels, nerves, glands and hair follicles
❑ Appendages of the skin	Sudoriferous glands (sweat glands) Sebaceous glands (oil glands) Hair and nails

B. Types of Skin Lesions

❑ Vesicle greater than 1 cm in diameter (e.g. pemphigus)	Bulla
❑ A raised, itchy lesion (e.g. hives)	Wheal
❑ Elevated, filled with serous fluid (e.g. varicella, shingles)	Vesicle
❑ Thickened, rough epidermal skin (e.g. chronic dermatitis)	Lichenification
❑ Tiny purple, red or brown spots on the skin	Petechiae
❑ Red or purple spots caused by bleeding	Purpura
❑ Discoloration due to bruising	Ecchymosis
❑ Flat, circumscribed lesions (e.g. freckles)	Macule
❑ Elevated, firm area (e.g. wart)	Papule
❑ Fine, red line due to vasodilation (e.g. rosacea)	Telangiectasis
❑ Elevated lesion containing pus (e.g. impetigo)	Pustule

***NCLEX Alert!** You should remember the characteristic lesions in every skin disorder!*

C. Integumentary System Disorders

Herpes Simplex

❑ Description	Herpes simplex type 1 (cold sore) Herpes simplex type 2 (genital herpes)
❑ Assessment	Painful, crusted vesicles
❑ Interventions	Antivirals, Analgesics, Warm compress
❑ Is there a cure for this condition?	No
❑ Is this disease transmissible even without symptoms?	Yes, during asymptomatic viral shedding

Herpes Zoster (Shingles)

❑ Description	Reactivation of **varicella** or **chickenpox** virus infection
❑ Transmission	Contact (*plus airborne for clients who are immunosuppressed or have disseminated type of infection*)
❑ Cause	Immunosuppression, chemotherapy
❑ Assessment	Burning pain, vesicles
❑ Interventions	Analgesics, Antiviral drugs, Cool compress
❑ Is this disease a danger to persons with no varicella immunity or negative titer levels?	Yes, the person can acquire chickenpox

Impetigo Contagiosa

❑ Description	Caused by staphylococcus
❑ Transmission	Contact
❑ Assessment	Red sores, **honey-colored** crust
❑ Interventions	Wound precautions, ATB ointment
❑ Complication	Acute glomerulonephritis

Furuncles and Carbuncles

❑ Description	Infection of the hair follicles caused by bacteria (staphylococcus) or fungus
❑ A boil	Furuncle
❑ Cluster of boils	Carbuncles
❑ Transmission	Contact
❑ Assessment	Swollen, red and painful lesion
❑ Interventions	Incision and drainage ATB, Warm soaks
❑ Can this disease spread to other body parts?	Yes

Dermatophytoses

❑ Description	A fungal skin infection
❑ Tinea corporis	Affects the body
❑ Tinea cruris	Affects the groin (Jock itch)
❑ Tinea pedis	Affects the feet (Athlete's foot)
❑ Assessment	Red rashes, scaly patches, Skin lesion emits a **blue-green** color in Wood's lamp exam (tinea capitis)
❑ Interventions	Antifungals - tolnaftate (Tinactin) Keep area dry, Avoid sharing towels

Eczema (Atopic Dermatitis)

❑ Description	Inflammation of the skin
❑ Risk factors	Allergies to chocolate, eggs, milk, soy wheat, fish, peanuts and orange juice
❑ Assessment	Redness, crusted vesicles, pruritus
❑ Interventions	Hydrate the skin, Wet dressings, Eucerin

Acne Vulgaris

❑ Description	Hair follicles are clogged
❑ Causes	Heredity, diet, stress, hormones
❑ Assessment	Blackheads (comedo), pustules
❑ Interventions	Benzoyl peroxide gel, Vitamin A acids Tetracycline, isotretinoin (Accutane)

Psoriasis

❑ Description	Skin cells divide more rapidly than normal
❑ Assessment	Red, **silvery scaly plaques**, pruritus
❑ Interventions	Hydrocortisone, Tar preparations, Salicylic acid, Methotrexate, adalimumab (Humira), Photochemotherapy
❑ Is this disease infectious?	No

Scabies

❑ Description	Caused by female itch mite
❑ How long can a mite survive without a host?	2-3 days
❑ Transmission	Contact
❑ Assessment	Threadlike lines with burrows, pruritus
❑ Interventions	permethrin cream 5% (Elimite)

❑ How is the cream or lotion applied?	Apply to dry and cool skin from neck down Leave on for 12 hours
❑ Should close contacts be treated?	Family members and sexual contacts need treatment at the same time
❑ How should the clothes be washed?	Wash clothes in hot water or seal in a bag for 72 hours

Rosacea

❑ Description	Incurable, chronic acne-like skin condition
❑ Assessment	**Persistent blushing**, pimples, telangiectasis
❑ Interventions	Use sunscreen, Emollient, Avoid hot temperature, Laser and light therapy

Skin Cancer

❑ Most deadly type	Malignant melanoma
❑ What is ABCDE technique in skin assessment for identifying skin cancer?	A - symmetry (other half does not match) B - orders (uneven and irregular) C - olor (lesion shows a variety of colors) D - iameter (larger than a pencil eraser) E - nlarging (change in size or shape)
❑ Assessment	A new skin lesion or a change in appearance or size of an existing lesion
❑ Interventions	Surgical excision, Chemotherapy, Radiation
❑ Use sunscreens with SPF ___ or higher	15
❑ Avoid sun exposure from ____ am to ____ pm	10, 4

D. Stages of Pressure Sores

❑ Intact skin with **non-blanchable** redness	Stage 1
❑ Shallow ulcer with a red or pink wound bed, no sloughing	Stage 2
❑ Usually presents as an intact or ruptured blister	Stage 2
❑ Undermining, slough and tunneling may be present	Stage 3 or 4
❑ Subcutaneous fat is exposed but bone, tendon or muscles cannot be seen	Stage 3
❑ Slough or eschar may be present	Stage 3 or 4
❑ Full thickness tissue loss in which the ulcer is covered by black eschar	Unstageable

> ***NCLEX Alert!*** *The most effective way to prevent pressure sores is to reposition the client every 2 hours.*

E. Caring for Clients with Burns

Pathophysiology of Burns

1st 24-48 Hours (Plasma to Interstitial Fluid Shifting)
❑ Immediately after a major burn injury → vasodilation → increased capillary permeability → plasma to interstitial fluid shifting → decreased blood volume → decreased cardiac output → decreased renal circulation → **acute renal failure** ❑ Destruction of cells → release of potassium → **hyperkalemia** → dysrhythmias → cardiac arrest
48-72 Hours Post-Burn (Interstitial to Plasma Fluid Shifting)
❑ Interstitial to plasma fluid shifting → Increased blood volume → increased renal circulation → polyuria → **hypokalemia**

Stages of Burns

HYPOVOLEMIC STAGE 1st 24-48 Hours (Plasma to the interstitial fluid shifting)	DIURETIC STAGE 48-72 Hours Post-Burn (Interstitial to the plasma fluid shifting)
❑ Hypovolemia ❑ Shock ❑ Hyperkalemia ❑ Oliguria ❑ Hemoconcentration (↑ hematocrit) ❑ Hyponatremia ❑ Metabolic acidosis	❑ Hypervolemia ❑ Heart failure ❑ Hypokalemia ❑ Polyuria ❑ Hemodilution (↓ hematocrit) ❑ Hyponatremia ❑ Metabolic acidosis

Classification of Burns (based on depth)

FIRST DEGREE (Superficial)	SECOND DEGREE (Partial Thickness)	THIRD DEGREE (Full Thickness)
❑ Involves the epidermis ❑ Red ❑ Dry ❑ Painful	❑ Involves the epidermis and part of the dermis ❑ Red ❑ **Blistered** ❑ Very painful	❑ Involves the epidermis, dermis, bones, muscles and tendons ❑ White or charred ❑ Painless due to nerve damage

❑ What are the signs and symptoms of smoke inhalation?

Hoarse voice, singed nasal hairs and sooty, black sputum

❑ What are the signs and symptoms of carbon monoxide (CO) poisoning?

Vomiting, headache, ataxia, weakness, blurred vision, confusion, dyspnea

❑ What is the emergency treatment for CO poisoning?

Give 100% oxygen
Hyperbaric oxygen therapy

Rule of Nines

❑ What is the purpose of Rule of Nines?

A method to quickly estimate the percentage of burn area and is used as a basis to calculate the amount of fluid resuscitation in a major burn injury

BODY AREA	PERCENTAGE
Head and neck	9%
Right arm	9%
Left arm	9%
Trunk	36% - anterior = 18% *(chest = 9%; abdomen = 9%)*
	- posterior = 18% *(upper back = 9%; lower back = 9%)*
Right lower extremity	18%
Left lower extremity	18%
Perineum	1%

Total	100 %

❑ Lund and Browder Chart

Preferred in pediatric burns as it considers age with different percentages of Body Surface Area (BSA) for the head and lower extremities

❑ What is **Parkland Formula**?

Estimates the amount of fluid replacement for the first 24 hours after a burn injury
Formula: 4 mL /kg /% of burned surface

❑ How do you administer IV fluids for the first 24 hours after a major burn injury?

Give 50% in the first 8 hours
Give 25% in the second 8 hours
Give 25% in the third 8 hours

Interventions for Burns

❑ Emergency management	Ensure own safety Use stop, drop and roll technique if clothing is on fire Smother the flames with a blanket or coat Remove clothing and jewelry if possible Do not use ice, ice water or very cool water Rinse with cool water (chemical burn) Do not touch unless safe (electrical burn) Open the airway and control bleeding
❑ Monitor intake and output	To monitor the effect of fluid therapy
❑ Monitor BUN and creatinine	To assess for acute renal failure
❑ Diet	High calorie, high protein diet
❑ Protective isolation	To prevent infection
❑ Antacids	To prevent **Curling's ulcer**
❑ Use bed cradle	To prevent wound pain from heavy sheets
❑ Monitor bowel sounds	To assess for the presence of paralytic ileus
❑ Escharotomy	Incision of eschar to improve circulation
❑ Autograft	Implanted tissue from self
❑ Homograft/allograft	Implanted tissue from same species
❑ Heterograft/xenograft	Implanted tissue from another species

F. Integumentary System Drugs

1. Drugs for Psoriasis

tazarotene (Tazorac, Avage, Fabior)

❑ Description	Vitamin A derivative
❑ Side effects	Photosensitivity, burning, stinging, itching
❑ Contraindication	Pregnancy (**teratogenic**)
❑ Interventions	Use sunscreen Requires a negative pregnancy test

acitretin (Soriatane)

❑ Description	Vitamin A derivative; For severe psoriasis
❑ Side effects	Redness, itching, scaling
❑ Contraindication	Pregnancy (**teratogenic**)
❑ Interventions	Requires a negative pregnancy test Avoid alcohol and vitamin A supplements

ustekinumab (Stelara PFS)

❑ Description	A biologic or immunomodulatory drug Increases cancer risk
❑ Side effects	Infections, headache, joint pain
❑ Contraindications	BCG within the past year, active TB
❑ Interventions	Avoid live virus vaccines (risk for infection)

Photochemotherapy

❑ Description	Combination of radiation with methoxsalen
❑ Side effects	Photosensitivity
❑ Interventions	Avoid consecutive days of therapy

2. Drugs for Acne

isotretinoin (Accutane)

❑ Description	Vitamin A derivative Prescribed on I-Pledge Program
❑ Side effects	Dry skin, itchiness
❑ Contraindication	Pregnancy (**teratogenic**)
❑ Interventions	Avoid pregnancy during treatment

spironolactone (Aldactone)

❑ Description	Treats hormonal acne by decreasing androgen activity
❑ Contraindication	Pregnancy (**teratogenic**)
❑ Side effects	Dizziness, **hyperkalemia**, gynecomastia
❑ Interventions	Avoid a high potassium diet

3. Drugs for Burns

mafenide acetate (Sulfamylon)

❑ Description	Antimicrobial, Painful to apply
❑ Side effects	**Metabolic acidosis,** skin rash
❑ Interventions	Stop drug if client is hyperventilating (indicates metabolic acidosis)

Silver nitrate

❑ Description	Debridement agent, Antiseptic, Less painful
❑ Side effects	**Staining of the skin**, burning, irritation
❑ Interventions	Apply with caution (highly corrosive)

Musculoskeletal System 7

A. The Musculoskeletal System

- ❑ Functions
  Movement, Protection, Support, Hematopoiesis, Calcium storage

- ❑ Types of Bone Cells
  Osteoblasts (bone-building)
  Osteocytes (mature osteoblasts)
  Osteoclasts (breaks down bony tissue)

- ❑ Types of Bone Tissues
  COMPACT (CORTICAL BONE)
  - Dense tissue in shaft of long bones
  - Contains yellow bone marrow

  SPONGY (CANCELLOUS BONE)
  - Contains red bone marrow

- ❑ Types of Joints
  SYNARTHROSIS
  - no movements (e.g. sutures of the skull)

  AMPHIARTHROSIS
  - slight movement (e.g. spinal column)

  DIARTHROSIS
  - free movement (e.g. elbow joint)

- ❑ Vertebral Column
  Cervical (C_1-C_7)
  Thoracic (T_1-T_{12})
  Lumbar (L_1-L_5)
  Sacrum
  Coccyx

- ❑ Types of muscles
  SKELETAL/VOLUNTARY MUSCLES
  - Under conscious control

  SMOOTH MUSCLES
  - Involuntary or visceral
    (e.g. digestive tract & blood vessels)

  CARDIAC MUSCLES
  - Cannot be controlled

❑ Tendon	Anchors muscles to the bones
❑ Ligament	Fibrous tissue that attaches bones to bones
❑ Acetylcholine	Neurotransmitter at the neuromuscular junction for skeletal muscle contraction
❑ Cholinesterase	Breaks down acetylcholine

B. Musculoskeletal Devices

Casts

❑ What are the 6 P's of neurovascular assessment?	P-ulselessness, P-ain, P-aralysis, P-oikilothermia, P-aresthesia, P-allor
❑ Elevate casted extremity and support with pillows	To prevent edema
❑ Handle wet cast with the palms of the hands	To prevent indentation and pressure sore
❑ Is it normal if the cast feels warm while drying?	Yes, the drying cast generates heat
❑ Is use of heat lamp or hair dryer allowed?	No, a fan may be used to circulate air
❑ Can the cast be covered?	No, it prevents the escape of moisture
❑ Report the presence of odor or drainage	It indicates infection (e.g. osteomyelitis)
❑ Petal the cast edges with moleskin or tape	To prevent skin irritation
❑ What should you do if you notice a blood spot on the cast?	Circle with a pen to monitor bleeding
❑ What should you do if the client complains of pruritus?	Give antihistamines; Use a hair dryer on a cool setting and aim it under the cast
❑ What is the purpose of windowing?	To inspect a of "hot spot" or infection
❑ What is the purpose of bivalving?	To relieve pressure from a tight cast
❑ What device should be prepared at the bedside at all times?	Cast cutter

Skeletal Traction

❑ What is the purpose of a skeletal traction?	Reduce (realign) a fracture
❑ What is the difference between a skin and skeletal traction?	Skeletal traction uses pins and wires attached to the bones; Skin traction applies pressure on the skin using bandages and tapes
❑ What is a Balanced Suspension Traction?	A traction that allows changes in client position without interfering with traction (Thomas Splint with Pearson attachment)

Skin Traction

❑ What is a Bucks Traction?	Maintains reduction of a hip fracture Usually applied temporarily to reduce painful **muscle spasms** before surgery

❑ What is a Russel Traction?

Used for hip and knee fractures
Allows more movement and knee flexion
Check the **popliteal area** for signs of pressure from the knee sling (e.g. redness)

❑ What is a Bryant's Traction?

Used for children with fractured femurs
Legs are suspended at a 90° angle
Body weight acts as the source of traction
Buttocks should not touch the mattress

> ***NCLEX Alert!*** *CARE OF THE CLIENT IN TRACTION*
>
> *Weights should not touch the floor or bed; Ropes should hang freely; Never remove the weights; Clean pin sites per protocol using one cotton-tip swab per pin; Increase fluid intake*

Crutch Safety and Measurement

❑ Bear weight on the ____________, not the axillae — Hands

❑ Allow a 2-inch width between the axillary fold and the arm piece of the crutches — To prevent nerve damage in armpit area

❑ Should the elbow be slightly flexed? — Yes

❑ Crutch tip should be ___ inches away from side of feet — 6

Types of Crutch Walking

TYPE	DESCRIPTION	
Two-Point Gait	❑ Requires partial weight-bearing on both feet	❑ Right leg and left crutch move forward followed by the left leg and right crutch
Three-Point Gait	❑ Used when one foot is non-weight-bearing	❑ Crutches with **bad leg** move forward followed by **good leg**
Four-Point Gait	❑ Requires partial weight-bearing on both feet	❑ Right crutch moves forward followed by left leg then left crutch moves forward followed by right leg
Swing-To Gait	❑ Requires weight-bearing on both feet (or one foot)	❑ Both crutches are advanced individually or together, followed by swinging the feet slightly off the floor to an imaginary line just **behind** the crutches
Swing-Through Gait	❑ Requires weight-bearing on both feet (or one foot)	❑ Both crutches are advanced together, followed by swinging the feet **beyond** the crutches

NCLEX Alert! *GOING UPSTAIRS - Good leg first; GOING DOWNSTAIRS - Bad leg first with crutches*

NCLEX Alert! *Remember COAL and WWAL*
Cane OPPOSITE Affected Leg; Walker WITH Affected Leg

C. Diagnostic Tests

Nuclear Scanning

❑ Description	Scanners record the images on film
❑ Are special precautions needed?	No, dosages of radioisotopes are low

Computerized Tomography (CT) Scan

❑ Description	Uses x-rays to produce detailed pictures
❑ How is this procedure different from MRI?	It exposes the client to radiation
❑ Interventions	Ask for iodine allergy, NPO, Lie still

Bone Scan

❑ Description	Nuclear imaging test that detects metastatic and inflammatory bone disease

Arthroscopy

❑ Description	Direct endoscopic exam of the joint using a large needle and saline instillation

Endoscopic Spinal Surgery

❑ Description	Small incisions that require using a scope to diagnose for herniated disc and scoliosis

Synovial Fluid Aspiration

❑ Description	Aspiration of synovial fluid to diagnose osteoarthritis and gout

Electromyogram

❑ Description	Insertion of needle electrodes into the muscles to assess electrical activity Determines the cause of muscle weakness

D. Musculoskeletal System Disorders

RHEUMATOID ARTHRITIS	OSTEOARTHRITIS	GOUTY ARTHRITIS
Inflammation of synovial membranes	Bones and joints degenerate due to thinning of cartilage	Accumulation of uric acid in the blood and deposition in joints
Cause: Autoimmune, genetics	Cause: Obesity, repetitive joint use Can occur related to weather	Cause: metabolic disease, chemotherapy, genetics
Assessment ❑ Fever ❑ Subcutaneous nodules ❑ **Morning stiffness** ❑ **Symmetrical joint pain** ❑ Hand deformities: ▪ Swan-neck deformity ▪ Boutonniere deformity ▪ Ulnar deviation	Assessment ❑ Joint pain, swelling, stiffness and tenderness ❑ Crepitus ❑ Hand deformities: ▪ Heberden's nodes ▪ Bouchard's nodes	Assessment ❑ Tophi formation in joints (uric acid crystal deposits) ❑ Excruciating pain on great toe ❑ Kidney stones ❑ Sudden painful attack at night
Interventions ❑ Warm and cold application ❑ Exercise ❑ Disease-modifying antirheumatic drugs (DMARDs) ❑ NSAIDs, Steroids ❑ Biologic agents ▪ abatacept (Orencia) ▪ adalimumab (Humira) ▪ etanercept (Enbrel)	Interventions ❑ NSAIDs ❑ Warm application ❑ Exercise ❑ Hip joint replacement	Interventions ❑ Increase fluid intake ❑ Low purine diet ❑ Avoid **high-purine** foods - organ meats and fish such as anchovies, herring, sardines, mussels, scallops, trout, haddock, mackerel and tuna ❑ colchicine, NSAIDs ❑ allopurinol (Zyloprim)

Osteoporosis

- ❑ Description — Bone loss due to a sedentary lifestyle, steroids and caffeine
- ❑ Incidence — Small-framed, thin and menopausal women
- ❑ Assessment — Backache, **height loss,** lordosis, kyphosis
- ❑ Diagnostic Test — Bone densitometry (DEXA)
- ❑ Interventions — Calcium with vitamin D, Weight-bearing exercises, Hormonal replacement, Bone resorption inhibitor drugs

Osteomyelitis

❑ Description	Bone infection
❑ Cause	Trauma such as compound (open) fracture
❑ Assessment	Bone pain, drainage, fever
❑ Interventions	Aggressive IV ATBs, Wound irrigation
❑ Why is this condition hard to treat?	Bone has poor circulation

Fibromyalgia

❑ Description	Chronic pain in muscles and joints
❑ Assessment	Generalized pain (**11/18 tender points**), fatigue, depression, insomnia
❑ What will make this condition worse?	Cold weather, fatigue, stress
❑ Interventions	Relaxation techniques, Exercise Antidepressant - amitriptyline (Elavil) Anticonvulsant - pregabalin (Lyrica)

Ankylosing Spondylitis

❑ Description	Chronic, progressive disorder → stiffness of hip joints and spine
❑ Assessment	Kyphosis, backache, dyspnea
❑ Interventions	NSAIDs, Exercise, Firm mattress, Braces

Rhabdomyolosis

❑ Description	Breakdown of muscle tissue → releases myoglobin → kidney damage
❑ Causes	**Statins**, severe heat, marathon
❑ Assessment	**Cola-colored urine**, oliguria, muscle pain
❑ Interventions	Diuretics, Bicarbonate, Dialysis

> ***NCLEX Alert!*** *Proper hydration and rest can prevent rhabdomyolosis during intense exertion.*

Bone cancer

❑ Description	Osteochondroma is the most common benign tumor
❑ Assessment	Spontaneous fractures, bone pain
❑ Interventions	Amputation, Radiation, Chemotherapy

Sprains

❑ Description	Tearing of ligaments
❑ What is sprain of the cervical spine called?	Whiplash
❑ Assessment	Pain, swelling, bruising
❑ Interventions	Immobilization, Analgesics

Strains

❑ Description	Overstretching of muscles and tendons
❑ Assessment	Pain, soreness, weakness
❑ Interventions	Analgesics, Muscle relaxants, Ice compress

Dislocations

❑ Description	Tearing of the joint
❑ Common sites	Shoulder, hips and knee
❑ Assessment	Pain, loss of function, edema, **shortening** of the extremity
❑ Interventions	R.I.C.E., Splint, Surgery
❑ What is the meaning of RICE?	R-est, I-ce, C-ompression, E-levation

Carpal Tunnel Syndrome

❑ Description	Compression of the median nerve
❑ Assessment	Pain on the wrist and hand, inability to grasp or hold small objects, burning and tingling pain
❑ What is a positive Tinel's Test?	Tapping over the wrist → paresthesia
❑ What is a positive Phalen's Test?	Hold wrists in palmar flexion → paresthesia
❑ Interventions	Exercises, Splinting, Cortisone injection Surgery, Decompression of median nerve

Fractures

❑ Types	COMPOUND – open fracture SIMPLE – closed fracture GREENSTICK – bone bends and breaks COMMINUTED – fragmented fracture

❑ Colle's fracture is a fracture of the ______.	Wrist
❑ Pott's fracture is a fracture of the ______.	Distal end of the fibula
❑ Interventions	R.I.C.E., Analgesics
❑ What is the meaning of **reduction** of a fracture?	Realignment of bones
❑ What is the meaning of **fixation** of a fracture?	Stabilizing fractured bones using metal plates, pins, rods, wires or screws
❑ What is the meaning of ORIF?	Open reduction and internal fixation
❑ What device is important to prepare at the bedside if client has a wired jaw due to mandibular fracture?	Wire cutter → in case the client vomits or has dyspnea

Hip Fracture

❑ Description	A break in the femur due to falls or trauma
❑ Assessment	Severe pain, crepitus, shock, **shortening** or **external rotation** of the leg
❑ Interventions	Skin traction, Arthroplasty, Hip replacement
❑ Why is it important to place the legs in **abducted** position after hip replacement surgery?	To prevent hip dislocation
❑ What instructions are important to teach the client after hip replacement surgery in order to prevent hip dislocation?	Avoid crossing of legs and flexion of hips beyond 90°, Use raised toilet seats, Sit up when dressing, Avoid bending, Avoid internal and external rotation of the hip
❑ Complications of hip joint replacement surgery	Bleeding, **thrombosis**, anemia, infection

Complications of Fractures

COMPARTMENT SYNDROME	FAT EMBOLISM
Pressure (fractures, tight cast) → compression of arteries, nerves and tendons → muscle hypoxia → paralysis and sensory loss → disability of extremity	Fractures of the pelvis or **long bones** → release of fat globules → occlusion of pulmonary circulation → pulmonary embolism → respiratory distress
Assessment ❑ Unrelenting pain **unrelieved** by analgesics ❑ Numbness or tingling ❑ Volkmann's contracture (claw-like hand deformity)	Assessment ❑ Confusion, restlessness, dyspnea ❑ Chest pain, fever ❑ Petechial rash
Interventions ❑ Elevate the limb, Fasciotomy (relieves the pressure)	Interventions ❑ Oxygen, Steroids, Immobilization

Amputation

❑ Elevate the extremity for the first 24-48 hours	To reduce swelling
❑ Avoid Semi-Fowler's position in above-the-knee amputation (AKA)	To prevent hip flexion contracture
❑ Place client in prone position several times a day	To prevent hip flexion contracture
❑ Remove and reapply compression bandage when healed	To control swelling and shape the stump
❑ Wash, rinse and dry the stump daily	To prevent infection and promote healing
❑ Do not apply anything to the stump	To prevent skin breakdown and infection
❑ What is phantom limb sensation?	Sensation that the amputated limb exists
❑ What is the management for phantom limb pain?	Gently massage the area, Give analgesics
❑ What item should be prepared at the bedside at all times?	Tourniquet to stop severe bleeding

E. Musculoskeletal System Drugs

1. Drugs for Arthritis

Non-Steroidal Anti-Inflammatory Drugs (NSAIDs)

❑ Description	Reduces swelling and inflammation
❑ Drugs	Examples: ▪ aspirin ▪ naproxen (Naprosyn) ▪ indomethacin (Indocin)
❑ Side effects	Gastric upset, **bleeding**
❑ Interventions	Give with food or milk

Disease-Modifying Antirheumatic Drugs (DMARDs)

❑ Description	Reduces swelling, pain and stiffness and slows effects of rheumatoid arthritis
❑ Drugs	Examples: ▪ azathioprine (Imuran) ▪ cyclophosphamide (Cytoxan) ▪ sulfasalazine (Azulfidine) ▪ cyclosporine (Neoral) ▪ tofacitinib (Xeljanz) ▪ methotrexate (Rheumatrex, Trexall)
❑ Side effects	Gastric upset, nausea, diarrhea, alopecia, fatigue, liver damage
❑ Interventions	Monitor for infection (immunosuppressant)

- Combined with Biologics or Immunomodulators — Examples:
  - etanercept (Enbrel)
  - abatacept (Orencia)
  - infliximab (Remicade)
  - adalimumab (Humira)

2. Skeletal Muscle Relaxants

- Description — Relieves painful muscle spasm
- Drugs — Examples:
  - carisoprodol (Soma)
  - cyclobenzaprine (Flexeril)
  - baclofen (Lioresal)
  - diazepam (Valium)
  - methocarbamol (Robaxin)
  - dantrolene (Dantrium)
- Side effects — **Dizziness**, ataxia, dry mouth, nausea
- Interventions — Avoid alcohol and sedatives

3. Drugs for Gout

allopurinol (Zyloprim)

- Description — Reduces the production of uric acid. Also used for clients on chemotherapy
- Side effects — Drowsiness, kidney stones
- Interventions — Increase fluid intake, Avoid alcohol. Avoid excessive intake of Vitamin C to prevent kidney stones

colchicine (Colcrys, Mitigare)

- Description — Reduces pain and swelling of joints
- Side effects — Nausea, vomiting, abdominal pain
- Interventions — Give at the first sign of attack. **Stop when GI symptoms occur**
- Why should the client avoid grapefruit? — Grapefruit juice may increase the amount of colchicine the body absorbs

probenecid (Benemid)

- Description — Excretes uric acid through the urine (uricosuric)
- Side effects — Polyuria, headache, joint pain
- Interventions — Increase fluid intake, **Avoid aspirin**

sulfinpyrazone (Anturane)

❑ Description	Excretes uric acid through the urine
❑ Side effects	Gastric upset
❑ Contraindications	Peptic ulcer disease
❑ Interventions	Increase fluid intake

febuxostat (Uloric)

❑ Description	A xanthine oxidase inhibitor Reduces production of uric acid
❑ Side effects	Nausea, joint pain, swelling, stiffness
❑ Interventions	Teach client that gout may briefly flare up

4. Drugs for Osteoporosis

Biphosphonates

❑ Description	Inhibits bone resorption or breakdown
❑ Drugs	Examples: ▪ ibandronate (Boniva) ▪ alendronate (Fosamax) ▪ risedronate (Actonel)
❑ Contraindications	Esophageal disease, hypocalcemia, clients who cannot sit/stand for 30 minutes
❑ Side effects	**Heartburn**, esophagitis, muscle pain
❑ Interventions	Take first thing in the morning then NPO and **sit upright** for 30 minutes thereafter

raloxifene (Evista)

❑ Description	Inhibits bone resorption or breakdown Risk for stroke and **thrombosis**
❑ Contraindications	Breastfeeding women, pregnancy, male
❑ Side effects	Hot flashes, swelling in hands, leg cramps
❑ Interventions	Avoid prolonged immobile periods

teriparatide (Forteo)

❑ Description	Promotes new bone formation For clients at high-risk for fractures Risk for bone cancer; Injected for 2 years
❑ Side effects	Hypotension, dizziness, hypercalcemia
❑ Interventions	Change positions slowly

Gastrointestinal System 8

A. The Gastrointestinal System

❑ Structures of the Digestive System	Mouth, Pharynx, Esophagus, Stomach Small intestine ▪ Duodenum, Jejunum, Ileum Large intestine ▪ Cecum ▪ Colon ▪ Ascending colon ▪ Transverse colon ▪ Descending colon ▪ Sigmoid colon ▪ Rectum ▪ Anus
❑ Accessories	Teeth and gums, tongue, liver, gallbladder, pancreas, salivary glands Stomach ▪ Cardiac and pyloric sphincter ▪ Gastric juices ▪ Protein digestion occurs
❑ What cells produce hydrochloric acid?	Parietal cells
❑ What protects the stomach lining from acidity?	Mucin
❑ What is chyme?	Semi-liquid, partially digested food
❑ What physiologic process occurs in the small intestine?	Carbohydrate and protein metabolism Bile and pancreatic juices enter duodenum Microvilli absorb the nutrients
❑ What are the 3 pancreatic enzymes?	Amylase (carbohydrates digestion) Lipase (fat digestion) Trypsin (protein digestion)

- ❑ The bacteria in the large intestines are involved in the synthesis of ___________. — Vitamin K
- ❑ What is cholecystokinin? — Hormone that stimulates contraction of the gallbladder to release bile
- ❑ What are the functions of the liver? — Bile production and excretion
  Activation of Vitamin D
  Converting ammonia to urea
  Processing old red blood cells
  Detoxification of harmful substances
  Formation of cholesterol
  Storage of glucose as glycogen
  Synthesis of albumin and clotting factors

B. Diagnostic Tests

Upper and Lower GI Series

UPPER GI SERIES (BARIUM SWALLOW)	LOWER GI SERIES (BARIUM ENEMA)
X-ray of the esophagus, stomach and duodenum using barium; Gastrografin dye may be added	X-ray of the colon through rectal instillation of barium
Interventions ❑ Low fiber diet 2-3 days before test ❑ NPO after midnight	Interventions ❑ Magnesium citrate the evening before procedure ❑ NPO after midnight ❑ Cleansing enema in the evening or morning ❑ May be used as treatment for intussusception
After the procedure ❑ Stool will be **light-colored** or **chalky**; Milk of Magnesia may be ordered; Increase fluid intake to prevent constipation; Monitor bowel movement; Report severe abdominal cramping and vomiting (barium enema)	

Esophagogastroduodenoscopy

- ❑ Description — Detects polyps, ulcers and H. pylori
- ❑ Interventions — NPO, Sedation, Assess for perforation

> ***NCLEX Alert!*** *To assess for the return of gag reflex, slightly touch the back of the throat with a tongue depressor and observe for gagging response.*

Colonoscopy

- ❑ Description — Visualization of the entire large intestine
- ❑ Interventions — Clear liquid diet, NPO, Enema, Laxatives

❑ What is Golytely?	An osmotic electrolyte solution Mix with lemonade to mask taste Given with metochlopramide (Reglan) Give 250 mL every 15 minutes Provide blankets to prevent chilling Will cause **clear, watery** stools

Esophageal Function Studies (Bernstein Test)

❑ Description	An acid-perfusion test Differentiates angina versus GERD by irrigating the esophagus with an acid solution to mimic heartburn
❑ How is GERD diagnosed?	Pain is present during instillation of HCl acid through NGT; saline relieves the pain
❑ Interventions	Avoid antacids and proton-pump inhibitors

Tube Gastric Analysis

❑ Description	Aspiration of gastric contents to assess acid production or cancer
❑ Interventions	Avoid smoking and anticholinergic drugs

Occult Blood Test (Guaiac, Hemoccult, Hematest)

❑ Description	Detects hidden blood in the stool
❑ Interventions	Should be done before any barium study Avoid **red meat** 24-48 hours prior Avoid eating radishes, bean sprouts, turnips, beets, mushrooms, broccoli, artichokes and cauliflower Avoid aspirin, NSAIDs and iron drugs

Endoscopic Retrograde Cholangiopancreatography (ERCP)

❑ Description	Examines the biliary and pancreatic duct with a scope inserted from the stomach to the duodenum
❑ Interventions	Keep on NPO until the gag reflex returns

Oral Cholecystography (Gallbladder Series)

❑ Description	X-ray of the gallbladder after ingestion of radiopaque, iodinated dye tablets

❑ Interventions	Ask for allergy to iodine Give 6 telepaque tablets (one per hour) after a low fat evening meal NPO post-midnight after taking tablets High-fat meal may also be given

Needle Liver Biopsy

❑ What laboratory tests are ordered?	PT, INR, platelet, clotting and bleeding time
❑ Position during the procedure	Supine position with right hand above head or left lateral position
❑ During needle insertion	Hold breath to prevent lung puncture
❑ After the procedure	Right side-lying position Avoid heavy lifting

H. Pylori Testing

❑ Urea Breath Test	H. pylori converts the urea into carbon dioxide, which is then recorded in breath Avoid ATB and PPI drugs before the test
❑ Stool Test	Traces of H. pylori in feces Confirms success of treatment
❑ Blood Test	Identifies H. pylori antibodies in blood

C. Gastrointestinal Interventions

Colostomy

❑ Description	Performed for colon cancer and Crohn's disease or ulcerative colitis
❑ Location and Consistency	Ascending colostomy - liquid Transverse colostomy - semi-liquid Descending colostomy - soft Sigmoid colostomy - formed
❑ Forms	Single/double barrel, loop colostomy

Ileostomy

❑ Non-continent ileostomy	Collecting bag is needed; has liquid stool
❑ Continent Ileostomy (Kock pouch, Ileoanal Reservoir)	Collecting bag not needed; has liquid stool

Stoma Care

❑ Stoma should be ________ and __________.	Moist, shiny, and dark pink to red
❑ Dark blue and painful stoma	Abnormal, indicates lack of circulation
❑ Minimal bleeding and swelling	Normal
❑ Wash peristomal skin with _______________.	Soap and water
❑ Empty the pouch when it is _____ full	1/3
❑ Opening of the ostomy appliance should be ______ larger than the stoma	1/8-inch
❑ What foods should be eaten in limited amounts?	Raw vegetables, skins of fruit, wheat bran cereals and bread, milk, beans, peas, lentils, corn and popcorn, brown and wild rice, nuts and seeds

Colostomy Irrigation

❑ Purpose	To stimulate peristalsis and prevent constipation by instilling water into colon
❑ Best location	Toilet
❑ Irrigating bag should be placed at the level of the ________ or _______ above the stoma	Shoulder, 18 inches
❑ What should you do if abdominal cramping occurs during the instillation of solution?	Clamp the tubing temporarily then resume when the cramping stops
❑ When is the best time to perform colostomy irrigation?	Same time daily 1 hour after meals

Rectal Tube Insertion

❑ Description	Relieves abdominal distention and flatus
❑ Position during procedure	Sim's position
❑ Insert tube ______ inches	4-6
❑ Leave the tube for no more than ____ minutes	30

Types of Enema

❑ Cleansing enema	Uses tap water, normal saline and soap suds solution; maximum of 3 times only
❑ Hypertonic	Distends the colon with fluid to stimulate bowel movement
❑ Oil retention enema	Softens the feces by instillation of mineral oil retained for a few hours

❑ Fleet enema	A saline laxative that attracts fluid into the colon to soften the stool
❑ Harris flush (return flow enema)	Relieves flatus and abdominal distention by alternating flow of fluid in and out of the rectum and sigmoid colon

D. Gastrointestinal System Disorders

Gastroesophageal Reflux Disease (GERD)

❑ Description	Relaxation of the cardiac sphincter → reflux of stomach acids
❑ Assessment	Heartburn, nausea, chest pain
❑ Untreated GERD leads to ____________	Barret's esophagus
❑ Interventions	Stop smoking, Lose weight Small, frequent low fat meals Antacids, Proton-Pump Inhibitors
❑ Remain _______ 1-2 hours after meals	Upright
❑ What should be avoided to prevent reflux?	Eating 2-3 hours before sleep, caffeine, alcohol, constrictive clothing, bending, lying down after eating
❑ What is fundoplication?	Tightening of the cardiac sphincter

> ***NCLEX Alert!*** *Barrett's esophagus increases the client's risk of developing esophageal cancer.*

Achalasia

❑ Description	Spasm of the cardiac sphincter → foods cannot enter the stomach
❑ Assessment	Dysphagia, regurgitation, weight loss
❑ Interventions	Elevate the head, Avoid bending
❑ Surgery	Esophageal dilatation

Acute Gastritis

❑ Description	Inflammation of the stomach lining
❑ Causes	Alcoholism, stress, burns, NSAIDs
❑ Assessment	Epigastric pain, anorexia, vomiting, melena
❑ Interventions	NPO, IVF, Antiemetics, Antacids, H_2 blockers, ATBs

Peptic Ulcer

- ❑ Description — Painful sores in the stomach or duodenum

- ❑ Causes — NSAIDs, aspirin, steroids, tobacco, coffee
  Severe burns (Curling's ulcer)
  Brain injury (Cushing's ulcer)

- ❑ Why does H. pylori cause peptic ulcer? — H. pylori depletes the mucus that protects the gastric lining

- ❑ Why does stress ulcer develop in severe burns or brain injury with increased ICP? — Severe stress causes gastric ischemia that leads to ulcer formation

- ❑ Assessment

GASTRIC ULCER	DUODENAL ULCER
❑ Pain with **food intake** or pain 30 minutes-1 hour after meals	❑ Pain 2-3 hours after meals or pain when the stomach is **empty** (pain relieved by food)
❑ Weight loss	❑ Weight gain
❑ Hematemesis	❑ Melena

- ❑ Interventions — Antacids, H_2 Blockers, PPI, ATBs
- ❑ What is gastroduodenostomy (Billroth 1)? — Partial gastrectomy for gastric ulcers
- ❑ What is gastrojejunostomy (Billroth 2)? — Partial gastrectomy and doudenectomy
- ❑ What is vagotomy? — Removing part of the vagus nerve to decrease acid production

- ❑ What is **Dumping Syndrome**? — Occurs with gastric resection surgery
  Distention of the duodenum due to rapid gastric emptying and hypertonic food

- ❑ What are the signs and symptoms of Dumping Syndrome? — **Dizziness**, **sweating**, epigastric pain, vomiting, diarrhea, borborygmi, dyspepsia, tachycardia, tremors

- ❑ Management for Dumping Syndrome — Small, frequent meals
  High protein, high fat diet
  Low carbohydrate diet
  Avoid fluid intake during meals
  Anticholinergic agents
  Lie flat after meals

- ❑ What is pernicious anemia?

Deficiency of intrinsic factor (due to stomach removal) necessary for vitamin B_{12} absorption

Cancer of the Stomach

- ❑ Description

Stomach cancer due to smoking, eating processed foods, hypochlorhydria, gastric ulcer, low fiber diet or H. pylori infection

- ❑ Assessment

Vague epigastric discomfort, anorexia, heartburn, bloating

- ❑ Interventions

Chemotherapy, Radiation, Gastrectomy

Inflammatory Bowel Disease

	ULCERATIVE COLITIS	CROHN'S DISEASE
Causes	Unknown, stress, genetic, immune-related	Unknown, immune-related; Common among Jewish ancestry
Sites	Colon and rectum	Entire gastrointestinal tract
Inflammation	Continuous pattern	Skip lesions (granulomas)
Diarrhea	Yes (**blood and mucus**)	Yes (**fatty stool/steatorrhea**)
Malabsorption	Rare	Yes
Weight loss/malnutrition	Yes	Yes
Abdominal pain/discomfort	Yes	Yes
Bloody stool (hematochezia)	Yes	Rare
Risk for colon cancer	Yes	Rare
Remissions/exacerbations	Yes	Yes

- ❑ Interventions

5-Aminosalicylic Acid Anti-Inflammatory Drugs

- sulfasalazine (Azulfidine)
- azathioprine (Imuran)
- balsalazide (Colazal)
- olsalazine (Dipentum)
- mesalamine (Rowasa, Asacol)

High protein, high calorie diet, TPN

Low fat diet (Crohn's disease)

Colon resection, Kock pouch, Ileostomy

❑ What is a free elemental diet?	A diet that replaces all foods with a liquid formula made up of nutrients in their simplest, most absorbable form

Appendicitis

❑ Description	Inflammation of the appendix → rupture → peritonitis
❑ Assessment	Vague, generalized abdominal pain, **rebound tenderness**, low-grade fever, vomiting, absent bowel sounds, RLQ abdominal pain (Mc Burney's point)
❑ What is rebound tenderness?	Pain when removing pressure on abdomen
❑ What is a positive Rovsing's sign?	Palpation of the LLQ causes pain on RLQ
❑ Interventions	NPO, Bed rest, ATB Laparoscopic or open appendectomy
❑ What should be avoided?	Opioids, laxatives, enema, hot water bag
❑ Post-operative position for a ruptured appendix	Semi-Fowler's to localize the infection

> ***NCLEX Alert!*** *Report sudden absence of pain as it indicates rupture of an inflamed appendix.*

Irritable Bowel Syndrome (IBS)

❑ Description	Disorder in intestinal motility
❑ Types	Diarrhea or constipation dominant
❑ Causes	Unknown, genetics, brain-gut dysfunction, stress, bacteria
❑ Assessment	Alternating **diarrhea** or **constipation**, bloating, urgency, cramping, indigestion, sensation of incompletely passing stools
❑ Interventions	Lifestyle and diet modifications Antispasmodics, Laxatives, Antidiarrheals Anxiolytics, Probiotics, ATBs
❑ What are examples of alternative treatments?	Cognitive Behavioral Therapy, Acupuncture, Hypnosis, Herbal, Yoga

Diverticulosis

- ❑ Description — Pouch-like herniations in the colon
- ❑ Causes — Aging, low fiber and residue diet
- ❑ Assessment — Asymptomatic, pain the LLQ, flatus, nausea
- ❑ What should be avoided in acute diverticulitis? — **High fiber, high residue diet,** colonoscopy
- ❑ Interventions — Stool softeners, High fiber diet
  Colectomy with anastomosis

> ***NCLEX Alert!*** *Instruct the client to avoid fruits with small seeds during an attack of diverticulitis.*

Peritonitis

- ❑ Description — Inflammation of the peritoneal membrane
- ❑ Causes — Ruptured appendix, peritoneal dialysis
- ❑ Assessment — Severe abdominal pain, fever, nausea, vomiting, absent bowel sounds, **board-like**, rigid, tender abdomen, sepsis
- ❑ Interventions — ATB, IVF, NGT, Semi-Fowler's position

Hernia

- ❑ Description — Organ protrusion due to muscle weakness
- ❑ Common sites — Inguinal, umbilical, femoral
- ❑ What aggravates the condition? — Increased intra-abdominal pressure from coughing or straining
- ❑ Types

REDUCIBLE	IRREDUCIBLE/INCARCERATED	STRANGULATED
❑ Flattens and can be replaced back into the abdominal cavity	❑ Cannot be manipulated or replaced back into the abdominal cavity	❑ Painful ❑ Emergency as blood supply is cut off

- ❑ Assessment — Tenderness on palpation, obvious presence of a mass, bulging around the umbilicus
- ❑ Report pain, vomiting and abdominal distention — Indicates strangulated hernia
- ❑ Interventions — Apply the truss device over site
  Avoid heavy lifting
- ❑ Surgery — Hernioplasty/herniorrhaphy
- ❑ Interventions after inguinal hernia repair — Elevate scrotum on a rolled pad, apply ice pack or jockstrap to prevent scrotal edema

Hiatal Hernia

❑ Description	Protrusion of the stomach through an opening where the food enters the esophagus
❑ Assessment	GERD-like symptoms
❑ Interventions	Similar to GERD

Intestinal Obstruction

❑ Description	Obstruction → build-up of fluid, air and bacteria → fluid shifting → abdominal distention → peritonitis
❑ Types	MECHANICAL ▪ Due to intussusception or volvulus NON-MECHANICAL ▪ Due to paralytic ileus
❑ Assessment	Severe abdominal pain, vomiting, **high-pitched bowel sounds** (mechanical), **absent bowel sounds** (paralytic ileus)
❑ Interventions	NGT to decompress the abdomen, enema IVF, Analgesics, Surgery

Colon Cancer

❑ Description	Cancer in the colon or rectum
❑ Causes	**Heredity**, ulcerative colitis, low fiber diet
❑ Assessment	Unexplained change in bowel habits, feeling of full bowel, weight loss, **rectal bleeding**, flat ribbon-like stools
❑ Diagnostic Tests	Colonoscopy, occult blood exam, increased serum carcinoembryonic antigen (CEA)
❑ Interventions	Radiation, Chemotherapy
❑ Surgery	Colon resection with anastomosis
❑ When is colorectal cancer screening recommended?	At age 50-75 years-old; Tests include fecal occult blood test, fecal immunochemical test (FIT) and colonoscopy every 10 years

Hemorrhoids

❑ Description	Swollen veins in the rectum or anus
❑ Causes	Increased intra-abdominal pressure, diarrhea, constipation, portal hypertension, prolonged sitting and standing, straining
❑ Assessment	Prolapse, bleeding, itchiness, pain during swelling or flare-ups, painful lumps (external hemorrhoids), painless bleeding (internal hemorrhoids)
❑ Interventions	Ointments (Anusol, Preparation H) Psyllium (Metamucil) Sitz bath Rubber-band ligation Sclerotherapy, Cryotherapy, Laser excision, Hemorrhoidectomy

Liver Cirrhosis

❑ Description	Chronic, progressive degenerative disease → liver replaced with scar or fibrous tissues
❑ Obstruction of portal vein leads to ________	Portal hypertension
❑ Portal hypertension leads to ________	Esophageal Varices
❑ Portal hypertension, hypoalbuminemia, and hyperaldosteronism leads to ________	Ascites
❑ Increased ammonia leads to ________	Hepatic encephalopathy
❑ Lack of Vitamin K leads to ________	Bleeding
❑ Types	Alcoholic (Laennec's) Post-necrotic (hepatitis) Biliary (gallstones) Cardiac (heart failure)
❑ Assessment: Later Stage	Weight loss, pruritus, ascites, splenomegaly, anemia, jaundice gynecomastia, **fetor hepaticus** (ammonia-like breath), **spider telangiectasis** (spider veins), **palmar erythema** (pink palms)
❑ Diagnostic Tests	Elevated bilirubin, AST, ALT, LDH prolonged PT, INR

- ❑ Interventions — Eliminate alcohol
  Weigh daily
  Measure abdominal girth
  High calorie, moderately high protein, low fat, low sodium diet
- ❑ Monitor the level of consciousness — To detect hepatic encephalopathy
- ❑ What should be monitored after giving laxatives? — Monitor the bowel movements to ensure that ammonia is flushed out
- ❑ Complications

ASCITES	ESOPHAGEAL VARICES	HEPATIC ENCEPHALOPATHY
Abnormal accumulation fluid in the abdominal (peritoneal) cavity	Abnormal veins in the esophagus	Severe accumulation of ammonia that leads to neurologic symptoms such as **behavior change**, confusion, **asterixis** (flapping tremors of the hands) and coma
Interventions ❑ Fluid and sodium restriction ❑ Potassium-sparing diuretic - spironolactone (Aldactone) ❑ Albumin replacement ❑ Paracentesis - Ask client to void to prevent bladder puncture - Monitor for hypotension	Interventions ❑ Avoid sneezing and coughing ❑ Avoid harsh foods (e.g. tacos) ❑ Vasopressin ❑ Sengstaken-Blakemore Tube - a 3-lumen tube with balloons inflated to control GI bleeding	Interventions ❑ Goal: Reduce ammonia level ❑ **Low protein diet** ❑ Lactulose ❑ Neomycin orally or rectally to destroy colonic bacteria that helps produce ammonia

> ***NCLEX Alert!*** *When caring for a client who has a Sengstaken-Blakemore tube, a pair of scissors must be kept at the bedside at all times to cut the tube in case of respiratory distress.*

Hepatitis

- ❑ Infectious hepatitis — Hepa A
- ❑ Serum hepatitis — Hepa B
- ❑ Fecal-oral transmission — Hepa A, E
- ❑ Blood transmission — Hepa B, C, D, G
- ❑ Co-infects with Hepatitis B — Hepa D
- ❑ Leads to cancer — Hepa B, C
- ❑ Leads to cirrhosis — Hepa B, C, D
- ❑ Leads to a carrier state — Hepa B
- ❑ Vaccines available — Hepa A, B

- ❑ Assessment — Malaise, pruritus, hepatomegaly, jaundice, **dark tea-colored** urine, **clay-colored** stools
- ❑ Diagnostic Tests — Elevated bilirubin, AST, ALT; Prolonged PT, INR
- ❑ Interventions — Promote rest, Gamma globulins; High protein, high calorie, low fat diet

Cholelithiasis and Cholecystitis

- ❑ Description — Bile stones → obstruction of bile flow → irritation of gallbladder → inflammation → swelling → rupture → peritonitis
- ❑ Risk factors — Remember 6 F's!
  - F - emale
  - F - orty
  - F - ertile
  - F - latulent
  - F - air-skinned
  - F - at
- ❑ Assessment — May be asymptomatic, discomfort or indigestion after eating **fatty foods** such as french fries, RUQ pain that radiates to right scapula
- ❑ What is a positive Murphy's sign? — Palpation of subcostal region causes increased pain when breathing deeply
- ❑ What are the signs of acute cholecystitis? — Fever, vomiting, jaundice, clay-colored stool, dark urine
- ❑ Diagnostic Tests — Ultrasound, Oral cholecystogram
- ❑ Interventions — NPO, NGT, Antispasmodics, Low fat diet
- ❑ What drug should be avoided? — Morphine sulfate because it causes spasm of the sphincter of Oddi and leads to pain
- ❑ Why is cholestyramine (Questran) given? — To relieve pruritus
- ❑ What is Extracorporeal Shock Wave Lithotripsy? — Uses shock waves to crush the stones; Client lies on a water-filled cushion; No incision is made
- ❑ Surgery — Laparoscopic or open cholecystectomy

- ❑ What should the client expect after surgery? — Presence of Jack-Pratt drains
- ❑ What is the purpose of T tube insertion? — A T tube drains excess bile and allows the bile ducts to heal after removal of stones
- ❑ What is the normal color of drainage? — Initially blood-tinged to greenish brown
- ❑ What is the normal amount of T tube drainage? — 500-1000 mL for the first 24 hours
- ❑ What is a sign of successful bile drainage? — Stool returns to normal color

Pancreatitis

- ❑ Description — Blockage of pancreatic duct → backflow of enzymes → enzymes destroy the pancreas (autodigestion) → inflammation
- ❑ Causes — Alcoholism, gallbladder stones, smoking
- ❑ Assessment — Upper abdominal pain radiating to the back aggravated by eating **fatty** foods
- ❑ What are the signs of acute pancreatitis? — Vomiting, fever, steatorrhea, severe pain
- ❑ What is Cullen's sign? — Bluish discoloration around the umbilicus
- ❑ What is Grey-Turner's sign? — Bluish discoloration on the flank
- ❑ What do Cullen's and Grey-Turner's signs indicate? — Retroperitoneal hemorrhage
- ❑ Diagnostic Tests — Increased serum amylase and lipase
- ❑ Interventions — NPO, IVF replacement, ATB
  Low fat diet, meperidine (Demerol)
- ❑ Why is propantheline (Probanthine) given? — To decrease gastric motility and pain
- ❑ What complications should be monitored? — Alcohol withdrawal and hyperglycemia
- ❑ What should the client avoid? — Caffeine and alcohol

Cancer of the Pancreas

- ❑ Causes — Genetics, diabetes, smoking, obesity
- ❑ Assessment — Vague symptoms, nausea, bloating, dull epigastric pain, fatigue
- ❑ What is the prognosis? — Very poor; Usually diagnosed late
- ❑ Diagnostic Tests — carcinoembryonic antigen (CEA) test, ultrasound, ERCP
- ❑ Interventions — Radiation, Chemotherapy
- ❑ Surgery — WHIPPLE PROCEDURE
  - Removal of the gallbladder, common bile duct, part of the duodenum and the head of the pancreas

E. Gastrointestinal Drugs

1. Drugs for Peptic Ulcer

Antacids

❑ Description — Neutralizes the stomach acid

ALUMINUM HYDROXIDE (AMPHOJEL)	MAGNESIUM HYDROXIDE	CALCIUM CARBONATE	SODIUM BICARBONATE
Lowers phosphorus level	Combination with aluminum hydroxide	Used for osteoporosis	Used for metabolic acidosis
Side effects ❑ **Constipation** ❑ **Hypophosphatenemia**	Side effects ❑ **Diarrhea**	Side effects ❑ Constipation, flatulence	Side effects ❑ **Systemic alkalosis**, nausea, bloating
Interventions ❑ Give antacids 1-3 hours after meals or at bedtime ❑ Give 1 hour between other drugs to prevent drug interactions			

Other Drugs for Peptic Ulcer

CYTOPROTECTIVE AGENT	GASTRIC ACID PROTECTANT	HISTAMINE 2 (H_2) RECEPTOR ANTAGONIST	PROTON PUMP INHIBITORS (PPI)
Prevents ulcer caused by high doses of NSAIDs or aspirin use	Coats the stomach and esophageal lining to provide protection from gastric acids	Suppresses secretion of gastric acid	Suppresses secretion of gastric acid
Drugs ❑ misoprostol (Cytotec)	Drugs ❑ sucralfate (Carafate)	Drugs ❑ nizatidine (Axid) ❑ ranitidine (Zantac) ❑ cimetidine (Tagamet)	Drugs ❑ lansoprazole (Prevacid) ❑ esomeprazole (Nexium) ❑ pantoprazole (Protonix)
Side effects ❑ Nausea, abdominal cramps, diarrhea	Side effects ❑ Constipation, dry mouth, stomach upset	Side effects ❑ Headache, constipation, diarrhea	Side effects ❑ Headache, nausea, diarrhea
Interventions ❑ Give with meals	Interventions ❑ Give on empty stomach or 2 hours after meals and at bedtime	Interventions ❑ Give with meals and at bedtime	Interventions ❑ Give before meals

2. Drugs for Helicobacter Pylori Infection

Multi-Drug Regimen

TRIPLE DRUG THERAPY	QUADRUPLE DRUG THERAPY
❑ amoxicillin (Amoxil) ❑ esomeprazole (Nexium) ❑ clarithromycin (Biaxin)	❑ metronidazole (Flagyl) ❑ ranitidine (Zantac) ❑ tetracycline ❑ bismuth subsalicylate

3. Bile Acid Sequestrants (Lipid-Lowering Drugs)

- ❑ Description: Binds with bile acids in the intestines → bile excreted in feces
  Treats biliary obstruction and pruritus
  Lowers low density lipoprotein (LDL) levels
- ❑ Drugs: Examples:
  - cholestyramine (Questran)
  - colesevelam (Welchol)
  - colestipol (Colestid)
- ❑ Side effects: Bloating, constipation, fecal impaction
- ❑ Interventions: Monitor bowel movement

> ***NCLEX Alert!*** *Mix powdered drug with juice to improve taste.*

4. Drugs for Inflammatory Bowel Disease

CORTICOSTEROID	IMMUNOSUPPRESSANTS	IMMUNOMODULATOR	ANTIBIOTICS	AMINOSALICYLATES
❑ Prednisone	❑ cyclosporine (Sandimmune, Neoral, Gengraf) ❑ azathioprine (Imuran) ❑ mercaptopurine (Purinethol)	❑ infliximab (Remicade) ❑ adalimumab (Humira) ❑ certolizumab (Cimzia)	❑ ciprofloxacin (Cipro) ❑ metronidazole (Flagyl)	❑ sulfasalazine (Azulfidine) ❑ olsalazine (Dipentum) ❑ mesalamine (Rowasa,Pentasa)

> ***NCLEX Alert!*** *Immunomodulators are drugs which either suppress or stimulate the immune system.*

5. Drugs for Irritable Bowel Syndrome

lubiprostone (Amitiza)

- ❑ Description — Treats constipation-dominant IBS and opioid-induced constipation
- ❑ Contraindication — **Diarrhea**
- ❑ Side effects — Nausea, vomiting, flatulence
- ❑ Interventions — Monitor for dehydration

alosetron (Lotronex)

- ❑ Description — Treats diarrhea-dominant IBS
- ❑ Contraindication — **Constipation**
- ❑ Side effects — Fecal impaction, colitis
- ❑ Interventions — Monitor bowel movement

6. Drugs for Nausea and Vomiting

Anti-Motion Sickness Drugs

- ❑ Drugs — Examples:
  - dimenhydrinate (Dramamine)
  - meclizine HCl (Bonine, Antivert)
- ❑ Side effects — **Drowsiness**, constipation, dry mouth

Antihistamines

- ❑ Drugs — Examples:
  - diphenhydramine (Benadryl)
  - hydroxyzine (Atarax, Vistaril)
- ❑ Side effects — **Drowsiness**, sleepiness, dry mouth

Serotonin Antagonists

- ❑ Drugs — Examples:
  - ondansetron (Zofran)
  - dolasetron (Anzemet)
- ❑ Side effects — Headache, lightheadedness, **dizziness**

Phenothiazines

- ❑ Drugs — Examples:
  - chlorpromazine (Thorazine)
  - promethazine (Phenergan)
  - prochlorperazine (Compazine)
- ❑ Side effects — Drowsiness, hypotension

Other drugs for nausea and vomiting — metochlopramide (Reglan); scopolamine transdermal

7. Laxatives

Bulk-Forming Laxatives

- ❑ Description — Attracts water to increase the bulk of stools
- ❑ Drugs — Examples:
  - psyllium (Metamucil)
  - methylcellulose (Citrucel)
  - polycarbophil (FiberCon)
- ❑ Side effects — **Abdominal cramps**, laxative dependency

Stimulants

- ❑ Description — Stimulates peristalsis
- ❑ Drugs — Examples:
  - cascara sagrada, senna (Senokot)
  - bisacodyl (Dulcolax)
- ❑ Side effects — **Abdominal cramps**, diarrhea

Stool Softener

- ❑ Description — Softens the feces
- ❑ Drugs — Examples: docusate sodium (Colace)
- ❑ Side effects — **Diarrhea**, bloating, abdominal cramps

Osmotic Agents

- ❑ Description — Stimulates intestinal motility
- ❑ Drugs — Examples:
  - polyethylene (GoLYTELY, MiraLAX)
  - magnesium hydroxide (Milk of Magnesia)
  - magnesium citrate
  - sodium phosphates (Fleet enema)
- ❑ Side effects — **Abdominal cramping**, diarrhea

8. Drugs for Diarrhea

- ❑ Drugs — Examples:
  - diphenoxylate and atropine (Lomotil)
  - bismuth subsalicylate (Pepto-Bismol, Kaopectate)
  - loperamide (Imodium)
- ❑ Side effects — Dizziness, constipation

Respiratory System 9

A. The Respiratory System

❑ Upper Airway	Nose, paranasal sinuses, turbinate bones, pharynx, larynx
❑ Lower Airway	Trachea, bronchi and bronchioles, lungs and alveoli, accessory structures
❑ 4 paranasal sinuses	Frontal, ethmoid, sphenoid, maxillary
❑ 3 divisions of the pharynx	Nasopharynx, oropharynx, laryngopharynx
❑ What structures are found in the nasopharynx?	Adenoids and eustachian tubes
❑ What structures are found in the larynx?	Epiglottis (valve flap covering the larynx) Glottis (opening between vocal cords) Vocal cords (produces sound)
❑ Trachea divides at the ___________	Carina
❑ Structures that sweep mucus	Cilia
❑ Smallest part of the bronchus	Bronchioles
❑ Site of gas exchange	Alveoli (air sacs)
❑ Substance that prevents collapse of the lungs	Surfactant
❑ Major muscle of respiration	Diaphragm
❑ Space between the lungs	Mediastinum
❑ Membrane that covers the lung surface	Visceral pleura
❑ Membrane that covers the chest wall	Parietal pleura
❑ Thin space between the visceral and parietal pleura	Pleural space
❑ Normal pressure in the pleural space	Negative pressure
❑ What will happen if air invades the pleural space?	Pressure becomes **positive** which can lead to the collapse of the lungs (atelectasis)
❑ Receptors that respond to changes in CO_2 levels and H^+ ion concentrations	Chemoreceptors
❑ Regulates respiration	Medulla oblongata

B. Respiratory Assessment

Normal Breath Sounds

VESICULAR	BRONCHIAL	BRONCHOVESICULAR
Soft, blowing sounds	Louder, high-pitched, hollow-sounding	Softer than bronchial breath sound
Heard throughout most of the lung fields	Heard over the trachea and larynx	Heard on the posterior chest between the scapulae and in the middle of anterior chest

Abnormal/Adventitious Breath Sounds

WHEEZING	CRACKLES (RALES)	STRIDOR	FRICTION RUB
Caused by narrowed airways due to broncho-spasm or secretions	Caused by fluid in the airways (e.g. pulmonary edema in heart failure)	Caused by airway obstruction (e.g. croup)	Caused by inflammation of pleural membranes (e.g. pleuritis)
Sibilant Rhonchi High-pitched whistling sound caused by passage of air in narrowed airways (e.g. asthma) **Sonorous Rhonchi** Lower-pitched sounds with a snoring quality due to secretions	**Fine Crackles** Soft, **high-pitched** sounds like rolling hair strands between fingers in front of ear **Coarse Crackles** Louder, **low-pitched** and lasts longer like opening a Velcro	High-pitched harsh sound heard during inspiration; emergency due to respiratory distress	Rubbing sound of inflamed pleural surfaces that causes chest pain especially during breathing

Percussion of the Chest Wall

SOUND	DESCRIPTION	IMPLICATIONS
Resonant	Low pitched, hollow sounds	Considered as a normal lung sound
Hyperresonant	Louder, lower pitched	Lungs hyperinflated with air (e.g. pneumothorax, asthma)
Tympanic	Hollow, drum-like sound	Indicates excessive air (e.g. pneumothorax)
Dull	Medium pitch and intensity	Absence of air or fluid is present (e.g. effusion)
Flat	Short duration, high-pitched	Heard over solid areas (e.g. bones)

C. Diagnostic Tests

Tuberculin Skin Test

- ❑ Description — Mantoux or PPD Skin Test (Purified Protein Derivative)
0.1 mL in tuberculin syringe, intradermally
- ❑ When is the result interpreted? — After 48-72 hours
- ❑ What does a positive result mean? — Exposure or contact with TB
- ❑ What is being measured? — **Induration** (hard area), not erythema

TB SKIN TEST RESULTS		
5 or > millimeters is positive	**10 or > millimeters is positive**	**15 or > millimeters is positive**
❑ HIV-infected persons ❑ A recent contact of a person with TB disease ❑ Persons with fibrotic changes on chest radiograph consistent with prior TB ❑ Clients with organ transplants ❑ Persons who are **immunosuppressed** for other reasons (e.g. taking the equivalent of >15 mg/day of prednisone for 1 month or longer, taking TNF-a antagonists)	❑ Recent immigrants (< 5 years) from high prevalence countries ❑ Injection drug users ❑ Residents and employees of high-risk congregate settings ❑ Mycobacteriology laboratory personnel ❑ Persons with clinical conditions that place them at high risk ❑ Children < 4 years of age ❑ Infants, children, and adolescents exposed to adults in high-risk categories	❑ Any person, including persons with **no known risk factors** for TB.

Reference: Centers for Disease Control and Prevention

Pulmonary Function Test

- ❑ Description — Measures the functional ability of the lungs
- ❑ Tidal volume — Volume of air inhaled & exhaled with every normal breath
- ❑ Residual volume — Volume of air remaining in the lungs after maximum expiration
- ❑ Vital capacity — Maximum amount of air that can be exhaled after a maximum inhalation

Pulmonary Angiography

❑ Description	Radioisotope study involving contrast medium injection into the femoral artery **Detects pulmonary embolism**
❑ Interventions	Ask for allergy to iodine
❑ After the procedure	Assess puncture site for bleeding Bedrest, Apply pressure dressing

Lung Scans (V-Q Scan)

❑ Description	Use of radioisotopes and scanning machine Identifies pulmonary emboli, COPD, and pulmonary edema
❑ How is the test performed?	Radioactive contrast is **injected IV** for perfusion scan while radioactive gas is **inhaled** for ventilation scan Scan results will be compared for "match"
❑ Interventions	Ask for iodine allergy

Bronchoscopy

❑ Description	Direct visualization of the larynx, trachea, bronchi using a flexible fiberoptic scope
❑ Interventions	NPO before procedure, Neck anesthesia,
❑ Why is atropine given?	To dry the secretions (antimuscarinic effect)
❑ After the procedure	Semi-Fowler's position to prevent aspiration, Check the gag reflex

Thoracentesis

❑ Description	Performed to aspirate fluid or air in pleura (effusion and empyema)
❑ Position during the procedure	Sitting on edge of bed leaning over the bedside table or side-lying on the unaffected side
❑ After the procedure	Side-lying position on unaffected side Report hemoptysis or dyspnea

D. Respiratory Interventions

Postural Drainage

❑ Description	Performed before meals and at bedtime to prevent vomiting and aspiration
❑ Perform chest percussion and vibration	To promote drainage of secretions
❑ Discontinue if dyspnea, chest pain and hemoptysis occur	Indicates hypoxia or trauma
❑ Contraindications	Head injury, increased ICP, glaucoma

Suctioning

❑ Steps:	
1. Hyperoxygenate with ___________	100% O_2
2. Place on _____________ position	Semi-Fowler's
3. Lubricate catheter with __________	Normal saline
4. Do not apply _______ when inserting catheter	Suction
5. Do not force the suction catheter into the airway beyond resistance	
6. Apply intermittent suction for ____ seconds	10-15
7. Withdraw the catheter in a rotating motion while applying intermittent ____________	Suction
8. Allow _____ minutes of rest between suctioning	1-2

Oxygen Delivery Systems

❑ What is the normal Fraction of Inspired Oxygen (FIO_2) with normal breathing or breathing in room air?	21%

DEVICE	DESCRIPTION
Nasal Cannula	❑ Low flow system ❑ Provides flow rates of 1-6 L/min. (24% - 44% FIO_2) ❑ Provide humidification if giving more than 4L/min.
Simple Face Mask	❑ Low flow system ❑ Provides flow rates of 5-8 L/min. (40-60% FIO_2) ❑ For short-term, emergency use only
Partial Rebreather Mask	❑ High-flow system ❑ Provides flow rates of 6-15 L/min (70-90 % FIO_2) ❑ Has reservoir bag that allows the client to "rebreathe" oxygen to provide high FIO_2 ❑ Keep the reservoir inflated 2/3 full during inspiration

DEVICE	DESCRIPTION
Non-Rebreather Mask	❑ Provides the highest flow rates of 10-15 L/min (60-100% FIO_2) ❑ Has a reservoir bag attached but does not allow for the rebreathing of exhaled air because it escapes through the side ports ❑ Keep the reservoir inflated 2/3 full during inspiration ❑ Used for worsening respiratory status
Venturi Mask	❑ Provides flow rates 4-10 L/min (24-55% FIO_2) ❑ Delivers accurate percentage of oxygen concentration ❑ Favorable for COPD clients
Oxygen Concentrator	❑ Electrical device that takes in and filters air to produce oxygen

Ventilator Alarms

- ❑ What does a high-pressure alarm indicate?

  Secretions
  Bronchospasm
  Coughing
  Displaced endotracheal tube

- ❑ What does a low-pressure alarm indicate?

  Disconnection
  Respiratory arrest

NCLEX Alert! *Remember HOLD*

H – igh pressure alarm, O – bstruction, L – ow pressure alarm, D - isconnection

CPAP versus BIPAP

- ❑ Description

  These devices deliver positive pressurized air through a mask to the client's airways. Positive air pressure keeps the airway from collapsing.

- ❑ BIPAP (Bilevel Positive Airway Pressure)

  With 2 pressure settings: pressure for inhalation and exhalation to allow the client to get more air in and out of the lungs

- ❑ CPAP (Continuous Positive Airway Pressure)

  Set to a single pressure that delivers steady pressurized air to the airways

E. Respiratory System Disorders

Sleep Apnea

❑ Description	Pharyngeal obstruction during sleep → apnea → hypoxemia
❑ Causes	Obesity, septal deviation, polyps
❑ Assessment	Severe, loud **snoring** with apnea episodes, insomnia, hypertension, depression
❑ Diagnostic Test	Polysomnography
❑ Interventions	Lose weight, Oral devices, CPAP or BIPAP
❑ Surgery	UPPP (Uvulopalatopharyngoplasty) LAUP (Laser assisted uvulopalatoplasty)

> ***NCLEX Alert!*** *The client should avoid alcohol and sedatives.*

Cancer of the Larynx

❑ Causes	Smoking, laryngitis, alcohol, vocal abuse
❑ Assessment	Persistent **hoarseness** (> 2 weeks) sore throat, ear pain, dysphagia, odynophagia, lump in the throat
❑ Diagnostic Test	Laryngoscopy with biopsy
❑ Interventions	Radiation, Chemotherapy, Surgery
❑ Surgery	Partial or total laryngectomy Radical neck dissection
❑ What are the consequences of total laryngectomy?	Creation of a permanent tracheostomy Reduced sense of smell, Aphonia

Acute Rhinitis (Colds or Coryza)

❑ Description	Infection of the airways due to rhinoviruses
❑ Transmission	Droplet/indirect contact
❑ Incubation period	Within 24-48 hours
❑ Assessment	Sore throat, dyspnea, nasal congestion
❑ Interventions	Self-limiting, Fluids, Warm Compress, Rest

Influenza (Flu)

❑ Description	Infection of the airways due to a flu virus
❑ Transmission	Droplet or indirect contact
❑ Is this disease transmissible even without symptoms?	Yes, flu is infectious 1 day before symptoms appear and 5-7 days after

- ❑ Assessment — Remember FACTS!
  - F - ever
  - A - ches
  - C - hills
  - T - iredness
  - S - udden onset of symptoms
- ❑ Interventions — Self-limiting, Rest, Hydration, Analgesics,

Tonsillitis

❑ Description	Inflammation of tonsils usually caused by Group A beta-hemolytic streptococci
❑ Assessment	Edematous, red tonsils, dysphagia, dyspnea
❑ Complications	**Rheumatic fever**, carditis, nephritis
❑ Diagnostic Tests	Throat cultures (Rapid Strep Test)
❑ Interventions	ATB, analgesics, Warm saline gargles
❑ Surgery	Tonsillectomy, Adenoidectomy
❑ Interventions after tonsillectomy	Prone or side lying position Provide ice cold liquids and ice cream Apply ice collar

> ***NCLEX Alert!*** *Frequent swallowing after tonsillectomy indicates bleeding.*

Laryngitis

❑ Description	Inflammation of the larynx
❑ Causes	Bacterial, viral, vocal abuse
❑ Assessment	Hoarseness, aphonia
❑ Interventions	Voice rest, Analgesics, Lozenges

Pharyngitis (Sore Throat)

❑ Description	Inflammation of the pharynx
❑ Causes	Viral, bacterial (streptococcal sore throat)
❑ Is this disease contagious?	Contagious for 2-3 days after onset
❑ Assessment	Red and painful throat, fever, enlarged cervical lymph glands
❑ Diagnostic Tests	Throat culture Rapid Antigen Detection Test (RADT)
❑ Interventions	Penicillin, Analgesics, Warm saline gargles

Sinusitis

❑ Description	Infection of the sinuses
❑ Causes	Colds, allergy
❑ Assessment	Headache, tenderness, purulent exudate
❑ Diagnostic Tests	Sinus x-ray, transillumination
❑ What is transillumination?	Reflecting light through the sinus tissues to detect infection
❑ Interventions	Steam inhalation Warm, moist packs Irrigate nasal passages with saline ATBs, Analgesics, Antihistamines Vasoconstrictors – nasal sprays (Afrin)
❑ Surgery	CALDWELL-LUC OPERATION (involves incision under the upper lip)

Legionnaire's Disease

❑ Description	Legionella pneumophilia in **water reservoirs** (air conditioners, purifiers) → airborne transmission → pneumonia
❑ Assessment	**High fever**, flu-like symptoms nonproductive cough, muscle aches
❑ Is this disease transmissible from human to human?	No
❑ Interventions	ATBs, Mechanical ventilation

Tuberculosis

❑ Description	Due to inhalation of droplet nuclei containing tubercle bacillus
❑ What does TB infection mean?	It means exposure to TB
❑ What does active TB mean?	It means clinical disease
❑ Assessment	May be asymptomatic, vague symptoms, **low-grade afternoon fever**, weight loss, productive cough, chills, night sweats, hemoptysis
❑ Diagnostic Tests	Mantoux skin test QuantiFERON blood test Chest x-ray Acid-fast bacilli testing/sputum smear Sputum culture

- ❑ What does a positive Mantoux test mean? — Indicates infection or exposure only
- ❑ What does a positive QuantiFERON blood test mean? — Indicates infection or exposure only
- ❑ What does a positive sputum culture mean? — Definitive test for active TB
- ❑ Why is chest x-ray ordered? — Assesses presence and extent of lesions
- ❑ Interventions — Isolation using negative pressure room
- ❑ What are the drugs in TB Multidrug Therapy? — Remember RIPES!
  - R - ifampin (RIF)
  - I - soniazid (INH)
  - P - yrazinamide (PZA)
  - E - thambutol (EMB)
  - S - treptomycin (SM)
- ❑ What drug is used for prophylaxis? — Isoniazid (INH)
- ❑ How long is the TB prophylaxis? — 9-12 months
- ❑ What client education is highly important? — Compliance with ATB therapy to prevent development of antibiotic resistance

Pneumonia

- ❑ Description — Inflammation of the lungs
- ❑ Causes — Viruses, fungi, streptococcus, HIV/AIDS
- ❑ Assessment — Severe chills, high-grade fever, productive cough, **pleural friction rub,** rusty sputum (streptococci)
- ❑ Diagnostic Tests — Blood and sputum culture, chest x-ray
- ❑ Interventions — Penicillin, Erythromycin, Chest percussion
  Postural drainage, Splint the chest
- ❑ Who should receive pneumococcal conjugate vaccine? — All children younger than 2 years old
  All adults 65 years or older
  People 2-64 years-old with certain medical illness

Pleurisy (Pleuritis)

- ❑ Description — Inflammation of the pleural membranes
- ❑ Causes — Pneumonia, trauma, lung cancer
- ❑ Assessment — **Chest pain** during breathing, fever, pleural friction rub
- ❑ Diagnostic Test — Chest x-ray
- ❑ Interventions — ATB, analgesics, antipyretics
  Place on **affected** side to splint the chest
  Thoracentesis, Water-seal chest drainage

Atelectasis

❑ Description	Collapse of the lungs
❑ Causes	Pneumothorax, mucus, foreign body
❑ Assessment	Dyspnea, **decreased/absent** breath sounds
❑ Interventions	Incentive spirometry, Suctioning Chest physiotherapy, Bronchodilators, Mucolytics, Deep breathing and coughing

Pneumothorax

❑ Description	Air enters the pleural space → pressure becomes positive → atelectasis
❑ Causes	Open chest injury, ruptured bleb
❑ Assessment	Chest pain, dyspnea, decreased breath sounds, sucking sound on inhalation Mediastinal shift to the **unaffected** side
❑ Interventions	Chest tube insertion

> ***NCLEX Alert!*** *The classic sign of tension pneumothorax is tracheal deviation.*

Lung Cancer

❑ Description	Lung cancer due to smoking or pollution
❑ Assessment	**Chronic cough**, hemoptysis, weight loss
❑ Diagnostic Tests	CT scan, bronchoscopy
❑ Interventions	Radiation, Chemotherapy
❑ Surgery	Segmental Resection, Pneumonectomy
❑ What is expected after pneumonectomy?	No chest tubes are inserted Place on **operative** side (ex. right pneumonectomy → right side)
❑ What is expected after lobectomy?	With chest tubes inserted for drainage Place on **non-operative** side (ex. right lobectomy → left side)

Pulmonary Embolism

❑ Description	Clot, air, fat or amniotic fluid → blocks the pulmonary artery → hypoxia
❑ Assessment	Sudden, sharp chest pain, dyspnea, hemoptysis, decreased breath sounds
❑ Diagnostic Test	Pulmonary arteriogram

- ❑ Interventions: Umbrella filter device insertion; Anticoagulants, Thrombolytics; Elastic stockings, Elevate lower extremities

Chronic Obstructive Pulmonary Disease (COPD)

- ❑ Description: Chronic, irreversible lung disease
- ❑ Causes: Smoking, chemicals, air pollution, alpha-1 antitrypsin deficiency
- ❑ What is alpha-1 antitrypsin? Alpha-1 antitrypsin is a protein that protects the lungs from inflammation. Alpha-1 antitrypsin deficiency (AAT) increases the risk for lung (emphysema) and liver disease.
- ❑ Assessment: Cough, exertional dyspnea, wheezing, white, yellow or greenish sputum, fatigue, weight loss, finger-clubbing
- ❑ Why is finger clubbing present? Due to chronic hypoxia
- ❑ What is common among COPD conditions? Hypercapnia due to chronic retention of CO_2 → respiratory acidosis
- ❑ What is **cor pulmonale**? Hypertrophy of the right ventricle due to pulmonary hypertension

Types of COPD

EMPHYSEMA	CHRONIC BRONCHITIS	BRONCHIECTASIS
Damage to the alveolar walls	Inflammation of the bronchus	Chronic dilation of the bronchi
Destruction of the alveoli → air trapping (bleb/bullae) → alveolar distention → rupture → hypercapnia	Increased mucus → bronchospasm → hypercapnia	Infections, tumor, increased mucus, cystic fibrosis → blockage → hypercapnia
Assessment ❑ Known as the "**pink puffer**" ❑ Dyspnea on exertion ❑ **Barrel-chest**	Assessment ❑ Known as the "**blue bloater**" ❑ Chronic cough for a minimum of 3 months a year for at least 2 years ❑ Productive cough	Assessment ❑ Dyspnea ❑ Finger clubbing ❑ Foul-smelling sputum

- ☐ Interventions — Chest physiotherapy, Hydration, Bronchodilators, Corticosteroids, Antibiotics, Pursed-Lip Breathing, Rest periods, Smoking cessation

- ☐ What is the purpose of pursed-lip breathing? — To exhale excess CO_2

- ☐ What is the hypoxic drive theory? — The hypoxic drive theory is due to chronic CO_2 retention in COPD. As the body becomes used to chronic CO_2 retention, **low O_2** becomes the drive to breath.

> ***NCLEX Alert!*** *Maintain low-flow (1-2 L/min) oxygen to avoid elimination of hypoxic drive to breath.*

Asthma

- ☐ Description — Allergen → release of histamine → bronchospasm, mucus, inflammation

- ☐ Types — EXTRINSIC - pollens, dust
INTRINSIC - fatigue, stress, URTI

- ☐ Assessment — Severe dyspnea, **inspiratory wheezing**, use of accessory muscles, nasal flaring

- ☐ What is status asthmaticus? — Asthma attacks follow one another without pause and can lead to death

- ☐ Interventions — Bronchodilators, Corticosteroids, Epinephrine, Prophylactic drugs

- ☐ What is a peak-flow meter device? — Handheld device that measures how well air moves out of the lungs
Indicates success of therapy

- ☐ How to Use a Metered Dose Inhaler (MDI) with Spacer
  1. Remove cap
  2. Shake the inhaler well
  3. Attach inhaler to the spacer
  4. Exhale deeply
  5. Purse lips around the mouthpiece
  6. Take a slow breath in

7. Hold breath for at least ___ seconds	10
8. Wait __ minute between puffs	1

- ❑ What is a spacer? — Device attached to the MDI that helps the inhaled medication reach the lungs instead of the mouth

> ***NCLEX Alert!*** *When using two inhaled drugs, allow 5 minutes after the first inhaler before inhaling the second medication.*

Acute Respiratory Distress Syndrome (ARDS)

❑ Description	A complication following another disease
❑ Causes	Sepsis, pneumonia, traumatic injury
❑ Assessment	Rales, respiratory distress
❑ What is the main problem in this condition?	**Pulmonary edema**
❑ Interventions	Treat the cause, Oxygen, Ventilator

Cystic Fibrosis

❑ Description	Thick, viscous mucus → blockage of pancreatic ducts → dilation and fibrosis → decrease in pancreatic enzymes → malabsorption of nutrients Bronchial obstruction → infection, bronchiectasis, cystic dilations → respiratory failure
❑ Transmission	Autosomal recessive
❑ Assessment	**Steatorrhea**, **salty sweat**, failure to thrive, rectal prolapse, vitamin K deficiency, clubbing of fingers, barrel-chest, respiratory infections, **meconium ileus** in infants
❑ Diagnostic Test	+ Sweat Test (> 60 meq/L of chloride)
❑ Interventions	Chest physiotherapy, Expectorants, ATBs Mucolytics, Water-soluble vitamin ADEK High calorie, high protein, high salt diet

❑ What is the action of dornase alfa (Pulmozyme)?	Decreases the stickiness of mucus secretions
❑ When is the best time to give pancreatic enzyme replacements?	With meals or snacks to aid digestion

F. Respiratory System Drugs

1. Nasal Decongestants

❑ Description	Dries the nasal mucous membranes Treats colds and hay fever
❑ Drugs	Examples: ▪ oxymetazoline (Afrin) ▪ phenylephrine (Neo-Syneprhine) ▪ pseudoeophedrine (Sudafed)
❑ Side effects	**Hypertension**, nervousness
❑ Interventions	Monitor for arrhythmias, Avoid caffeine

2. Expectorants and Mucolytic Agents

❑ Drugs	Examples: EXPECTORANT ▪ guaifenesin (Mucinex) MUCOLYTIC ▪ acetylcysteine (Mucomyst)
❑ Expectorants are given for which type of cough?	Productive cough
❑ Interventions	Increase fluids to prevent dehydration

3. Antitussives

❑ Description	Suppresses cough
❑ Drugs	Examples: OPIOIDS ▪ codeine sulfate, hydrocodone NON-OPIOIDS ▪ benzonatate (Tessalon) ▪ dextromethorphan (Vicks DayQuil) ▪ diphenhydramine HCl (Benadryl)
❑ Antitussives are given for which type of cough?	Non-productive
❑ Side effects	**Sedation**, drowsiness, dizziness
❑ Interventions	Avoid alcohol, Monitor for CNS depression

4. Bronchodilators

❑ Description	Relaxes the smooth muscle of the bronchi Treats bronchospasm (e.g. asthma, COPD)
❑ Side effects	**Arrhythmias**, palpitations, nervousness, mouth dryness
❑ Interventions	Monitor for dysrhythmias Avoid caffeine

Beta$_2$ – Adrenergic Agonists

❑ Drugs	Examples: INHALED ▪ salmeterol (Serevent Diskus) ▪ albuterol (Proventil HFA) ▪ pirbuterol (Maxair Autohaler) ORAL ▪ terbutaline (Brethine) ▪ albuterol (VoSpire)

Methylxanthines

❑ Drugs	Examples: ▪ theophylline, oral (Theo-24)

Anticholinergics

❑ Drugs	Examples: ▪ tiotropium, inhaled (Spiriva) ▪ ipratropium, inhaled (Atrovent HFA)

> ***NCLEX Alert!*** *Always administer the bronchodilator first before the steroid inhaler. This allows the steroid to penetrate the lungs effectively. Rinse the mouth after administering a steroid inhaler to prevent fungal infections.*

5. Glucocorticoids

❑ Description	Reduces inflammation in asthma
❑ Drugs	Examples: INHALED ▪ triamcinolone acetonide (Azmacort) ▪ fluticasone propionate (Flovent HFA) ▪ beclomethasone dipropionate (Qvar) ORAL ▪ prednisone
❑ Side effects	Oral thrush (candidiasis)
❑ Interventions	Rinse the mouth, Use a spacer device

6. Leukotriene Modifiers

❑ Description	For prophylaxis against asthma Blocks bronchospasm
❑ Is this drug effective for acute asthma attack?	No
❑ Contraindications	Breastfeeding; may pass into breastmilk
❑ Drugs	Examples: ▪ montelukast, oral (Singulair) ▪ zileuton, oral (Zyflo CR) ▪ zafirlukast, oral (Accolate)
❑ Side effects	Headache, nausea, vomiting, diarrhea
❑ Interventions	Take the drug even if symptom-free

7. Monoclononal Antibodies

❑ Description	Monoclonal antibodies are biological drugs used to treat cancers, several types of arthritis, lupus, multiple sclerosis and IBD Treats allergic asthma Given SQ every 2-4 weeks
❑ Drugs	Example: omalizumab (Xolair)
❑ Side effects	Injection site reactions, allergy
❑ Interventions	Check for allergic reaction Avoid live virus vaccines

8. Inhaled Nonsteroidal Anti-Allergy Agent

❑ Description	For prophylaxis against asthma
❑ Drugs	Example: cromolyn sodium (Intal) A mast cell inhibitor
❑ Is this drug effective for acute asthma attack?	No
❑ Side effects	Itchy nose, sneezing, dry throat
❑ Interventions	Take a few sips of water for dry throat

9. Antihistamines

❑ Description	Histamine antagonists or H_1 blockers compete with histamine receptor sites → blocks a histamine response Treats colds and motion sickness
❑ Drugs	Examples: ▪ cetirizine (Zyrtec) ▪ diphenhydramine (Benadryl) ▪ desloratadine (Clarinex) ▪ dimenhydrinate (Dramamine)

- ❑ Side effects — CNS depression, **drowsiness**, dizziness, urinary retention, dry mouth
- ❑ Interventions — Avoid alcohol, Ice chips for dry mouth

10. Opioid Antagonist

- ❑ Description — Reverses respiratory depression
- ❑ Drugs — Examples:
  - nalmefene (Revex), naloxone (Narcan)
  - naltrexone (Revia), alvimopan (Entereg)
  - methylnaltrexone (Relistor)
- ❑ Side effects — Hypo/hypertension, arrhythmia, diarrhea
- ❑ Interventions — Monitor for acute opioid withdrawal

> ***NCLEX Alert!*** *Naloxone will not reverse respiratory depression and overdose resulting from non-opioid drugs such as benzodiazepines, cocaine or alcohol.*

11. Tuberculosis Drugs

- ❑ Description — Multidrug regimen to prevent the development of drug resistance; 9-12 months treatment duration but may take longer depending on response
- ❑ Drugs

FIRST-LINE DRUGS	SECOND-LINE DRUGS
❑ isoniazid (INH)	❑ streptomycin (injectable)
❑ rifampin (Rifadin)	❑ kanamycin (injectable)
❑ rifapentine (Priftin)	❑ amikacin (injectable)
❑ rifabutin (Mycobutin)	❑ capreomycin (injectable)
❑ pyrazinamide	❑ p-aminosalicylic acid (Paser)
❑ ethambutol (Myambutol)	❑ levofloxacin (Levaquin)
	❑ ethionamide
	❑ cycloserine

> ***NCLEX Alert!*** *Isoniazid, rifampicin and pyrazinamide are severely hepatotoxic. Liver functions tests must be done before the client takes these medications!*

TB DRUGS	SIDE EFFECTS	INTERVENTIONS
isoniazid (INH)	❑ **Peripheral neuritis** due to Vitamin B_6 (pyridoxine) deficiency ❑ Hepatotoxicity	❑ Avoid alcohol ❑ Monitor for tingling and numbness ❑ Give 1 hour before or 2 hours after meals
rifampin (Rifadin)	❑ **Reddish-orange/brown** body secretions ❑ Antagonistic effects to the following drugs: ▪ digoxin ▪ phenytoin ▪ oral anticoagulants ▪ oral hypoglycemic agents ▪ oral contraceptive pills ❑ Hepatotoxicity	❑ Avoid alcohol ❑ Use birth control methods other than pills ❑ Give on an empty stomach 1 hour before meals
ethambutol (Myambutol)	❑ Neurotoxicicity ❑ **Optic neuritis**	❑ Monitor for visual changes ❑ Give with food
pyrazinamide	❑ **Hyperuricemia** ❑ Photosensitivity ❑ Hepatotoxicicity	❑ Avoid alcohol ❑ Give with food ❑ Avoid sunlight exposure
streptomycin	❑ **Ototoxicity** ❑ **Nephrotoxicity**	❑ Assess hearing and renal function

12. Influenza Drugs

Antiviral Prophylaxis

❑ Drugs

Examples:
- zanamivir (Relenza)
- oseltamivir (Tamiflu)

❑ Give within __ days of onset of symptoms

2

Inactivated Vaccine (IM Injection)

❑ Drugs

Examples:
- Fluzone, Afluria

❑ Who should receive the vaccine given?

Ages 6 months and above

❑ Contraindications

Severe illness, **active fever**, chicken egg allergy, Guillain-Barre syndrome

Cardiovascular System

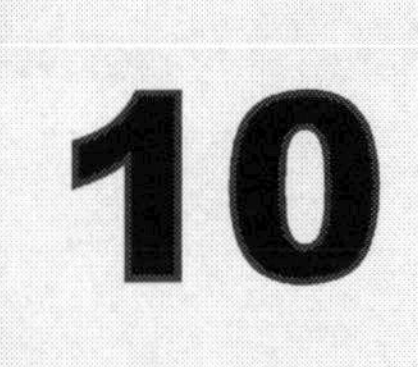

A. The Cardiovascular System

Systemic and Pulmonary Circulation

Superior vena cava → Right atrium → Tricuspid valve → Right ventricle → Pulmonary valve → Pulmonary artery → capillaries in the lungs → CO_2 and O_2 exchange → Pulmonary veins → Left atrium → Bicuspid/Mitral valve → Left ventricle → Aortic valve → Aorta

Cardiac Conduction System

SA node → AV node → Bundle of his → Right and left bundle branches → Purkinje fibers

❑ Stroke volume x heart rate = __________	Cardiac output; normally 4-8 L/minute
❑ Systole means __________________	Contraction/depolarization of the ventricles
❑ Diastole means __________________	Relaxation/repolarization of the ventricles
❑ Myocardial stretch before contraction	Preload
❑ Preload is affected by the ______________	Amount of blood volume
❑ Left ventricular resistance to pump blood	Afterload
❑ Afterload is affected by ______________	Peripheral vascular resistance
❑ Vasoconstriction increases the ______________	Afterload
❑ Increased preload and afterload will increase _________	Cardiac workload
❑ What drugs are given to decrease the preload?	Diuretics
❑ What drugs are given to decrease the afterload?	Vasodilators
❑ What is erythropoietin?	A hormone produced by the kidney to stimulate the bone marrow to form RBC
❑ Types of granulocytes	Basophils, Eosinophils, Neutrophils
❑ Types of nongranulocytes	Monocytes, B and T cell lymphocytes
❑ Stimulation of $beta_1$ receptor cells will lead to _______	Increased heart rate
❑ Stimulation of $beta_2$ receptor cells will lead to _______	Bronchodilation
❑ Stimulation of $alpha_1$ adrenergic cells will lead to _______	Vasoconstriction

B. Cardiovascular Assessment

❑ Best location of apical pulse	5th intercostal space, left midclavicular line; 60-100 beats/minute
❑ The difference between radial and apical pulse	Pulse deficit
❑ The difference between systolic and diastolic BP	Pulse pressure (e.g. 120/80 mmHg = 40)
❑ When is pulse pressure **widened**?	Increased intracranial pressure (IICP)
❑ When is pulse pressure **narrowed**?	Shock (e.g. 90/80 mmHg = 10)
❑ How is postural hypotension assessed?	Lay client down for 5 minutes, take a baseline BP. Then have the client stand and immediately take another BP
❑ When is postural hypotension present?	A drop in SBP >20 mmHg
❑ What is the normal pulse oximetry reading?	95-100%
❑ What are the signs of arterial occlusion?	Remember 6 P's! ▪ P-ulselessness, P-erishing cold, ▪ P-ain, P-allor, P-aresthesia, P-aralysis

The Renin-Angiotensin-Aldosterone Mechanism

Decreased blood volume and BP → kidney → release of renin → angiotensinogen → angiotensin 1 → converting enzyme in lungs → **angiotensin 2** → potent vasoconstriction → increased BP → adrenal cortex → **aldosterone** → sodium reabsorption → increased BP

Five Areas for Heart Sound Auscultation

❑ Aortic valve area	Right 2nd intercostal space
❑ Pulmonic valve area	Left 2nd intercostal space
❑ Erb's point	Left 3rd intercostal space
❑ Tricuspid area	Left sternal border, 4th intercostal space
❑ Mitral (or apical) area	Left 5th intercostal space, midclavicular line

Heart Sounds

❑ Atrioventricular valves close (lubb)	S_1 heart sound; loudest in apex
❑ Semilunar valves close (dubb)	S_2 heart sound; loudest in aortic area
❑ S_3 (ventricular gallop) heart sound	Abnormal; present in heart failure
❑ S_4 (atrial gallop) heart sound	Abnormal; present in hypertension
❑ Abnormal whooshing sound due to a valve problem	Murmurs
❑ Abnormal short, high-pitched sounds due to a valve problem	Clicks

Peripheral Edema

1+	2+	3+	4+
2 mm or less; mild indentation; no visible distortion; disappears fast	2-4 mm; slightly deeper indentation; disappears in 10-15 seconds	4-6 mm; noticeably deep indentation; may last >1 minute; swelling visible	6-8 mm; severely deep indentation; lasts 2-5 minutes; obviously malformed appearance

C. Diagnostic Tests

Magnetic Resonance Imaging

- ❑ Description — Uses magnetic field and radio waves
- ❑ Contraindications — Clients with metal or electronic devices
  - implantable heart defibrillator
  - cardiac pacemaker
  - joint prosthesis
  - artificial heart valves
- ❑ Interventions — Remove dentures, jewelry and hearing aids. Assess for claustrophobia, Lie still

Cardiac Catheterization

- ❑ Description — Visualizes the heart chambers, valves and coronary arteries
- ❑ Interventions — Ask for iodine allergy
- ❑ Feeling of warmth, salty taste and flushing — Normal reaction to the dye
- ❑ Report dyspnea and chest pain — Indicates an allergic reaction
- ❑ After the procedure — Increase fluid intake to flush the dye. Monitor insertion site for bleeding

> ***NCLEX Alert!*** *Palpate the distal pulses after the procedure to check for peripheral circulation.*

Electrocardiography

- ❑ Description — Graphic recording of the electrical activity of the heart
- ❑ What is a normal sinus rhythm? — Regular
- ❑ P wave — Depolarization (contraction) of atria
- ❑ PR interval — Travel time between atria to ventricles *(0.12 -.0.20 seconds)*

- ❑ QRS complex — Depolarization (contraction) of ventricles *(< 0.12 seconds)*
- ❑ T wave — Repolarization (relaxation) of ventricles
- ❑ What is a Holter monitor? — A 24- hour portable ECG monitoring device

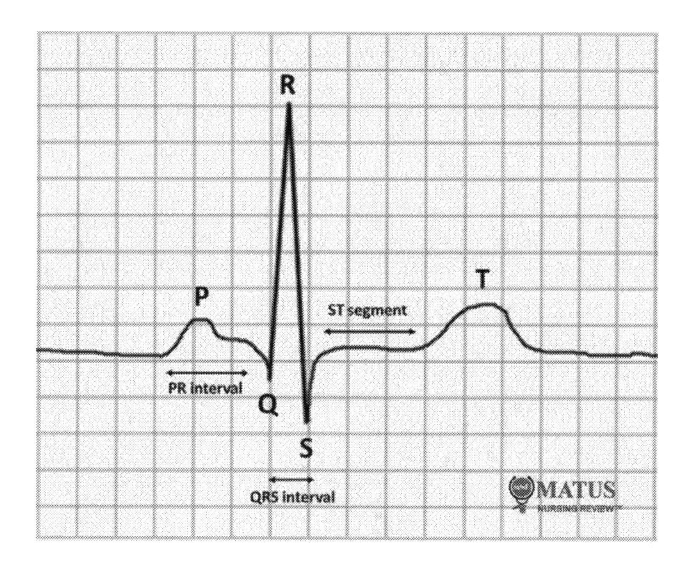

Calculating Heart Rate

1. Rule of 300 (for regular rhythm)

Count the number of large squares between 2 R waves and divide the number into 300 (R-R interval). Find an R wave on a dark line. Note the next block as 300, the second block 150, the third block 100, then 75, then 60, then 50, then 43, then 37, then 30.

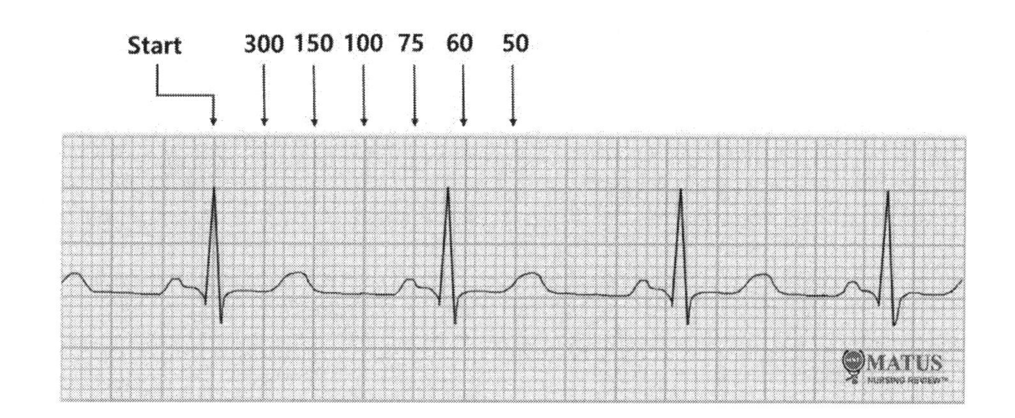

2. Six-Second Method (for irregular rhythm)

Count the number of complete R waves within a period of 6 seconds (30 large squares) and multiply the total by 10

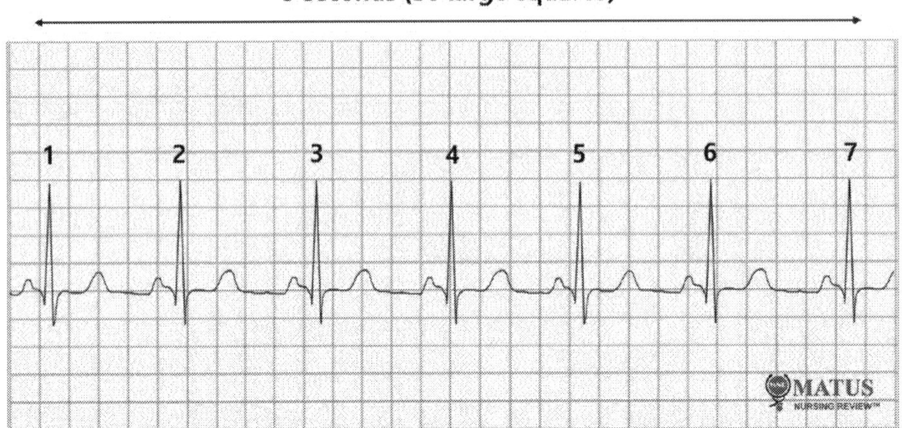

Heart Rate – 7 R waves X 10 = 70/minute

3. The Three-Second Method

Count the number of R waves in a period of three seconds and multiply the total by 20

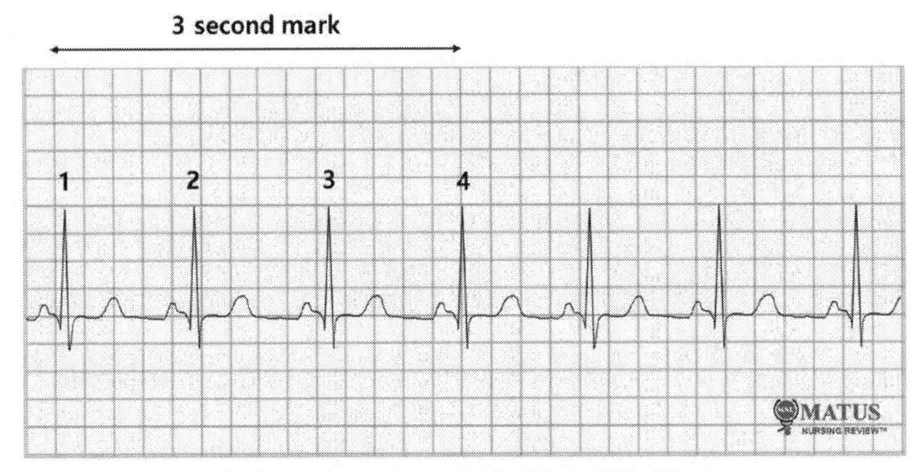

Heart Rate – 4 R waves X 20 = 80/minute

Exercise/Stress Test ECG

❑ Description

Treadmill or drug stress test
May be done with thallium scanning
Radioisotope injected IV while exercising

Echocardiography

- ❑ Description — A high-frequency ultrasound that measures the ejection fraction (EF)
- ❑ What is ejection fraction (EF)? — Percentage of blood leaving the ventricle per contraction
- ❑ 55-70% EF — Normal
- ❑ 40-55% EF — Below normal
- ❑ Less than 40% EF — Heart failure
- ❑ Less than 35% EF — Prone to arrhythmias and cardiac arrest

Multigated Acquisition (MUGA) Scan

- ❑ Description — Creates video images of the ventricles to assess the pumping action
Provides a more precise measure of EF

D. Cardiovascular System Disorders

Dysrhythmias

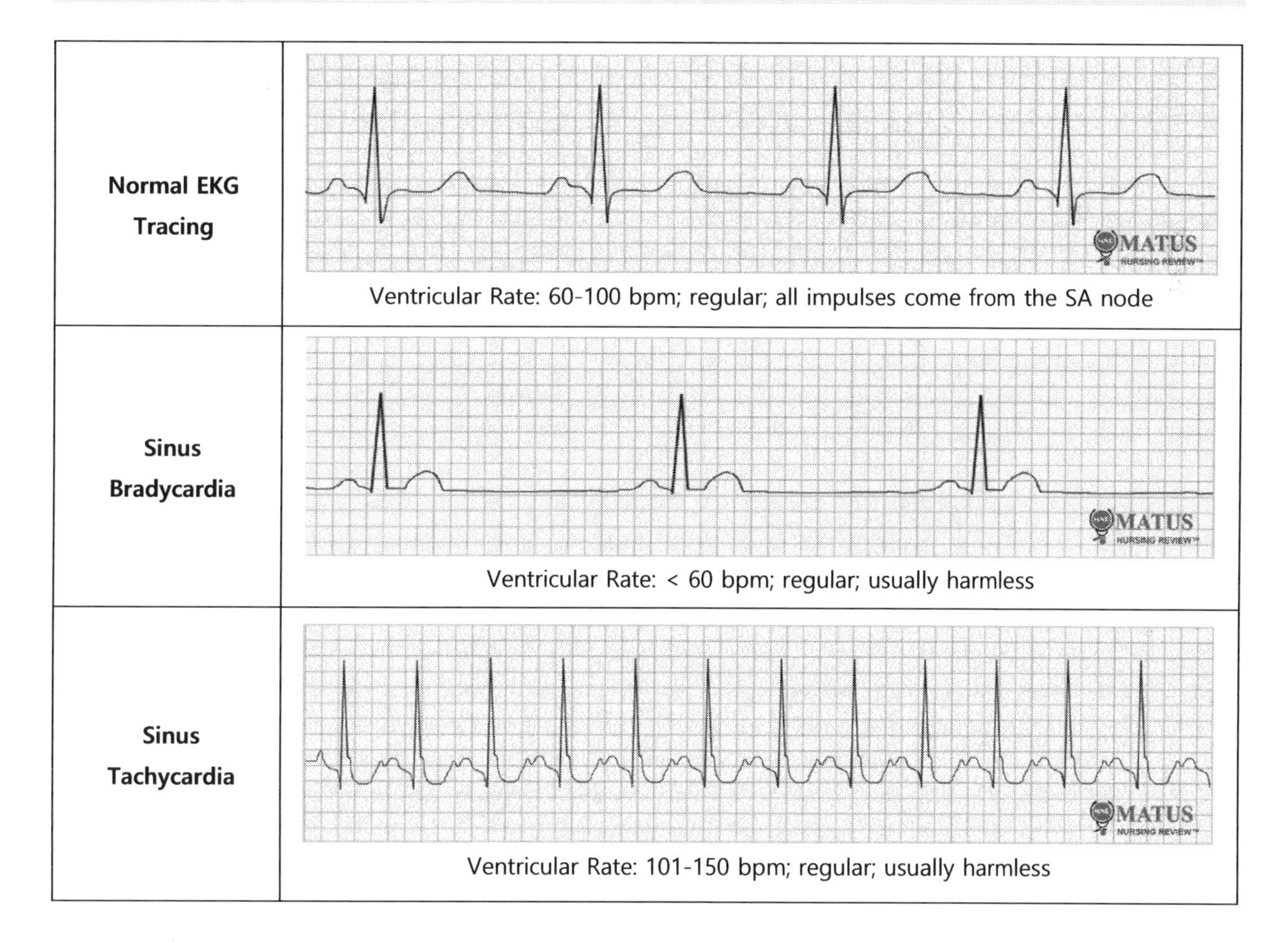

Normal EKG Tracing	Ventricular Rate: 60-100 bpm; regular; all impulses come from the SA node
Sinus Bradycardia	Ventricular Rate: < 60 bpm; regular; usually harmless
Sinus Tachycardia	Ventricular Rate: 101-150 bpm; regular; usually harmless

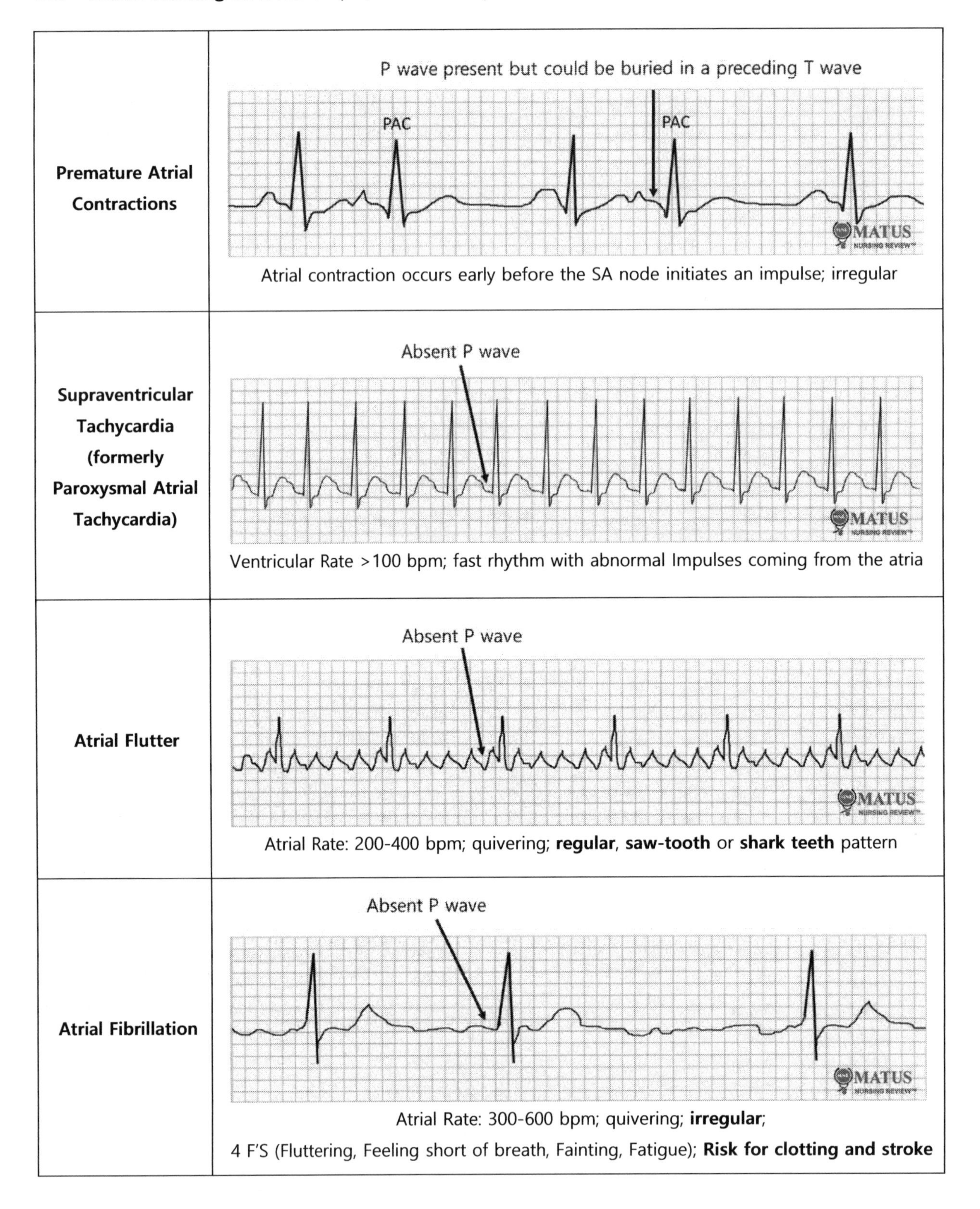

Premature Atrial Contractions	Atrial contraction occurs early before the SA node initiates an impulse; irregular
Supraventricular Tachycardia (formerly Paroxysmal Atrial Tachycardia)	Ventricular Rate >100 bpm; fast rhythm with abnormal Impulses coming from the atria
Atrial Flutter	Atrial Rate: 200-400 bpm; quivering; **regular**, **saw-tooth** or **shark teeth** pattern
Atrial Fibrillation	Atrial Rate: 300-600 bpm; quivering; **irregular**; 4 F'S (Fluttering, Feeling short of breath, Fainting, Fatigue); **Risk for clotting and stroke**

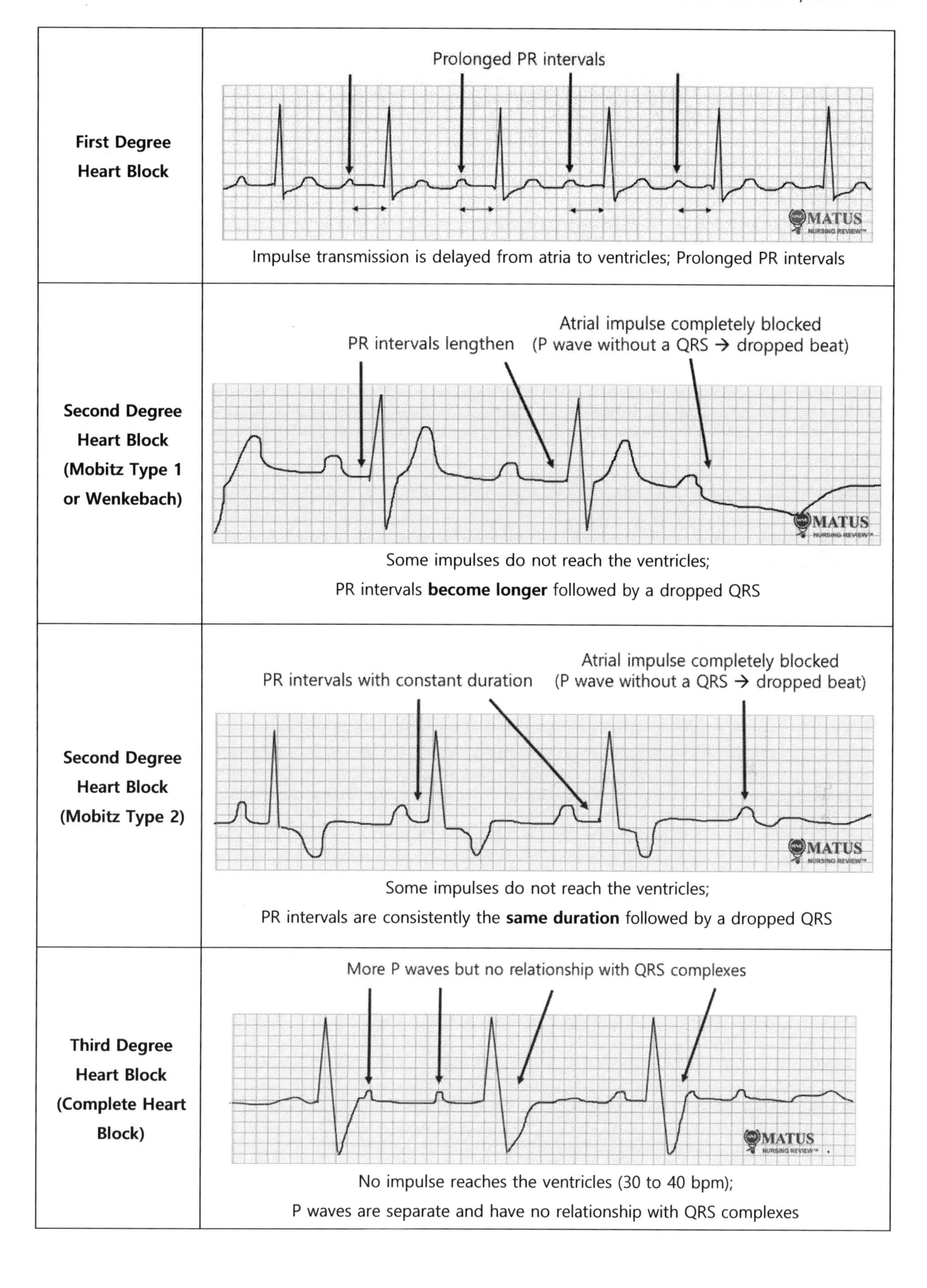

First Degree Heart Block	Prolonged PR intervals Impulse transmission is delayed from atria to ventricles; Prolonged PR intervals
Second Degree Heart Block (Mobitz Type 1 or Wenkebach)	PR intervals lengthen Atrial impulse completely blocked (P wave without a QRS → dropped beat) Some impulses do not reach the ventricles; PR intervals **become longer** followed by a dropped QRS
Second Degree Heart Block (Mobitz Type 2)	PR intervals with constant duration Atrial impulse completely blocked (P wave without a QRS → dropped beat) Some impulses do not reach the ventricles; PR intervals are consistently the **same duration** followed by a dropped QRS
Third Degree Heart Block (Complete Heart Block)	More P waves but no relationship with QRS complexes No impulse reaches the ventricles (30 to 40 bpm); P waves are separate and have no relationship with QRS complexes

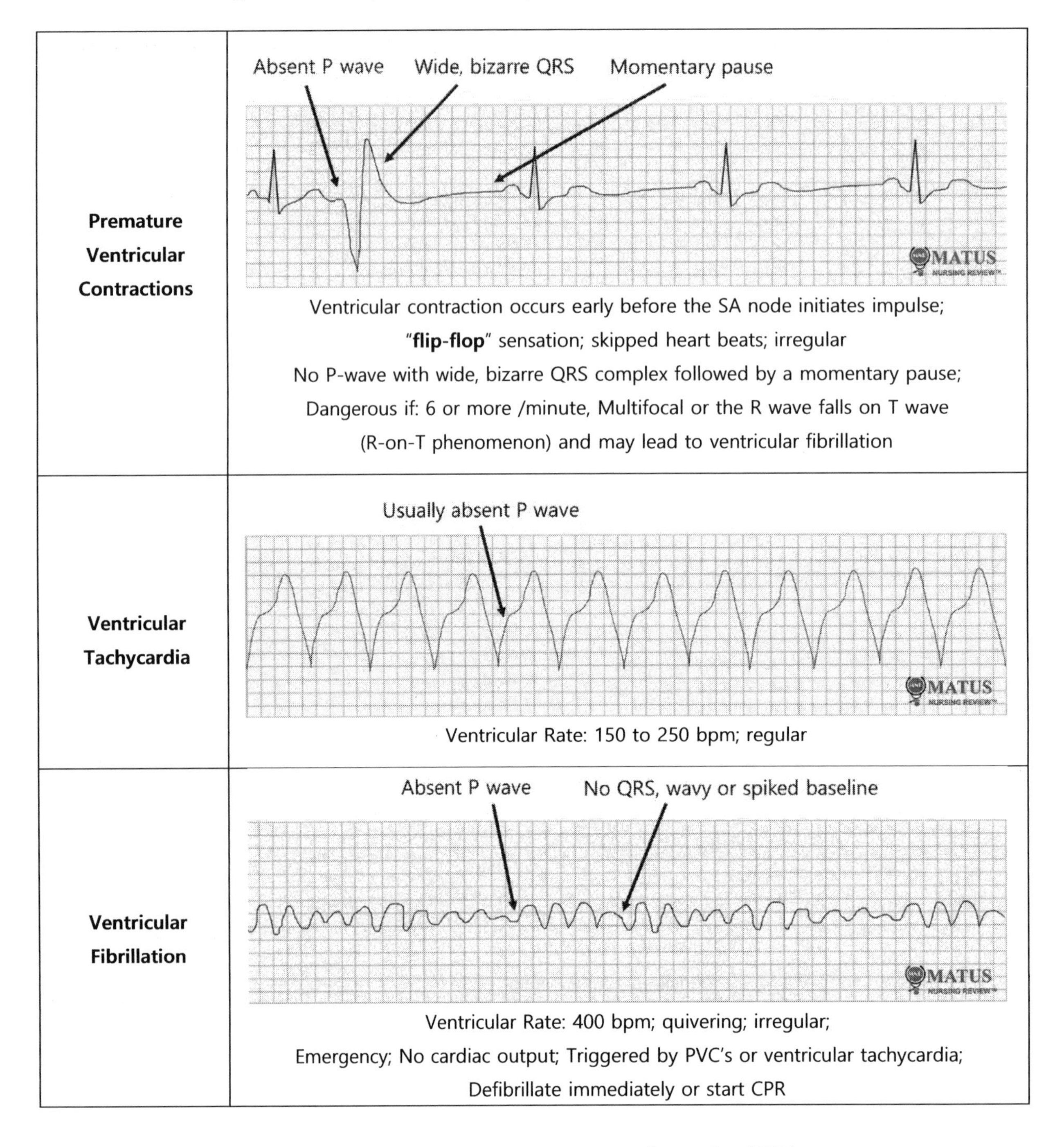

Premature Ventricular Contractions	Absent P wave; Wide, bizarre QRS; Momentary pause Ventricular contraction occurs early before the SA node initiates impulse; "**flip-flop**" sensation; skipped heart beats; irregular No P-wave with wide, bizarre QRS complex followed by a momentary pause; Dangerous if: 6 or more /minute, Multifocal or the R wave falls on T wave (R-on-T phenomenon) and may lead to ventricular fibrillation
Ventricular Tachycardia	Usually absent P wave Ventricular Rate: 150 to 250 bpm; regular
Ventricular Fibrillation	Absent P wave; No QRS, wavy or spiked baseline Ventricular Rate: 400 bpm; quivering; irregular; Emergency; No cardiac output; Triggered by PVC's or ventricular tachycardia; Defibrillate immediately or start CPR

❑ Drugs for bradycardia

Remember IDEA!

- I - soproterenol
- D - opamine
- E - pinephrine
- A - tropine sulfate

❑ Drugs for tachycardia

Remember ABC!

- B - eta-Blockers
- C - alcium-channel Blockers
- D – igoxin

❑ What is cardiac ablation?	Procedure that scars or destroy cardiac tissue to restore a normal heart rhythm
❑ What is a maze procedure?	Usually performed to treat atrial fibrillation by creating small incisions and use of radio waves, freezing, or ultrasound energy to form a scar tissue

Cardioversion versus Defibrillation

❑ Treats ventricular tachycardia and atrial fibrillation	Cardioversion
❑ Treats ventricular fibrillation and **pulseless** ventricular tachycardia	Defibrillation
❑ Emergency treatment (asynchronized)	Defibrillation
❑ Elective procedure; Machine fires on R wave (synchronized)	Cardioversion
❑ Client is sedated before the procedure	Cardioversion
❑ Client is unresponsive or unconscious	Defibrillation

Artificial Cardiac Pacemakers

❑ Device fires the impulses at pre-set rate	Fixed-rate mode
❑ Device fires the impulse when heart rate falls below pre-set rate	Demand mode
❑ What will be seen on the cardiac monitor or ECG strip when the pacemaker fires the impulse?	Spike (straight vertical line)
❑ Weakness, vertigo, chest pain and abnormal pulse	Indicates malfunction
❑ What items may interfere with pacemaker function?	Battery-operated toothbrushes, battery powered cordless tools, MRI
❑ At least how many inches should cellphones and headphones be away from the pacemaker?	6 inches to prevent pacemaker interference
❑ What instructions are important to teach the client?	Count the radial pulse regularly Avoid contact sports Wear a Medic-Alert bracelet for emergency

Angina Pectoris

❑ Description	Hypoxia of the heart muscle → chest pain
❑ Chest pain disappears with rest; predictable	Stable
❑ Unpredictable and more serious; leads to MI	Unstable
❑ Occurs at rest due to coronary spasm	Prinzmetal (Variant)
❑ Occurs when the client lies down	Angina decubitus
❑ Difficult to treat	Intractable angina

❑ Assessment	Substernal or retrosternal pain **relieved** by rest and nitroglycerin, radiates to the left inner arm, little finger, shoulder and jaw
❑ What are the EKG findings?	ST depression, T-wave inversion (hypoxia)
❑ What are the 5 E's that trigger angina pectoris?	E - xertion E - xcessive emotional response (anxiety) E - xcessive exposure to cold E - xcessive smoking E - xcessive eating
❑ Interventions	Aspirin, Beta-blockers, Calcium-channel blockers, Nitroglycerin
❑ Coronary Artery Bypass Graft (CABG)	Graft from saphenous or mammary veins bypasses the blocked coronary artery
❑ Percutaneous Transluminal Coronary Angioplasty (PTCA)	Uses balloon-catheter to widen the artery
❑ Coronary stent	Metal mesh that keeps the artery open
❑ What is a complication of stent placement?	Thrombosis

Myocardial Infarction

❑ Description	Blockage of coronary artery → hypoxia and necrosis of myocardium
❑ Causes	Thrombosis, embolus
❑ What is the most common complication?	Arrhythmia (tachycardia, PVC's)
❑ Assessment	Severe crushing pain **unrelieved** by rest and nitroglycerin, dyspnea, vomiting, diaphoresis, ashen color, a sense of doom
❑ Most specific protein for diagnosis	Troponin
❑ What are the EKG findings?	Inverted T wave → indicates hypoxia ST segment elevation → indicates injury Pathologic Q wave → indicates necrosis
❑ Interventions	Remember MONA! M-orphine, O-xygen,N-itroglycerin, A-spirin Low fat, low cholesterol, low sodium diet

❑ Why is morphine sulfate not given intramuscularly? — Muscle injury will falsely elevate the blood enzymes especially creatine kinase (CK)

❑ How soon should thrombolytics be given? — Within 6 hours

❑ Why are laxatives given? — To prevent Valsalva maneuver (straining)

❑ When can the client resume sexual activities? — If the client is able to climb 2 flights of stairs without dyspnea or chest pain

Heart Failure

❑ Description — Chronic, progressive disease → decreased cardiac output → hypoxia

❑ Assessment

RIGHT-SIDED HEART FAILURE (Systemic Congestion)	LEFT-SIDED HEART FAILURE (Pulmonary Congestion)
❑ Distended jugular veins	❑ Dyspnea
❑ Anorexia, nausea	❑ Paroxysmal nocturnal dyspnea
❑ Hepatomegaly, cirrhosis, ascites	❑ Orthopnea
❑ Splenomegaly	❑ Crackles
❑ Edema in ankles, feet and sacrum	❑ Frothy, blood tinged sputum
❑ Increased central venous pressure (CVP)	❑ Increased pulmonary artery pressures (PAP)

❑ What are the 2 types of left-sided heart failure?

Systolic heart failure
- Has reduced ejection fraction
- Loss of ability to contract or pump blood

Diastolic heart failure
- Has preserved ejection fraction
- Loss of ability to relax due to stiffness

❑ Interventions — Diuretics, Weigh daily, Rest periods
Low sodium, low cholesterol diet
digoxin (Lanoxin)

❑ What is the purpose of an Intra-Aortic Balloon Pump (IABP)? — Device that improves the cardiac output

Acute Pulmonary Edema

❑ Description — Sudden accumulation of fluid in the lungs

❑ Assessment — **Pink-tinged frothy sputum,** severe dyspnea, tachycardia, pallor

❑ Interventions — Morphine sulfate, Oxygen, Digoxin

❑ Why is morphine sulfate given? — To relieve anxiety and cause vasodilation

❑ What is the best position for this condition? — High-Fowler's position

Valvular Heart Disease

❑ Description	Stenosis (narrowing) and insufficiency (regurgitation) of the heart valves → backflow of blood → heart failure
❑ Causes	Rheumatic heart disease, endocarditis
❑ Assessment	Fatigue, angina, weight gain, fainting
❑ Interventions	Anticoagulants, Low sodium diet, Diuretics
❑ Surgery	Valve replacement, Balloon valvuloplasty

> ***NCLEX Alert!*** *The client should receive prophylactic antibiotics before invasive procedures to prevent infective endocarditis.*

Rheumatic Heart Disease

❑ Description	Group A beta-hemolytic strep throat → rheumatic fever → endocarditis → heart valve damage → heart failure
❑ Assessment	5 MAJOR SIGNS ▪ Carditis ▪ Polyarthritis ▪ Subcutaneous nodules ▪ Erythema marginatum (rash) ▪ Sydenham's chorea MINOR SIGNS ▪ fever, + ASO titer, arthralgia ▪ elevated ESR and +C-reactive protein
❑ Interventions	Bed rest, Pen G (Penadur) monthly IM
❑ What should be given before surgery?	Prophylactic antibiotics
❑ Surgery	Valve replacement

Pericarditis

❑ Description	Inflammation of the pericardium → effusion → cardiac compression → decreased cardiac output
❑ Assessment	**Chest pain upon movement,** pericardial friction rub
❑ Diagnostic Tests	Chest x-ray, Pericardiocentesis
❑ Interventions	Antibiotics, Analgesics, Bed rest

❑ Complication

CARDIAC TAMPONADE

- Compression of the heart due to fluid accumulation in the pericardium

❑ What is **pulsus paradoxus**?

A large drop in SBP >10 mmHg during inspiration (indicates cardiac tamponade)

Infective Endocarditis

❑ Description

Infection of the inner lining of the heart

❑ Assessment

Fever, murmur, dyspnea, Osler node, Roth spots, splinter hemorrhages, Janeway lesions, pulmonary embolism

❑ Diagnostic Tests

Increased WBC and ESR, Blood cultures

❑ Interventions

ATBs before invasive procedures

❑ Surgery

Valve replacement

Cardiomyopathy

❑ Description

Changes in myocardium → heart failure

❑ Causes

Alcohol, cocaine, chemotherapy drugs

❑ Types

DILATED – stretching
HYPERTROPHIC - thickening
RESTRICTIVE – stiffening

❑ Assessment

Fainting, fatigue, exertional dyspnea

❑ Diagnostic Tests

Echocardiogram, cardiac biopsy

❑ Interventions

Same management as heart failure

❑ Surgery

Myotomy, Myectomy, Heart Transplant

Hypertension

❑ Description

Systolic BP >130, diastolic BP >80 mmHg

❑ What is the normal BP?

<120/80 mm Hg

❑ Stages of Hypertension

PREHYPERTENSION	STAGE 1	STAGE 2	HYPERTENSIVE CRISIS
SBP 120 -129 mm Hg DBP <80 mm Hg	SBP 130-139 mm Hg DBP 80-89 mm Hg	SBP at least 140 mm Hg DBP at least 90 mm Hg	SBP 180 mm Hg DBP 120 mm Hg

Reference: American Heart Association

- ❑ Types — ESSENTIAL (PRIMARY) - unknown cause
  SECONDARY - heart failure, hypertension
  MALIGNANT – sudden, severe high BP
- ❑ Assessment — "Silent killer", occipital headache, chest pain, stroke, nephropathy
- ❑ Diagnostic Tests — Lipid profile, creatinine, BUN, chest x-ray
- ❑ Interventions — Lose weight, Stop smoking, Limit alcohol, sodium and caffeine, Stress management
- ❑ What are the main drugs for hypertension? — A - CE inhibitors
  B - eta-blockers
  C - alcium channel blockers
  D – iuretics
- ❑ Why are antihypertensive drugs not abruptly stopped? — To prevent rebound hypertension
- ❑ What instruction is important to teach the client? — Encourage early detection and screening

Arterial versus Venous Ulcers

ARTERIAL	VENOUS
❑ Intermittent claudication	❑ Heavy, dull, tired or achy legs
❑ Pain worsens with walking or running	❑ Pain worsens with standing
❑ Pain subsides when lowering the leg	❑ Pain subsides when elevating the legs
❑ Wound ulcers on the toes and feet	❑ Wound ulcers on the lower legs and ankles
❑ Deep, punched-out wound appearance	❑ Superficial and shallow wound
❑ Absent or minimal edema	❑ Marked edema and drainage
❑ Pulses are absent or diminished	❑ Pulses are present but may be hard to palpate
❑ Pale skin color and may have eschar	❑ Ruddy skin color

Arteriosclerosis Obliterans

- ❑ Description — Plaques → ischemia → gangrene ulcers
- ❑ Assessment — 6 P's of arterial occlusion
- ❑ What is **intermittent claudication**? — Cramping leg pain during exertion
- ❑ Diagnostic Tests — Treadmill testing, Doppler ultrasound
- ❑ Interventions — Anticoagulants, Fibrinolytics, Vasodilators
  Place legs in a **dependent** position
- ❑ Surgery — Embolectomy, Angioplasty, Amputation
- ❑ What should the client avoid? — Tight clothes, Crossing legs, Cold exposure

Aneurysm

❑ Description	Dilation of an artery usually the aorta
❑ Causes	Arteriosclerosis, congenital, hypertension
❑ Types	Saccular, Fusiform, Dissecting
❑ Palpable mass, low back pain	Abdominal aortic aneurysm
❑ Dysphagia, dyspnea	Thoracic aortic aneurysm
❑ Headache, visual changes	Cerebral aneurysm
❑ Diagnostic Tests	Fluoroscopy, Chest x-ray, Aortogram
❑ Interventions	Antihypertensive drugs Resection and replacement with Teflon
❑ Report severe back pain after surgery	Indicates retroperitoneal hemorrhage

Thromboangiitis Obliterans (Buerger's Disease)

❑ Description	Inflamed, thrombotic arteries of the hands and feet → hypoxia → gangrene leg ulcers
❑ What is the greatest risk factor?	Smoking
❑ Assessment	Intermittent or in-step claudication, 6 P's of arterial occlusion
❑ Interventions	Meticulous foot care, **Stop smoking** Sympathectomy, Amputation
❑ What is the purpose of Buerger-Allen exercise?	To promote circulation to the legs
❑ What are the steps in Buerger-Allen exercise?	1. Elevate feet for 2- 3 minutes 2. Sit on the edge of bed for feet exercises (pronation/supination) for 3 minutes 3. Lie flat for 5 minutes 4. Repeat cycle 4-5 times; 3x a day

Raynaud's Disease

❑ Description	Vasospasm → tissue ischemia
❑ Assessment	Coldness, pallor, pain, ulcers on fingers
❑ Diagnostic Test	**Cold Stimulation Test** (hands in ice)
❑ Interventions	Stop smoking, Calcium-channel blockers Wear warm socks, Stress management
❑ What is McIntyre maneuver?	Swinging the hands to reverse the symptoms
❑ Surgery	Sympathectomy

Thrombophlebitis

❑ Description	Clot formation → inflammation of the vein → dislodgement → pulmonary embolism
❑ 3 conditions that lead to clot formation (Virchow's triad)	3 V's: V-enostasis, V-essel injury, V-iscosity
❑ Types	Superficial thrombophlebitis Deep vein thrombosis (DVT)
❑ Assessment	Edema, warmth, erythema, tenderness
❑ What is a positive Homan's sign?	Pain in the calf during dorsiflexion
❑ Diagnostic Tests	Venous Doppler, Serum D-dimer
❑ What is D-dimer?	Product of blood clot formation
❑ Interventions	Bed rest, Moist heat, Elevate legs, Elastic stockings, Anticoagulants
❑ What is an umbrella filter device?	Device placed in the inferior vena cava to trap a dislodged clot from the legs and prevent pulmonary embolism
❑ How can thrombosis be prevented?	Remember 6 E's! E - levate legs E - ncourage ambulation E - ncourage fluids E - xtend the knees (Avoid crossing of legs) E - lastic stockings E - ncourage exercise
❑ What should be avoided during acute thrombosis?	Massaging the legs to prevent dislodging the clot that will lead to embolism

Varicose Veins

❑ Description	Dilation of the saphenous veins
❑ Causes	Congenital defect, obesity, pregnancy, prolonged standing/sitting, crossing legs
❑ Assessment	Dark, tortuous veins, fatigue, cramping, venous stasis ulcers
❑ Diagnostic Test	Trendelenburg Test

- ❑ What are the steps in Trendelenburg Test?
  1. Ask the client to lie down
  2. Elevate the leg
  3. Apply tourniquet in the upper thigh
  4. Ask the client to stand
  5. Observe the filling pattern
     → veins fill in 20-30 seconds (normal)
     → rapid filling (abnormal)
- ❑ Interventions — Elastic stockings, Elevate legs
  Sclerotherapy, Vein ligation and stripping
- ❑ What is the purpose of Hyperbaric Oxygen Therapy? — Treats non-healing wounds by placing client in a chamber while inhaling 100% O_2

Hodgkin's Disease

- ❑ Description — Cancer of the lymphocytes
- ❑ Causes — Unknown, **Epstein-Barr virus infection**, immune disorder, immunosuppression
- ❑ Assessment — **Painless enlargement** of the cervical, axillary or inguinal lymph nodes, cachexia
- ❑ Diagnostic Test — **Reed-Sternberg** cells on microscopy
- ❑ Interventions — Radiation, Chemotherapy

Pernicious Anemia

- ❑ Description — Lack of Vitamin B_{12} or intrinsic factor
  → immature RBC's → macrocytic anemia
- ❑ Assessment — Weakness, paresthesia, amnesia, ataxia
- ❑ Why are neurologic symptoms present? — Vitamin B_{12} maintains the myelin sheath
- ❑ Diagnostic Test — Schilling Test
- ❑ Steps in Schilling Test
  1. Avoid Vitamin B_{12} injections days before the test
  2. NPO (except water) 8 hours before the test
  3. Give oral **radioactive** Vitamin B_{12} supplement followed by IM injection of **non-radioactive** Vitamin B_{12}
  4. Collect urine for **24** hours
  5. Measure radioactive B_{12} in urine
  6. Result: High percentage of B_{12} in the urine — Negative
  7. Result: Low percentage of B_{12} in the urine — Positive
  8. Intrinsic factor will be added when the test is repeated to verify the cause

- ❑ Interventions — Monthly Vitamin B_{12} injections
- ❑ What foods are high in Vitamin B_{12}? — Milk products, meat, poultry, eggs, shellfish

Aplastic Anemia

- ❑ Description — Bone marrow fails to produce RBC, WBC and platelets → anemia, infection, bleeding
- ❑ Causes — Pesticides, radiation, chemotherapy, chloramphenicol, autoimmune
- ❑ Assessment — Fatigue, dizziness, fever, bruising
- ❑ Interventions — Colony-stimulating factors; Immunosuppressants, Antibiotics

E. Cardiovascular System Drugs

1. Anticoagulants

- ❑ Description — Prevents clots from forming by blocking clotting factors in the coagulation pathway
- ❑ Side effects — Bleeding, **osteoporosis** (long-term heparin)
- ❑ Interventions — Monitor for hematuria and bruising

	HEPARIN	WARFARIN
Effect	Rapid effect in minutes	Delayed effect (onset: 24 hours; full effect: 3-5 days)
Route and site of administration	IV or SQ; 25-28 gauge; 5/8-inch needle; abdomen; 2 inches away from umbilicus	Oral
Dose	Units	Milligrams
Lab monitoring	Monitor aPTT or PTT	Monitor PT and INR
Effect on pregnancy	Not passed via placenta or breastmilk	Passed via placenta (**teratogenic**)
Antidote	Protamine sulfate	phytomenadione (Vitamin K, Mephyton)
Interventions	Avoid aspirin and NSAIDs	Avoid aspirin and NSAIDs Avoid dark green, leafy vegetables

> ***NCLEX Alert!*** *To determine the effectiveness of heparin and warfarin therapy, the goal is to achieve lab results (aPTT, PTT, PT) that are* ***1.5 to 2.5 times*** *the control value. Ensure that the values are not excessively prolonged. Also, heparin and warfarin may be given together because the effect of warfarin is delayed. This is important to remember in the NCLEX!*

- ❑ Other anticoagulants: enoxaparin (Lovenox), lepirudin (Refludan), fondaparinux (Arixtra), argatroban (Acova) bivalirudin (Angiomax), dalteparin (Fragmin), dabigatran (Pradaxa), desirudin (Iprivask), tinzaparin (Innohep)

2. Antiplatelet Drugs

- ❑ Description — Blocks platelet aggregation
  Used as prophylaxis for stroke and MI
- ❑ Drugs — Examples:
  - clopidogrel (Plavix)
  - ticlodipine (Ticlid)
  - dipyridamole (Persantin)
  - tirofiban (Aggrastat)
- ❑ Side effects — Bleeding, hematuria, bruising
- ❑ Interventions — Monitor for signs of bleeding

3. Thrombolytic Drugs

- ❑ Description — Dissolves existing clots
- ❑ Drugs — Examples:
  - streptokinase (Streptase)
  - tenecteplase (TNKase)
  - alteplase (tPA)
- ❑ Side effects — Bleeding, arrhythmias
- ❑ Interventions — Check aPTT, PT, platelet count
- ❑ What is the antidote for thrombolytic toxicity? — aminocaproic acid (Amicar)

4. Cardiac Glycosides

Positive Inotropic Effect	Increases force of contraction to increase cardiac output
Negative Chronotropic Effect	Slows the heart rate to reduce oxygen demand
Negative Dromotropic Effect	Slows the conduction through the AV node

- ❑ Drug — digoxin (Lanoxin)
- ❑ Side effects — Nausea, vomiting, diarrhea, loss of appetite, weakness, dizziness, headache, anxiety, depression, bradycardia, tachycardia, arrhythmia
- ❑ What is the normal serum digoxin level? — 0.5-2.0 ng/mL
- ❑ What are the dangers of **hypokalemia**, hypomagnesemia, and hypercalcemia? — Digoxin toxicity

❑ What are the signs of digoxin toxicity?	**Anorexia**, **nausea**, **vomiting**, **diarrhea**, yellow-green halo vision, arrhythmias, **bradycardia** or tachycardia, photophobia

> ***NCLEX Alert!*** *The initial signs and symptoms of digoxin toxicity are gastrointestinal symptoms!*

❑ Check the ______ for 1 full minute before administration	Apical pulse
❑ Hold and report if HR is:	
Adult: < _____ or > _____	60, 100
Infants/young children: < ______-______	70, 90
Older children: < _____	100
❑ What is the antidote for digoxin toxicity?	digoxin immune fab (Digibind)

5. Antihypertensive Drugs

Alpha-Adrenergic Blockers

❑ Description	Blocks $alpha_1$ receptors → vasodilation → decreased BP
❑ Drugs	Examples: ▪ doxazosin (Cardura) ▪ prazosin (Minipress) ▪ terazosin (Hytrin)
❑ Side effects	Orthostatic hypotension

Sympatholytics

❑ Description	Causes vasodilation → decreased BP
❑ Drugs	Examples: ▪ clonidine (Catapres) ▪ guanabenz (Wytensin) ▪ methylodopa (Aldomet)
❑ Side effects	Orthostatic hypotension

> ***NCLEX Alert!*** *REMEMBER THE COMMON SIDE EFFECTS OF ANTIHYPERTENSIVE DRUGS!*
> *orthostatic hypotension, dizziness, cough, dry mouth, nocturia, diarrhea, constipation, erectile problems, nervousness, fatigue, drowsiness, headache, nausea, unintentional weight loss or gain, skin rash*

Angiotensin-Converting Enzyme (ACE) Inhibitors and Angiotensin II Receptor Blockers (ARBs)

ACE INHIBITORS	ARBs
Blocks the conversion of angiotensin 1 to angiotensin 2 → vasodilation → ↓ BP	Blocks the action of angiotensin 2 → vasodilation and inhibited aldosterone release → ↓ BP
❑ enalapril (Vasotec) ❑ captopril (Capoten) ❑ benazepril (Lotensin)	❑ losartan (Cozaar) ❑ valsartan (Diovan) ❑ irbesartan (Avapro)

❑ Side effects

ACE inhibitors – **dry cough**
ARBs – decreased taste

❑ What are the side effects of both drugs?

Hypotension, **hyperkalemia** (due to decreased aldosterone)

Diuretics

THIAZIDE DIURETICS	LOOP DIURETICS	POTASSIUM-SPARING
Potassium- wasting	Potassium-wasting	Potassium-sparing
Drugs ❑ hydrochlorothiazide (Diuril) ❑ hydroflumethiazide (Saluron) ❑ metolazone (Zaroxolyn)	Drugs ❑ furosemide (Lasix) ❑ bumetanide (Bumex) ❑ ethacrynic acid (Edecrin)	Drugs ❑ amiloride (Midamor) ❑ spironolactone (Aldactone) ❑ triamterene (Dyrenium) ❑ aldosterone-receptor blocker - eplerenone (Inspra)
Side effects ❑ **Hypokalemia** ❑ **Hyponatremia** ❑ Hypercalcemia ❑ Hyperuricemia ❑ Hyperglycemia	Side effects ❑ **Hypokalemia** ❑ **Hyponatremia** ❑ Hypocalcemia ❑ Hyperuricemia ❑ Hypomagnesemia	Side effects ❑ **Hyperkalemia** ❑ **Hyponatremia** ❑ Nausea ❑ Diarrhea
Interventions ❑ Take the drug in the morning to prevent nocturia and disruption in sleep. ❑ Eat foods high in potassium (potassium-wasting diuretics). ❑ Avoid potassium-rich foods (potassium-sparing diuretics). ❑ Monitor for postural hypotension. ❑ Change positions slowly. ❑ Avoid hot showers or excessive heat exposure.		

Beta-Adrenergic Blockers

- ❑ Description — Decreases the heart rate and BP
  Treats angina, arrhythmias and migraine
- ❑ Drugs

NON-CARDIOSELECTIVE AGENTS	CARDIOSELECTIVE AGENTS
Blocks both $beta_1$ and $beta_2$ cell receptors → **bradycardia** and **bronchospasm**	Blocks $beta_1$ cell receptors only → **bradycardia** only
❑ nadolol (Corgard) ❑ propanolol (Inderal) ❑ labetalol (Normodyne)	❑ acebutolol (Sectral) ❑ atenolol (Tenormin) ❑ metoprolol (Lopressor)

- ❑ Contraindications — **COPD**, **asthma**, bradycardia, diabetes
- ❑ Side effects — **Bradycardia, bronchospasm**
  hypotension, hyperglycemia,
  agranulocytosis, depression
- ❑ Interventions — Hold the drug if pulse rate is <60
  Monitor for respiratory distress

Calcium-Channel Blockers

- ❑ Description — Decreases the contractility of the heart
  → slows the HR → ↓ BP

  Causes vasodilation of the coronary
  artery and peripheral blood vessels → ↓ BP

  Treats angina, dysrhythmia or hypertension
- ❑ Drugs — Examples:
  - nifedipine (Adalat)
  - amlodipine (Norvasc)
  - verapamil (Calan)
  - felopidine (Plendil)
  - diltiazem (Cardizem)
- ❑ Side effects — **Bradycardia**, hypotension, edema
- ❑ Interventions — Monitor BP, Monitor for heart block

6. Drugs for Angina Pectoris

Nitrates

- ❑ Description — Causes vasodilation → increased O_2
- ❑ Drugs — Examples
  - isosorbide dinitrate (Isordil)
  - nitroglycerin, sublingual (Nitrostat)
  - nitroglycerin, transdermal (Minitran)
  - nitroglycerin, transmucosal (Nitrogard)
  - nitroglycerin ointment (Nitro-Bid)
  - IV nitroglycerin (Nitro-Bid IV)
- ❑ Side effects — **Headache**, orthostatic hypotension, dizziness, nausea, **flushing**, **tachycardia**
- ❑ Interventions — Change positions slowly, Monitor BP

SUBLINGUAL MEDICATIONS	TRANSDERMAL PATCH	TOPICAL OINTMENTS
❑ Give 1 tablet for chest pain, repeat every 5 minutes, for a total of 3 doses; call HCP if unrelieved ❑ Stinging sensation is expected; indicates potency ❑ Store in a dark, tightly closed bottle	❑ Apply to hairless area ❑ Rotate the sites ❑ Remove patch after 12-14 hours to prevent drug tolerance	❑ Spread ointment on chest, upper arm, abdomen, back, or thigh ❑ Rotate the sites ❑ Avoid touching the ointment to prevent self-absorption

7. Peripheral Vasodilators

- ❑ Description — Promotes circulation to the extremities; Treats Raynaud's disease
- ❑ Drugs — Examples:
  - pentoxifylline (Trental)
  - terazosin (Hytrin)
  - prazosin (Minipress)
- ❑ Side effects — Orthostatic hypotension
- ❑ Interventions — Monitor BP, Change positions slowly

8. Brain Natriuretic Peptide

- ❑ Description — Synthetic BNP that promotes diuresis and vasodilation in heart failure → ↓ BP
- ❑ Drugs — Example:
  - nesiritide (Natrecor)
- ❑ Side effects — Hypotension
- ❑ Interventions — Monitor BP, Drug will affect BNP levels

9. Drugs for Hyperlipidemia

HMG-CoA Reductase Inhibitors

- ❑ Description — Decreases low density lipoprotein levels
- ❑ Contraindications — Liver disease
- ❑ Drugs — Examples:
  - pravastatin (Pravachol)
  - lovastatin (Mevacor)
  - simvastatin (Zocor)
  - fluvastatin (Lescol)
  - atorvastatin (Lipitor)
- ❑ Side effects — **Muscle cramps, hepatoxicity**
  nausea, constipation
- ❑ Interventions — Monitor liver enzyme levels
  Monitor creatine kinase level
  Avoid alcohol and pregnancy
  Annual eye exam
  Report muscle pain → rhabdomyolosis

Bile Acid Sequestrants

- ❑ Description — Binds with intestinal acids
  → blocks reabsorption of lipids
- ❑ Drugs — Examples:
  - colesevalam (WelChol)
  - cholestyramine (Questran)
  - colestipol (Colestid)
- ❑ Side effects — Constipation, heartburn
- ❑ Interventions — Monitor for peptic ulcer disease

Other Drugs for Hyperlipidemia

- ❑ Drugs — Examples:
  - ezetimibe (Zetia)
  - nicotinic acid (Niacin)
  - gemfibrozil (Lopid)
  - ezetimibe/simvastatin (Vytorin)
- ❑ Contraindications — Liver and kidney disease
- ❑ Side effects — Mild stomach pain, nausea, vomiting, constipation, diarrhea, joint pain
- ❑ Interventions — Monitor liver and kidney function
  Report muscle pain → rhabdomyolosis

10. Drugs for Dysrhythmias

DRUGS	USES	SIDE EFFECTS	INTERVENTIONS
CLASS I (A, B, C) **(Na^+ channel blockers)** ❑ quinidine (Quinaglute) ❑ disopyramide (Norpace) ❑ lidocaine HCl (Xylocaine) ❑ procainamide (Pronestyl) ❑ phenytoin sodium (Dilantin)	❑ Atrial fibrillation ❑ Ventricular arrhythmias	❑ Hypotension ❑ Diarrhea ❑ Bradycardia ❑ Dizziness	❑ Monitor HR and ECG ❑ Assess for dizziness, drowsiness and altered mental status ❑ Monitor for digoxin toxicity
Class II (Beta-blockers) ❑ propranolol (Inderal) ❑ adenosine (Adenocard)	❑ Ventricular dysrhythmias	❑ Bradycardia ❑ Hypotension ❑ Bronchospasm	❑ Check HR before administration ❑ Contraindicated in COPD and asthma
Class III (K+ channel blockers) ❑ sotalol (Betapace) ❑ amiodarone HCl (Cordarone) ❑ ibutilide (Convert) ❑ bretylium tosylate (Bretylium)	❑ Ventricular dysrhythmias	❑ Hypo/hypertension ❑ Arrhythmias ❑ **Photophobia** (amiodarone)	❑ Assess vital signs and ECG
Class IV (Ca+ channel blockers) ❑ verapamil HCl (Calan, Isoptin)	❑ Supraventricular dysrhythmias	❑ Bradycardia ❑ Hypotension	❑ Check HR and BP before administration ❑ Monitor for postural hypotension
MISCELLANEOUS ANTIDYSRHYTHMIC AGENTS			
❑ epinephrine (Adrenaline)	❑ Asystole	❑ Hypertension ❑ Tachycardia	❑ Assess HR, BP and ECG
❑ atropine sulfate	❑ Bradycardia	❑ Dry mouth ❑ Constipation ❑ Urinary retention	❑ Assess HR and BP ❑ Contraindicated in glaucoma
❑ digoxin (Lanoxin) ❑ digitoxin (Crystodigin)	❑ Atrial fibrillation ❑ Supraventricular dysrhythmias	❑ Bradycardia ❑ Anorexia, diarrhea, nausea, vomiting	❑ Check HR before administration ❑ Monitor K^+ levels

NCLEX Alert! *You need to know the side effects of antidysrhythmic drugs. Most of them will cause hypotension and bradycardia!*

Endocrine System

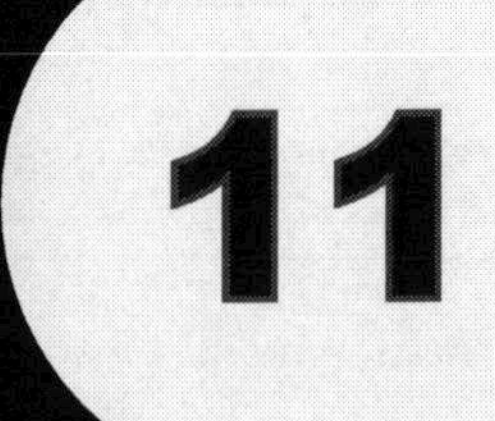

A. The Endocrine System

GLANDS	HORMONES	FUNCTIONS
Pituitary Gland	POSTERIOR PITUITARY GLAND ▪ Antidiuretic Hormone (ADH), Oxytocin ANTERIOR PITUITARY GLAND ▪ Somatotropin (Growth Hormone), Prolactin, Thyroid-Stimulating Hormone, (TSH), Adrenocorticotropic Hormone (ACTH), Follicle-Stimulating Hormone (FSH), Luteinizing Hormone (LH)	ADH: Reabsorbs water Oxytocin: Stimulates uterine contraction Somatotropin: Stimulates bone growth Prolactin: Stimulates milk production ACTH: Stimulates the adrenal cortex TSH: Stimulates the thyroid gland FSH: Stimulates development of ovum LH: Stimulates ovulation
Pineal Gland	Melatonin	Regulates sleep pattern
Thyroid Gland	Tetraiodothyronine (T_4), Triiodothyronine (T_3)	Regulates rate of body metabolism
	Calcitonin	Decreases calcium in the blood
Parathyroid Glands	Parathormone	Increases calcium in the blood
Adrenal Glands	CORTEX ▪ Glucocorticoids (cortisol) ▪ Mineralocorticoids (aldosterone) ▪ Androgens MEDULLA Epinephrine and Norepinephrine (also known as catecholamines)	 Increases blood glucose Maintains blood pressure Fights stress and inflammation Regulates Na^+, water and K^+ excretion Develops secondary sex characteristics Fights stress; Fight-or-flight response
Pancreas	Alpha cells: Glucagon Beta cells: Insulin	Increases blood glucose Decreases blood glucose
Ovaries	Estrogen, Progesterone	Develops female sex organs
Testes	Androgens (Testosterone)	Develops and maintains male sex organs

B. Endocrine System Disorders

Anterior Pituitary Disorders

ACROMEGALY (HYPERPITUITARISM)	SIMMOND'S DISEASE (PANHYPOPITUITARISM)
Increased production of growth hormone (GH)	Decreased production of anterior pituitary hormones
Causes ❑ Benign tumor (adenoma) of the pituitary gland	Causes ❑ Benign tumor of the pituitary gland, pituitary gland damage due to radiation or surgery
Assessment ❑ Huge lower jaw ❑ Thick lips and tongue ❑ Oversized hands and feet ❑ Painful and stiff joints ❑ Deepened voice ❑ Muscle weakness	Assessment ❑ Decreased thyroid and adrenal hormone levels ❑ Gonadal atrophy ❑ Hypoglycemia ❑ Adrenal insufficiency ❑ Weight loss ❑ Premature aging
Diagnostic Tests ❑ GLUCOSE TOLERANCE TEST → increased GH production → positive → decreased GH production → negative	Diagnostic Tests ❑ Decreased serum thyroid, steroids and reproductive hormone levels
Interventions ❑ Radiation therapy ❑ Hypophysectomy (removal of pituitary gland) ❑ Bromocriptine mesylate (Parlodel) → decreases GH production ❑ Physical changes **cannot** be reversed	Interventions ❑ Hormone replacements for life ❑ Comply with medication schedules ❑ Regular blood hormone level check-up ❑ Teach client disease is fatal if left untreated

Posterior Pituitary Disorders

SYNDROME OF INAPPROPRIATE ANTIDIURETIC HORMONE (SIADH)	DIABETES INSIPIDUS
Increased ADH → increased reabsorption of water → oliguria → **water retention**	Decreased ADH → decreased reabsorption of water → polyuria → **dehydration**
Causes ❑ head injury, stroke, vasopressin drug overdose	Causes ❑ head injury, brain tumors, hypophysectomy

SYNDROME OF INAPPROPRIATE ANTIDIURETIC HORMONE (SIADH)	DIABETES INSIPIDUS
Assessment ❑ Decreased urine output ❑ Concentrated urine ❑ Water retention ❑ Weight gain ❑ Cerebral edema	Assessment ❑ Increased urine output ❑ Colorless, diluted urine ❑ Dehydration ❑ Weight loss ❑ Thirst
Diagnostic Tests ❑ Decreased serum sodium level (dilutional hyponatremia) ❑ Increased specific gravity of urine	Diagnostic Tests ❑ FLUID DEPRIVATION TEST 1. Hold fluid intake for 12 hours 2. Measure the specific gravity of urine 3. Diluted urine → positive ❑ Decreased specific gravity of urine
Interventions ❑ Osmotic diuretics - mannitol (Osmitrol) ❑ Loop diuretics - furosemide (Lasix) ❑ IV 3% hypertonic NaCl solution ❑ Measure weight ❑ Monitor for pulmonary edema and heart failure	Interventions ❑ Desmopressin (DDAVP) nasal solution ❑ Lypressin (Diapid) nasal spray ❑ Monitor intake and output ❑ Measure weight ❑ Monitor for dehydration

Thyroid Disorders

HYPERTHYROIDISM (Grave's Disease, Basedow's Disease)		HYPOTHYROIDISM	
Increased T_3 and T_4 → increased metabolic rate		Decreased T_3 and T_4 → decreased metabolic rate	
Causes: Thyroid or pituitary tumor, increased TSH		Causes: Thyroid or pituitary tumor, decreased TSH	
Assessment ❑ Restlessness ❑ Intolerance to heat ❑ Increased appetite ❑ Weight loss ❑ Diarrhea ❑ Tachycardia ❑ Amenorrhea	❑ Fine hand tremors ❑ Fine hair ❑ Flushed, warm skin ❑ Goiter ❑ Exophthalmos ❑ THYROID STORM ▪ Fever ▪ Tachycardia ▪ Arrhythmias	Assessment ❑ Lethargy ❑ Intolerance to cold ❑ Anorexia ❑ Weight gain ❑ Constipation ❑ Bradycardia ❑ Forgetfulness ❑ Menorrhagia	❑ Coarse sparse hair ❑ Thick nails, dry skin ❑ Masklike face ❑ Large tongue ❑ Low-pitched voice ❑ MYXEDEMA COMA ▪ Hypothermia ▪ Hypotension ▪ Hypoventilation

HYPERTHYROIDISM (Grave's Disease, Basedow's Disease)	HYPOTHYROIDISM
Diagnostic Tests ❑ Increased Protein-Bound Iodine (PBI) and serum T_3 and T_4 levels ❑ Decreased TSH level ❑ Increased radioactive iodine (RAI) uptake	Diagnostic Tests ❑ Decreased Protein-Bound Iodine (PBI) and serum T_3 and T_4 levels ❑ Increased TSH level ❑ Decreased radioactive iodine (RAI) uptake
Interventions ❑ Antithyroid drugs ▪ propylthiouracil (PTU) ▪ methimazole (Tapazole) ❑ Lugol's solution - decreases the synthesis of thyroid hormones ❑ Radioactive iodine (I-131) - destroys the thyroid gland ❑ Subtotal thyroidectomy, total thyroidectomy ❑ High calorie, high protein diet ❑ Monitor pulse rate and BP	Interventions ❑ Lifetime thyroid hormone replacement therapy ▪ levothyroxine (Synthroid) ▪ liothyronine (Cytomel) ❑ Weight loss program ❑ High fiber, low cholesterol, low fat diet ❑ Provide warmth ❑ Monitor for constipation

Thyrotoxic Crisis (Thyroid Storm)

❑ Description

Sudden, excessive production of T_3 and T_4
→ increased metabolism
→ life-threatening hyperthyroidism

❑ Causes

Stress, infection, overmanipulation of the thyroid gland during assessment or surgery

❑ Assessment

High fever, tachycardia, dysrhythmias, restlessness, delirium, convulsions

❑ Interventions

IV steroid, IV sodium iodide
Antipyretics, IV fluid replacement, propranolol (Inderal) to decrease the HR

❑ How can this condition be prevented?

Give Lugol's solution or saturated solution of potassium iodide (SSKI) before thyroidectomy to ensure a euthyroid state, decrease the vascularity of the thyroid gland and inhibit hormone release.

Thyroidectomy

- ❑ What are the complications of this surgery?

  Hemorrhage, respiratory distress, accidental removal of parathyroid gland, laryngeal nerve damage, thyroid storm

- ❑ Interventions

  Semi-Fowler's or Fowler's position
  Ice pack to the neck to reduce swelling
  Support head during position change
  Report severe voice hoarseness
  Avoid hyperextension/flexion of the neck

- ❑ What are the signs of accidental removal of the parathyroid gland (hypocalcemic crisis)?

  Spasms of the fingers and toes, positive Chvostek's and Trousseau's signs

> ***NCLEX Alert!*** *Check the back of the neck for bleeding after thyroidectomy.*

Parathyroid Disorders

HYPERPARATHYROIDISM	HYPOPARATHYROIDISM
Increased parathyroid hormone production → ↑ CALCIUM, ↓ PHOSPHORUS	Decreased parathyroid hormone production → ↓ CALCIUM, ↑ PHOSPHORUS
Causes: Parathyroid tumor, severe vitamin D and calcium deficiency, chronic renal failure	Causes: Accidental removal of the parathyroid gland, autoimmune disease
Assessment ❑ **Muscle weakness** ❑ Fatigue ❑ Constipation ❑ Bone pain (due to bone demineralization) ❑ Renal stones ❑ Spontaneous fractures	Assessment ❑ **Muscle tetany** ❑ Numbness and tingling on toes, fingers and lips ❑ Laryngeal spasm ❑ **Chvostek's sign** ▪ Tap the facial nerve → the mouth jerks and jaw tightens ❑ **Trousseau's sign** ▪ Place a BP cuff and inflate between SBP and DBP and wait 3 minutes → spasm of hand flexing inward
Diagnostic Tests ❑ ↑ calcium = ↓ phosphorus in the blood	Diagnostic Tests ❑ ↓ calcium = ↑ phosphorus in the blood

Interventions ❑ Low calcium, high phosphorus diet ❑ Vitamin D supplements ❑ Increase fluid intake to prevent calculi ❑ Surgical removal of the parathyroid gland	Interventions ❑ IV calcium gluconate ❑ Endotracheal tube insertion ❑ Oral calcium supplements ❑ High calcium, low phosphorus diet ❑ Avoid carbonated drinks (high in phosphorus)

Adrenal Disorders

CUSHING'S SYNDROME	ADDISON'S DISEASE
Increased production of adrenal hormones	Decreased production of adrenal hormones
Causes: Pituitary adenoma, increased ACTH, prolonged use of high doses of steroids	Causes: Autoimmune destruction of the adrenal glands, decreased ACTH
Assessment ❑ ↑SODIUM, ↓POTASSIUM ❑ Hyperglycemia, hypertension ❑ Truncal obesity, buffalo hump ❑ Moon-face, masculinization ❑ Thin extremities, abdominal striae ❑ Delayed wound healing ❑ Hirsutism, amenorrhea, mood swings ❑ Muscle wasting, osteoporosis	Assessment ❑ ↑POTASSIUM, ↓SODIUM ❑ Hypoglycemia ❑ Hypotension ❑ Fatigue ❑ Weight loss ❑ Anorexia ❑ Bronze, dark skin pigmentation ❑ Depression
Diagnostic Tests ❑ DEXAMETHASONE SUPPRESSION TEST ▪ Administration of steroids → steroids remain increased → positive ❑ Increased plasma and urine cortisol levels	Diagnostic Tests ❑ ACTH STIMULATION TEST ▪ Stimulation of adrenal gland → low adrenal response → positive ❑ Decreased plasma and urine cortisol levels
Interventions ❑ Low sodium, high potassium diet ❑ Low calorie, low carbohydrate diet ❑ Diuretics ❑ Monitor blood sugar ❑ Taper steroid use after prolonged use ❑ Meticulous skin care for fragile skin ❑ Monitor for masked signs infection ❑ Bilateral adrenalectomy	Interventions ❑ High sodium, low potassium diet ❑ High protein, moderate carbohydrate diet ❑ fludrocortisone (Florinef) ❑ Adjust steroid dose during stressful events ❑ Report sore throat and fever ❑ Provide rest periods ❑ Do not give insulin

NCLEX Alert! *The symptoms of Cushing's syndrome are reversible with treatment.*

Acute Adrenal Crisis (Addisonian Crisis)

- ❑ Description — Sudden, fatal deficiency of steroids
- ❑ Causes — Stress, infection, sudden steroid withdrawal
- ❑ Assessment — **Hypotension**, severe weakness, nausea, vomiting, headache, shock
- ❑ Interventions — IV steroids, IV D_5 0.9% sodium chloride; Provide warmth, Glucose replacement, ATB

Pheochromocytoma

- ❑ Description — Benign tumor of the adrenal medulla → release of catecholamines → ↑ BP
- ❑ Assessment — Remember 5 P's!
  - P - ressure (hypertension)
  - P - alpitations
  - P - erspiration (diaphoresis)
  - P - allor
  - P - ain (headache)
- ❑ Diagnostic Test — Increased vanillylmandeleic acid (VMA) (metabolite of catecholamine)
- ❑ What is a positive (phentolamine) Regitine Test? — Drop in BP after injection of Regitine
- ❑ Interventions — Antihypertensive drugs, phentolamine, metyrosine (Demser), adrenalectomy
- ❑ What is the action of metyrosine (Demser)? — Decreases the secretion of catecholamines

Hyperaldosteronism (Conn's Syndrome)

- ❑ Description — Increased production of aldosterone → increased sodium and water retention → fluid and electrolyte imbalance
- ❑ Causes — Gland tumor, heart failure, liver cirrhosis
- ❑ Assessment — Decreased potassium, increased sodium, hypertension, headache, weakness
- ❑ Interventions — Antihypertensives, Low sodium diet, Monitor for edema, Adrenalectomy
- ❑ Why is spironolactone (Aldactone) prescribed? — It is a potassium-sparing diuretic that blocks the action of aldosterone

C. Diabetes Mellitus

TYPE 1 (INSULIN-DEPENDENT)	TYPE 2 (NON-INSULIN-DEPENDENT)
Absence of insulin production	Lack of insulin or insulin resistance
❑ Childhood condition ❑ Autoimmune-related disease ❑ At risk for Diabetic Ketoacidosis (DKA)	❑ Related to aging, genetics, **obesity** ❑ At risk for Hyperosmolar, Hyperglycemic, Non-Ketotic (HHNK) Syndrome

Pathophysiology

- ❑ Absence of insulin, lack of insulin, insulin resistance → increased glucose in the blood (hyperglycemia) → increased osmotic pressure in the blood → glycosuria → polyuria → polydipsia
- ❑ Lack of glucose in cells → polyphagia → breakdown of fats and proteins (gluconeogenesis) → weight loss → production of ketones → ketoacidosis

❑ Assessment
3 P's (P-olydipsia, P-olyphagia, P-olyuria)
weight loss, vaginal infections

❑ What is pre-diabetes?
Blood glucose levels that are higher than normal but not yet diagnosed

❑ HgbA1c results
Normal: < 5.7%
Prediabetes: 5.7% to 6.4%
Diabetes: 6.5% or higher

❑ Fasting Blood Glucose (FBG) results
Normal: < than 100 mg/dL
Prediabetes: 100 mg/dL to 125 mg/dL
Diabetes: 126 mg/dL or higher

❑ Oral Glucose Tolerance Test (also called the OGTT)
Normal: < than 140 mg/dL
Prediabetes: 140 mg/dL to 199 mg/dL
Diabetes: 200 mg/dL or higher

❑ Random (also called Casual) Plasma Glucose Test
Diabetes: 200 mg/dL of higher

❑ Interventions
Diet, Weight loss, Exercise,
Insulin, Oral antidiabetic agents

NCLEX Alert! *Metabolic syndrome (Syndrome X) is a condition characterized by having a combination of risk factors such as hypertension, hyperglycemia, hyperlipidemia and large waist circumference. This condition increases the risk of a client in developing diabetes mellitus, heart disease and stroke.*

Complications of Diabetes Mellitus

DIABETIC KETOACIDOSIS (DKA)	HYPEROSMOLAR, HYPERGLYCEMIC NON-KETOTIC SYNDROME (HHNK)
Hyperglycemia with metabolic acidosis and ketosis	Hyperglycemia **without** ketosis
Causes: infection, starvation, uncontrolled DM	Causes: uncontrolled or undiagnosed DM, TPN
Assessment ❑ Very high blood glucose (>300-1000 mg/dL) ❑ Drowsiness ❑ Severe thirst ❑ Dehydration ❑ Fever ❑ Fruity-scented (acetone) breath ❑ Kussmaul breathing (to blow off excess acids) ❑ Diagnostic Tests: glucose and ketones in urine, low pH, decreased HCO_3 (metabolic acidosis)	Assessment ❑ Very high blood glucose (>600-1000 mg/dL) ❑ Drowsiness ❑ Severe thirst ❑ Dehydration ❑ Diagnostic Test: Normal pH
Interventions ❑ IV Regular insulin, IV 0.9% NaCl, K^+ replacement	Interventions ❑ IV Regular insulin, IV 0.9% NaCl, K^+ replacement

Hypoglycemia

- ❑ Causes — Exercise, alcohol intake, overdose of insulin, anorexia, oral hypoglycemic agents

- ❑ Assessment — Weakness, nausea, tremors, headache, sweating, confusion, irritability, seizures

- ❑ Interventions — Give 15 grams of simple carbohydrates
  Examples:
  - glucose tablets or gel tube
  - 2 tablespoons of raisins, hard candies
  - orange juice or regular soda (not diet)
  - 1 tbsp sugar, honey or corn syrup
  - 8 ounces of nonfat or 1% milk

  If unconscious → Inject glucagon
  Give $D_{50\%}$ glucose IV

- ❑ What should be given after the hypoglycemic episode? — Give complex carbohydrates to maintain the blood glucose level
  (e.g. milk, potatoes, graham crackers,)

- ❑ How can hypoglycemic episodes be prevented? — Serve meals after giving insulin
  Eat snacks before intense activity

Hyperglycemia versus Hypoglycemia

HYPERGLYCEMIA	HYPOGLYCEMIA
Slow onset	Sudden onset
Hot, flushed, dry skin	Pale, cool, clammy skin
Drowsy	Confused
Hunger	Extreme thirst
Vomiting	Vomiting

NCLEX Alert! *A sign of nocturnal hypoglycemia is cold, clammy skin and diaphoresis.*

Peripheral Neuropathy

- ❑ Assessment — Pain, paresthesia, voiding problem, slow GI movement (gastroparesis)
- ❑ Interventions — Diet, Exercise, Non-narcotic analgesics
- ❑ What antidepressant is given to manage pain? — imipramine (Tofranil)
- ❑ What anticonvulsants are given? — gabapentin (Neurontin)
  carbamazepine (Tegretol)
- ❑ What instructions about foot care are important to teach? — Wash feet in warm water
  Cut nails **straight** across
  Apply moisturizer to feet
  Insert lamb's wool between toes

Diabetic Nephropathy

- ❑ Assessment — Worsening hypertension, edema, albuminuria, oliguria
- ❑ Interventions — Control blood glucose
  Maintain BP, ACE inhibitors

Diabetic Retinopathy

- ❑ Assessment — Blurred vision, blindness, floating spots
- ❑ Interventions — ACE inhibitors to dilate retinal vessels

D. Endocrine System Drugs

1. Parathyroid Drugs

VITAMIN D SUPPLEMENTS	BIPHOSPHONATES AND CALCIUM REGULATING DRUGS	ORAL CALCIUM SUPPLEMENTS
Drugs ❑ ergocalciferol (Vitamin D_2) ❑ cholecalciferol (Vitamin D_3)	Drugs ❑ alendronate (Fosamax) ❑ calcitonin salmon (Calcimar) ❑ zoledronate (Reclast) ❑ risedronate sodium (Actonel) ❑ ibandronate (Boniva) ❑ etidronate disodium (Didronel)	Drugs ❑ calcium carbonate (Tums) ❑ calcium acetate (PhosLo)
Side effects ❑ Hypervitaminosis D	Side effects ❑ Stomach pain, constipation, diarrhea, flatulence, nausea	Side effects ❑ Gastric upset

2. Drugs for Hyperparathyroidism and Hypercalcemia

- ❑ Drugs — Examples:
  - gallium nitrate (Ganite)
  - cinacalcet hydrochloride (Sensipar)
  - paricalcitol (Zemplar)
  - doxercalciferol (Hectorol)
- ❑ Side effects — Nausea, vomiting, diarrhea
- ❑ Interventions — Avoid foods rich in calcium
- ❑ What is the function of vitamin D? — Enhances absorption of calcium in the GI
- ❑ What is the function of calcitonin? — Decreases serum calcium and inhibits bone breakdown (resorption)

3. Drugs for Pituitary Disorders

Growth Hormones

- ❑ Description — Treats deficiency of growth hormones
- ❑ Drugs — Examples:
  - mecasermin (Increlex)
  - somatropin (Humatrope)
- ❑ Side effects — Headache, vomiting, fatigue, muscle pain

Growth Hormone Receptor Antagonist

- ❑ Description — Treats acromegaly
- ❑ Drugs — Examples:
  - pegvisomant (Somavert)
  - octreotide (Sandostatin)
- ❑ Side effects — Diarrhea, nausea, blurred vision

Antidiuretic Hormones

- ❑ Description — Treats diabetes insipidus
- ❑ Drugs — Examples:
  - vasopressin (Pitressin)
  - desmopressin acetate (DDAVP)
- ❑ Side effects — **Water intoxication**, hypertension
- ❑ Interventions — Monitor weight, intake and output

4. Drugs for Thyroid Disorders

DRUGS FOR HYPOTHYROIDISM	DRUGS FOR HYPERTHYROIDISM
Drugs ❑ levothyroxine sodium (Synthroid) ❑ liothyronine sodium (Cytomel) ❑ liotrix (Thyrolar)	Drugs ❑ propylthiouracil (PTU) ❑ methimazole (Tapazole) ❑ potassium iodide ❑ iodine solution (Lugol's solution) ❑ Iodine 131
Side effects ❑ Signs of **hyperthyroidism**	Side Effects ❑ Signs of **hypothyroidism**
Interventions ❑ Monitor T_3, T_4 and TSH levels ❑ Take drug in morning on an empty stomach ❑ Monitor pulse rate	Interventions ❑ Monitor T_3, T_4 and TSH levels ❑ Monitor weight ❑ Take with meals

- ❑ What foods block thyroid gland function? — Cruciferous vegetables, cauliflower, cabbage, turnips, strawberries, peaches, pears, spinach, kale, brussels sprouts, radish, peas

> ***NCLEX Alert!*** *PTU causes agranulocytosis. Monitor for fever and sore throat. Check the CBC with differential for neutropenia.*

5. Mineralocorticoids

❑ Description	Replaces hormones in Addison's disease
❑ Drugs	Example: fludrocortisone acetate (Florinef)
❑ Side effects	Signs of Cushing's syndrome, **GI bleeding**
❑ Interventions	Take drugs with foods or milk High potassium diet

6. Glucocorticoids

❑ Description	Fights inflammation, Treats allergy Helps cope with stress
❑ Drugs	Examples: ▪ dexamethasone ▪ prednisone ▪ hydrocortisone
❑ Side effects	Cushing's syndrome ▪ hypernatremia ▪ hypokalemia ▪ hyperglycemia ▪ osteoporosis ▪ weight gain ▪ mood swings ▪ cataracts ▪ acne
❑ Interventions	Monitor blood sugar High potassium diet Monitor for GI bleeding Take drug in the morning

7. Androgens

❑ Description	Replaces androgen hormones and treats certain types of breast cancers Risk for prostate cancer
❑ Drugs	Examples: ▪ methyltestosterone (Testred)
❑ Side effects	Masculinization, priapism, acne, menstrual irregularities, changes in libido
❑ Interventions	Take with foods or snacks

> ***NCLEX Alert!*** *Steroid drugs should not be stopped abruptly. It takes a while for the adrenal gland to produce its own steroids after it is shut down from prolonged steroid use. The dose must be tapered to prevent a fatal adrenal crisis!*

8. Estrogens and Progestins

❑ Description	Estrogen develops reproductive organs Progestin stimulates the endometrium Estrogen-progestin hormones are used for contraception and hormonal cancer
❑ Drugs	Examples of estrogens: ▪ estrogens (Premarin) Examples of progestins: ▪ medroxyprogesterone acetate (Depo-Provera) ▪ megestrol acetate (Megace)
❑ Side effects	**Hypertension** **Stroke** Mastalgia Menstrual changes Depression Thrombosis and migraine (estrogen)
❑ Interventions	Avoid smoking Monitor for swelling and weight gain

> ***NCLEX Alert!*** *Estrogens are contraindicated in clients with a history of thrombosis, breast and uterine cancer and are pregnant and breastfeeding. Progestins are contraindicated in clients with breast cancer and a history of thrombosis.*

9. Contraceptives

❑ Description	Prevents ovulation by combining estrogen and progestin hormones Comes in a 21 or 28-day packs
❑ Take for straight ___ days then pause for ____ days	21 (active pills), 7 (placebo)

- Contraindications — History of thrombosis and stroke, pregnancy, estrogen-dependent cancer
- Side effects — **Breakthrough bleeding**, headache
- Interventions — Full effect takes 7 days
  Sex should be resumed 2 months after cessation of pills

10. Drugs for Erectile Dysfunction

- Description — Treats erectile dysfunction by increasing blood flow to the penis
- Drugs — Examples:
  - vardenafil (Levitra)
  - sildenafil (Viagra)
  - taladafil (Cialis)
  - alprostadil (Caverject) injection
- Side effects — **Dizziness**, headache, flushing, photophobia
- Interventions — Monitor BP, Change positions slowly,
  Do not take more than once a day
  Report severe, prolonged priapism
  Avoid alcohol to prevent hypotension

> ***NCLEX Alert!*** *Clients taking nitrates or beta-blockers should avoid taking phosphodiesterase type-5 (PDE_5) inhibitor drugs (vardenafil, sildenafil, vardenafil) to prevent severe hypotension!*

11. Drugs for Infertility

- Description — Stimulates ovulation and pregnancy
- Drugs — Examples:
  - clomiphene citrate (Clomid)
- Contraindications — Pregnancy, liver disease, abnormal uterine bleeding, ovarian and adrenal diseases
- Side effects — **Multiple gestation**, vaginal bleeding

E. Drugs for Diabetes Mellitus

1. Insulin

INSULIN	NAMES	ONSET	PEAK	DURATION	IMPLICATIONS
Rapid-Acting (Clear)	insulin aspart (NovoLog) insulin glulisine (Apidra) insulin lispro (Humalog)	15 mins.	30-90 mins.	3-5 hours	▪ Given immediately before meals ▪ Given SQ or IV ▪ *May mix with NPH insulin*
Short-Acting (Clear)	insulin regular (Humulin R, Novolin R)	30-60 mins.	2-4 hours	5-8 hours	▪ Given 30 minutes before meals ▪ Given SQ or IV ▪ *May mix with NPH insulin*
Intermediate-Acting (Cloudy)	insulin NPH human (Humulin N, Novolin N)	1-3 hours	8 hours	12-16 hours	▪ Lowers blood glucose elevations when RA insulins stop working ▪ Given SQ ▪ *May mix with RA or SA insulin*
Long-Acting (Clear)	insulin glargine (Lantus, Toujeo) insulin detemir (Levemir)	1 hour	Lantus No peak Levemir 6-8 hours	20-24 hours	▪ Lowers blood glucose levels when RA insulins stop working ▪ Usually taken once daily ▪ Given SQ ▪ ***Do not mix with other insulins!***
Mixed Insulins (Cloudy)	Humulin 70/30 Novolin 70/30 Relion 70/30	30 mins.	2-12 hours	24 hours	▪ Usually taken once daily ▪ Given SQ ▪ ***Do not mix with other insulins!***

NCLEX Alert! *You should know the peak times of insulin medications. It is the period when clients are most likely to develop a hypoglycemic or insulin reaction!*

❑ Why is insulin not given orally?	It is destroyed by gastric secretions
❑ What are the sites for insulin injection?	Abdomen (preferred), posterior arm, anterior thigh, and hips
❑ Why do you rotate injection sites?	To prevent lipodystrophy that will result into erratic insulin absorption
❑ What is the needle gauge for insulin injection?	Gauge 27-29 needle, ½ inch
❑ Why do you roll the insulin vial between the palms before preparation?	It properly dissolves the insulin solution and restores appearance
❑ Can you shake insulin vials?	No, the bubbles will expand insulin volume
❑ What is important before drawing insulin?	Inject air to both vials (**cloudy** first then **clear**)
❑ How do you draw insulin?	Draw insulin from **clear** vial first then **cloudy** to maintain the purity and clarity of the clear solution
❑ What insulins are not compatible for mixing with other types of insulin (even though they are clear)?	glargine (Lantus), Insulin detemir (Levemir)
❑ How is insulin injected?	Give subcutaneously at 45-90 degree angle; 45-60 degrees in thin clients
❑ Is aspiration needed?	No
❑ Which insulins can be given IV?	Rapid-acting and short-acting insulins

DAWN PHENOMENON	SOMOGYI PHENOMENON
❑ "DOWN INSULIN" ❑ Due to decreased effect of bedtime insulin dose ❑ Hyperglycemia occurs between 2:00 and 8:00 AM (early morning) ❑ May need to **increase** the insulin dose	❑ "SO MUCH INSULIN" ❑ A "**rebound hyperglycemia**" in response to low blood glucose at night ❑ May need to **decrease** the insulin dose or provide snacks at bedtime

NCLEX Alert! *Check the blood glucose level between 2:00 to 3:00 AM. If hypoglycemia is consistently present, suspect Somogyi phenomenon. If blood glucose level is usually high or normal, suspect Dawn phenomenon.*

2. Oral Hypoglycemic Agents

SULFONYLUREAS (stimulator)	MEGLITINIDES (stimulator)	BIGUANIDES (sensitizer)	ALPHA GLUCOSIDASE INHIBITORS	THIAZOLIDINE-DIONES (sensitizer)
Stimulates pancreatic insulin secretion	Stimulates pancreatic insulin secretion	Increases insulin sensitivity	Blocks the metabolism of carbohydrates	Increases insulin sensitivity; Decreases glucose production by the liver
Drugs ❑ glipizide (Glucotrol) ❑ chlorpropamide (Diabenese) ❑ glimepiride (Amaryl) ❑ glyburide (DiaBeta) ❑ tolbutamide (Orinase)	Drugs ❑ nateglinide (Starlix) ❑ repaglinide (Prandin)	Drugs ❑ metformin (Glucophage)	Drugs ❑ acarbose (Precose) ❑ miglitol (Glyset)	Drugs ❑ pioglitazone (Actos) ❑ rosiglitazone (Avandia)

3. Non-Insulin Drugs for Diabetes Mellitus

Amylinomimetic

- ❑ Description — Reduces glucagon secretion after meals
- ❑ Drugs — Examples:
  - pramlintide (SymlinPen 120)
- ❑ Side effects — Anorexia, **weight loss,** hypoglycemia
- ❑ Interventions — Avoid drinking alcohol

DPP-4 Inhibitors

- ❑ Description — Reduces glucagon; Risk of pancreatitis
- ❑ Drugs — Examples:
  - ogliptin (Nesina)
  - saxagliptin (Onglyza)
  - sitagliptin (Januvia)
  - linagliptin (Tradjenta)
- ❑ Side effects — Headache, runny nose, chills
- ❑ Interventions — Report severe abdominal pain (pancreatitis)

Glucagon-Like Peptides (GLP-1 Receptor Agonists)

❑ Description	Increases insulin and decreases glucagon All are injectable (subcutaneous)
❑ What are incretins?	Incretins are hormones that stimulate increased insulin secretion after eating, before blood glucose levels become elevated
❑ Drugs	Examples; ▪ albiglutide (Tanzeum) ▪ exenatide (Byetta) ▪ liraglutide (Victoza) ▪ dulaglutide (Trulicity)
❑ Side effects	Nausea, vomiting, diarrhea, dizziness
❑ Interventions	Report severe abdominal pain (pancreatitis)

Sodium Glucose Transporter 2 (SGLT2) Inhibitors

❑ Description	Prevents the kidney from retaining glucose
❑ Drugs	Examples: ▪ dapagliflozin (Farxiga) ▪ empagliflozin (Jardiance) ▪ canagliflozin (Invokana)
❑ Side effects	Hypotension, dehydration, glycosuria, **weight loss**
❑ Interventions	Monitor for dehydration

Inhaled Insulin

❑ Description	Ultra-rapid acting insulin (faster than rapid-acting insulins)
❑ Drugs	Examples: Afrezza
❑ Side effects	Hypoglycemia, cough, sore throat,
❑ Interventions	Avoid in clients with asthma and COPD

Nervous System 12

A. The Nervous System

❑ Central Nervous System (CNS)	Brain and spinal cord
❑ Peripheral Nervous System (PNS)	Cranial nerves and spinal nerves Autonomic nervous system
❑ Basic functional unit of the nervous system	Neurons
❑ Transmits impulses toward the cell body	Dendrites
❑ Carries impulses away from the cell body	Axon
❑ Space between neurons	Synapse
❑ Neurotransmitters	Acetylcholine Serotonin (mood, happiness, sleep) Norepinephrine (mood) GABA (gamma-aminobutyric acid) - relaxation dopamine (motivation, anti-anxiety)
❑ What substance destroys acetylcholine?	Acetylcholinesterase

The Brain

❑ Outside layer of the cerebrum made up of gray matter	Cerebral Cortex
❑ Interior of the brain made up of myelinated axons	White Matter
❑ Crossing of nerve fibers at the medulla oblongata	Decussation
❑ Spatial perception, pictures, art and musical ability	Right brain hemisphere
❑ Analytical and verbal skills (e.g. reading and writing, words, symbols, math)	Left brain hemisphere
❑ Regulates the pituitary gland	Hypothalamus
❑ Regulates body temperature, water balance, sleep, appetite, sexual urges and emotions	Hypothalamus
❑ Controls balance and coordination	Cerebellum
❑ Seat of emotions	Thalamus
❑ Parts of the brain stem	Midbrain, Pons, Medulla oblongata
❑ Functions of the medulla oblongata	Cardiac, vasomotor, respiratory, swallowing, coughing, sneezing centers

Lobes of the Brain

❑ Sensory function	Parietal lobe
❑ Interprets touch, temperature and pain	Parietal lobe
❑ Visual interpretation	Occipital lobe
❑ Motor function	Frontal lobe
❑ Broca's area (ability to produce speech)	Frontal lobe
❑ Hearing and smell	Temporal lobe
❑ Wernicke's area (ability to understand spoken/written words)	Temporal lobe

Meninges

❑ Outer layer	Dura mater
❑ Middle layer	Arachnoid mater
❑ Inner layer	Pia mater
❑ Space between the arachnoid and pia mater and filled with cerebrospinal fluid	Subarachnoid space
❑ Acts as a cushion and blood-brain barrier	Cerebrospinal Fluid (CSF)

Spinal Nerves

❑ Spinal nerves	Total: 31 ▪ Cervical (8 pairs) ▪ Thoracic (12 pairs) ▪ Lumbar (5 pairs) ▪ Sacral (5 pairs) ▪ Coccygeal (1 pair)

Cranial Nerves

❑ Cranial nerves	Total: 12
❑ Smell	CN 1, Olfactory nerve
❑ Vision	CN 2, Optic nerve
❑ Eye movement	CN 3, Oculomotor nerve CN 4, Trochlear nerve CN 6, Abducens nerve
❑ Pupil constriction	CN 3, Oculomotor nerve
❑ Facial sensation, chewing	CN 5, Trigeminal nerve
❑ Facial expression, salivation, taste	CN 7, Facial nerve
❑ Balance and hearing	CN 8, Auditory nerve
❑ Taste, swallowing, salivation	CN 9, Glossopharyngeal nerve

- ❑ Taste, swallowing, coughing, speech, salivation, gastric secretion, bradycardia — CN 10, Vagus nerve
- ❑ Tongue movement — CN 11, Hypoglossal nerve
- ❑ Head and shoulder movement — CN 12, Spinal Accessory nerve

Autonomic Nervous System

	SYMPATHETIC NERVOUS SYSTEM (Fight or Flight Response)	PARASYMPATHETIC NERVOUS SYSTEM (Rest and Digest)
Effects	Stimulates body processes **except** the gastrointestinal and genitourinary tract	Slows down body processes **except** the gastrointestinal and genitourinary tract
Names with similar effects	Adrenergic, Anticholinergic, Sympathomimetic, Parasympatholytic	Cholinergic, Parasympathomimetic, Sympatholytic
Neurotransmitters	Epinephrine and norepinephrine	Acetylcholine
Heart rate	Increased	Decreased
Blood pressure	Increased	Decreased
Respiratory rate	Increased	Decreased
Pupils	Dilation (mydriasis)	Constriction (miosis)
Bronchioles	Dilation	Constriction
Blood vessels	Constriction	No effect
Bladder	Inhibition (retention)	Stimulation (incontinence)
Digestive system	Inhibition (dry mouth, constipation)	Stimulation (salivation, diarrhea)
Glucose release from liver	Stimulation	Inhibition
Adrenal medulla	Stimulation	Inhibition

B. Neurological Assessment

Levels of Consciousness

- ❑ Able to respond to time, person and place — Conscious
- ❑ Drowsy but easily arousable, mild reduction in alertness — Somnolent or lethargic
- ❑ Responds only by vigorous and repetitive stimulation — Stuporous
- ❑ Nonresponsive except to painful stimuli — Semi-comatose
- ❑ Responsive only to extremely painful stimuli — Comatose

Glasgow Coma Scale

EYE OPENING RESPONSE	BEST VERBAL RESPONSE	BEST MOTOR RESPONSE
Spontaneous - 4 To voice - 3 To pain - 2 None - 1	Oriented - 5 Confused - 4 Inappropriate words - 3 Incomprehensible sounds -2 None – 1	Obeys command - 6 Localizes pain - 5 Withdraws - 4 Flexion to pain stimulus - 3 Extension to pain stimulus - 2 None – 1
Scores: 15 = fully awake; <10 = emergency; 3 = deep coma		

Motor Assessment

- ❑ Arms are **flexed**, fists are clenched, and legs extended — Decortication
- ❑ Adduction and **extension** of the arms, with the wrists pronated and the fingers flexed — Decerebration
- ❑ Absence of motor response to pain; an ominous sign — Flaccidity
- ❑ How do you assess motor strength? — Push the palm or sole against the examiner's palm
  Have client grasp objects firmly
- ❑ How do you assess balance function? — ROMBERG'S TEST
  - Client stands first with both eyes open then closed for 20-30 seconds while raising the arms forward
  - Slight swaying → normal
  - Loss of balance/falling → positive

C. Diagnostic Tests

Lumbar Puncture (Spinal Tap)

- ❑ Description — Performed to obtain CSF specimen, culture and sensitivity and injection of ATBs
- ❑ Position during procedure — Knee-chest position
- ❑ After the procedure — Flat position to prevent spinal headache

Electroencephalogram

- ❑ Description — Graphic recording of the electrical impulses produced by the brain

- Interventions
  - Withhold sedatives, caffeine and soda
  - Client should eat
  - Shampoo hair to ensure a clean scalp
  - Ask if the client needs to be sleep-deprived
- After the procedure
  - Hair shampoo to remove scalp gels

Electromyography

- Description
  - Records the electrical activity of muscles
  - Needle electrodes are placed into muscles
  - Soreness may occur in insertion sites

Caloric Stimulation Test

- Description
  - Irrigation of ear with warm or cold water
  - Normal response → nystagmus
  - Severe dizziness → Meniere's disease
  - Absence of nystagmus → brain tumor

D. Nervous System Disorders

Increased Intracranial Pressure

- Description
  - Increased ICP → hypoxia → acidosis → vasodilation → brainstem herniation
- Causes
  - Bleeding, meningitis, tumor, edema
- Assessment

EARLY	LATE
Change or decrease in level of consciousness	Unresponsive
Drowsiness	Decortication or decerebration response
Confusion	Dilated or unequal pupils (anisocuria)
Nausea and vomiting	Cheyne-Stokes breathing
Slow or unequal pupillary response	Widened pulse pressure (*SBP increases but DBP remains the same*)

- What is **Cushing's Triad**?
  - A late sign of increased ICP characterized by:
    1. *Decreased respiration*
    2. *Decreased pulse rate*
    3. *Increased blood pressure*

❑ Interventions	Oxygen, Elevate head, Quiet room
❑ Is suctioning allowed?	Yes, suction gently
❑ What should be avoided?	Narcotics, noise and extreme hip flexion
❑ Why is diazepam (Valium) given?	To prevent seizures
❑ Why is mannitol (Osmitrol) given?	To reduce cerebral edema by promoting urination (osmotic diuretic)
❑ Why is a stool softener given?	To prevent straining during defecation
❑ Why is a histamine antagonist drug given?	To prevent Cushing's ulcer

> ***NCLEX Alert!*** *SIGNS OF INCREASED ICP ARE OPPOSITE OF SHOCK!*
> *INCREASED ICP: ↑ BP, ↓ HR, ↓ RR, widened pulse pressure*
> *SHOCK: ↓ BP, ↑ HR, ↑ RR, narrowed pulse pressure*

Meningitis

❑ Description	Inflammation of the meninges
❑ Causes	Meningococci, streptococci, otitis media
❑ Assessment	Increased ICP, fever, **nuchal rigidity**, nausea, vomiting, photophobia, severe headache, **opisthotonos** (extreme arching of the back)
❑ What is a positive Kernig's sign?	When the thigh is flexed at the hip and knee at 90° angle → extension in the leg is painful
❑ What is a positive Brudzinski's sign?	Flexion of the neck → flexion of the hip and lower extremities
❑ Diagnostic Test	Lumbar puncture for C/S
❑ Interventions	Droplet precautions Monitor for increased ICP Penicillin, Rifampicin, Vancomycin
❑ How is CSF leakage monitored?	1. Test fluid for **halo** sign ▪ Dip the leaked fluid on a gauze ▪ Blood will form in the middle surrounded by a ring of CSF 2. Test fluid for the presence of **glucose**

> ***NCLEX Alert!*** *Rifampicin is the drug of choice for prophylaxis against meningitis.*

Guillain-Barre Syndrome

❑ Description	Antibodies attack the Schwann cells of peripheral nerves → nerve inflammation
❑ Causes	Autoimmune, recent viral infection (flu)
❑ Assessment	**Ascending paralysis**, paresthesia, weakness
❑ Diagnostic Tests	Lumbar puncture
❑ Interventions	Respiratory support IV immune globulin amitryptyline (Elavil) gabapentin (Neurontin)
❑ What is plasmapheresis?	Removal of plasma to remove antibodies
❑ Will the client recover?	Yes, but recovery will be slow

Multiple Sclerosis

❑ Description	Degeneration of the myelin sheath → impaired impulse transmission → sensory and motor paralysis With remissions and exacerbations
❑ Causes	Unknown, autoimmune disorder, genetics
❑ Assessment	**Blurred vision**, diplopia, nystagmus **scotoma** (blind spots in vision), weakness, **numbness and tingling**, ataxia, slurred, hesitant speech, mood swings, amnesia, bowel and bladder incontinence
❑ What is **Charcoat's Triad**?	Remember SIN! ▪ S - canning speech ▪ I - ntention tremors ▪ N - ystagmus
❑ Diagnostic Tests	Electrophoresis of CSF (abnormal IgG)
❑ Interventions	Muscle relaxants, Tranquilizers, Steroids
❑ Why is oxybutinin (Ditropan) given?	To treat urinary incontinence
❑ Why is bethanechol (Urecholine) given?	To treat urinary retention
❑ Is there a cure for this condition?	No

> ***NCLEX Alert!*** *Instruct the client to avoid stress, fatigue, infection and warm showers to prevent exacerbation of symptoms.*

Myasthenia Gravis

❑ Description	Destruction of the acetylcholine receptor sites → muscle weakness With remissions and exacerbations
❑ Causes	Unknown, autoimmune, thymus tumor
❑ Assessment	Muscle weakness, **ptosis**, dysphagia, diplopia, aphonia
❑ Diagnostic Tests	**Tensilon Test**, Electromyography
❑ How is edrophonium HCl (Tensilon) Test performed?	IV administration of edrophonium HCl A short-acting anticholinesterase Relieved muscle weakness → positive
❑ Interventions	ANTICHOLINESTERASE DRUGS ▪ pyridostigmine (Mestinon) ▪ neostigmine (Prostigmin) ▪ ambemonium chloride (Mytelase) Surgical removal of tumor Prednisone Plasmapheresis Mechanical ventilation
❑ How do anticholinesterase drugs work?	Prevents destruction of acetylcholine
❑ What are the side effects of anticholinesterase drugs?	Parasympathetic effects such as incontinence, salivation and diarrhea
❑ What instructions are important to teach the client?	Take the medications on time especially 30 minutes before meals to prevent dysphagia and aspiration Avoid stress, fatigue and infection to prevent exacerbation of symptoms

NCLEX Alert! *Monitor for **myasthenic crisis** (undermedication) as manifested by profound weakness, respiratory distress and dysphagia. **Cholinergic crisis** (overmedication) is manifested also by weakness in addition to parasympathetic symptoms such as salivation, wheezing and diarrhea. These conditions are fatal!*

Parkinson's Disease

❑ Description	Decreased dopamine and increased acetylcholine → impaired movement
❑ Causes	Unknown, antipsychotics, head injury
❑ Assessment	EARLY SIGNS ▪ T - remors (non-intention, pill-rolling) ▪ R - igidity ▪ A – kinesia or bradykinesia Mask-like facial expression, dysphagia, **shuffling gait** (festination), propulsive or retropulsive gait, stooped posture, slurred speech, cogwheel rigidity (jerky movements)
❑ Interventions	ANTI-PARKINSONIAN DRUGS ▪ selegiline (Eldepryl) ▪ levodopa (Dopar, Larodopa) ▪ carbidopa-levodopa (Sinemet) ▪ benztropine (Cogentin) ▪ amantadine (Symmetrel) ▪ bromocriptine (Parlodel) Promote self-care activities Assess for dysphagia Prevent injury and falls Provide assistive devices
❑ Surgery	DEEP BRAIN STIMULATION ▪ Involves the implantation of wire electrodes (brain pacemaker) to reduce tremors STEREOTAXIC PALLIDOTOMY ▪ Destroys part of the thalamus STEM CELL TRANSPLANTATION

> ***NCLEX Alert!*** *REMEMBER WHICH TYPE OF TREMOR IS PRESENT!*
>
> *Parkinson's disease → non-intention (resting) tremor; Multiple sclerosis → intention tremor*

Amyotrophic Lateral Sclerosis (Lou Gehrig's Disease)

❑ Description	Degeneration of motor neurons in the brain and spinal cord
❑ Causes	Autoimmune disorder, viral infection
❑ Assessment	**Vague symptoms**, worsening weakness, muscle wasting, dysphagia, **fasciculation** (localized seizures), respiratory failure
❑ Diagnostic Test	Electromyography
❑ Interventions	Similar care to multiple sclerosis

Temporomandibular Joint Syndrome (TMJ)

❑ Description	Pain and dysfunction in the jaw joint
❑ Causes	Jaw arthritis, teeth malalignment
❑ Assessment	Similar to trigeminal neuralgia Sudden jaw pain, headache, clicking of jaw
❑ Diagnostic Test	Dental x-ray
❑ Interventions	Soft diet, Analgesic, Mouth guard, TENS device, Dental referral, Surgery

Bell's Palsy

❑ Description	Inflammation of the 7th cranial nerve
❑ Cause	Unknown, viral infection
❑ Assessment	Facial pain and paralysis, numbness, ptosis, dysphasia, difficult chewing, drooling, drooping mouth, smooth and unwrinkled forehead
❑ Interventions	Steroids, Analgesics, Electrotherapy Eye patch at night, Irrigate eye with NS

Trigeminal Neuralgia (Tic Douloureux)

❑ Description	Pain involving the 5th cranial nerve Aggravated by temperature change, loud noise, wind, chewing and brushing teeth
❑ Assessment	Sudden burning pain, facial twitching
❑ Interventions	Opioids, carbamazepine (Tegretol) Protect the face from passing breeze Chew slowly Avoid electric shaver and hot foods

Huntington's Chorea

❑ Description	Degeneration of the basal ganglia & cortex
❑ What is the greatest risk factor?	Genetic (autosomal dominant transmission)
❑ What is an **autosomal dominant** transmission?	Disease is transmissible with one gene
❑ Assessment	**Chorea** (jerky movements) dysphagia, aphasia, clumsiness, amnesia, depression, agitation, paranoia
❑ Diagnostic Test	Genetic testing
❑ Interventions	Supportive treatment, Physical therapy, Tranquilizers, Anti-Parkinsonian drugs

> ***NCLEX Alert!*** *Hallucinations, delusions and mental decline are late signs.*

Seizure Disorders

❑ Causes	Hypocalcemia, hyponatremia, fever, hypoglycemia, alcohol withdrawal

PARTIAL (FOCAL) SEIZURE Affects specific areas of the brain	GENERALIZED SEIZURE Affects the entire brain; Has loss of consciousness
Simple partial seizure ❑ Retains consciousness **Jacksonian seizure (Jacksonian march)** ❑ A type of simple partial seizure ❑ Begins in one area then progresses ❑ Starts with a twitching or tingling sensation in a finger then spreads to the hand and face **Complex partial seizure (Psychomotor seizure)** ❑ Involves the temporal lobe ❑ With loss of consciousness for a few minutes ❑ Makes bizarre behaviors (dressing, hair combing) ❑ Cannot recall the event	**Tonic-Clonic seizure** ❑ Involves an aura (warning sign), epileptic cry, stiffness and jerking and post-ictal phase **Absence seizure (Petit mal)** ❑ Brief, staring spells with loss of consciousness **Myoclonic seizure** ❑ Sudden, quick and involuntary muscle jerking **Atonic seizure (Drop attacks)** ❑ Sudden loss of muscle tone; Risk for falls **Status epilepticus** ❑ Seizure lasting for >5 minutes or 2 or > seizures within a 5-minute period without pause

❑ Interventions	Anticonvulsants, Suction machine Oxygen, Pad side rails, Bed in low position, Avoid blinking lights and lack of sleep
❑ How do you promote safety during a generalized seizure?	Assist client to the floor if sitting Cradle the head to prevent injury
❑ Is restraining and insertion of a tongue depressor allowed during the seizure?	No, these actions will cause injury

- ❑ What is a **ketogenic diet**? — A high fat, low carbohydrate diet that reduces incidence of seizures

Transient Ischemic Attack (Mini Stroke)

- ❑ Description — A brief decrease in cerebral blood flow
  A **warning sign** of an impending stroke
- ❑ Causes — Atherosclerosis, thrombus, hypertension
- ❑ Assessment — Dizziness, confusion, speech impairment, vision loss, diplopia, numbness, weakness
- ❑ Interventions — Lifestyle changes, Control BP, Lose weight, Quit smoking, aspirin, clopidogrel (Plavix), dipyridadamole (Persantin)
- ❑ What is carotid endarterectomy? — Scraping the lining of the artery to remove the plaque

Cerebrovascular Accident (Stroke)

- ❑ Description — Decreased cerebral flow → hypoxia → brain infarction → neurologic deficits
- ❑ Types — Ischemic (thrombotic), Hemorrhagic
- ❑ Assessment — Remember FAST!
  - F - acial drooping
  - A - rm weakness
  - S - lurred speech
  - T - ime to call 911 at first sign
- ❑ What type of paralysis occurs first? — Flaccid turning to spastic paralysis
- ❑ What is **expressive/motor/Broca's aphasia**? — Inability to speak or form words
- ❑ What is **receptive/sensory/Wernicke's aphasia**? — Inability to understand written/spoken language
- ❑ What is global aphasia? — Both Broca's and Wernicke's aphasia
- ❑ What are the effects of **right-sided** (right brain) stroke? — Agnosia, impulsive, impaired judgment, unilateral neglect
  left hemianopia, left hemiplegia
- ❑ What are the effects of **left-sided** (left brain) stroke? — Aphasia, cautious, memory deficits, poor problem-solving skills
  right hemianopia, right hemiplegia

❑ What is hemianopia?	Blindness over half the field of vision Loss of vision is on **same** side of paralysis
❑ Interventions	TIME IS BRAIN! Thrombolytics given within 3 hours Elevate head of bed to decrease ICP Thickening agent to prevent aspiration Place foods on unaffected side of mouth Approach objects within field of vision Thrombectomy

> ***NCLEX Alert!*** *Thrombolytics are not given if the cause of stroke is cerebral hemorrhage.*

Concussion

❑ Description	Heavy blow to the head
❑ Assessment	Brief lapse of consciousness, confusion
❑ Interventions	Analgesics, Neuro-assessment Monitor for increased ICP

Contusion

❑ Description	Severe brain injury due to trauma
❑ Assessment	Loss of consciousness, amnesia, coma
❑ Interventions	Monitor for increased ICP and CSF leak

Cerebral Hematomas

❑ Description	Accumulation of blood in the brain
❑ Types	Epidural, Subdural, Intracerebral
❑ Assessment	Increased ICP, changes in LOC
❑ Interventions	Similar to increased ICP Craniotomy, craniectomy, cranioplasty
❑ Position after craniotomy surgery	**Supratentorial** → Semi-Fowler's position **Infratentorial** → Flat position

Skull Fractures

❑ Description	Break in the skull due to trauma or fall
❑ Assessment	Basilar skull fracture (most dangerous type) rhinorrhea, otorrhea
❑ What is **Racoon's eyes**?	Periorbital ecchymosis or bruising
❑ What is **Battle's sign**?	Mastoid ecchymosis or bruising
❑ Interventions	Monitor for increased ICP and CSF leak

Spinal Cord Injury

SPINAL SHOCK	AUTONOMIC DYSREFLEXIA
Acute loss of sympathetic function characterized by the **absence of sensation and reflexes** below the level of injury; Occurs within 30-60 minutes to weeks after spinal cord trauma	Exaggerated sympathetic response that occurs suddenly after spinal shock phase; Occurs in spinal injuries **above the 6th** thoracic vertebrae
Assessment ❑ Severe **hypotension** ❑ Bradycardia ❑ Flaccid paralysis ❑ Warm skin	Assessment ❑ Severe **hypertension** ❑ Bradycardia, severe pounding **headache**, nausea, flushed skin, blurred vision, diaphoresis, goosebumps, convulsions, death
Interventions ❑ Atropine ❑ Steroids ❑ IV fluids	Interventions ❑ Elevate the head of the bed to decrease the BP ❑ Loosen tight clothing ❑ Antihypertensive drug - phentolamine (Regitine) ❑ Avoid triggers: *full bladder, impacted feces, pressure sores, sexual intercourse, UTI*

> ***NCLEX Alert!*** *Autonomic dysreflexia is a life-threatening emergency. The priority action is to elevate the head of the bed (High Fowler's position), determine the cause and administer an antihypertensive drug.*

❑ Interventions

Immobilize head and neck, Intubation
Logroll method when turning to maintain spine alignment

❑ What is a Stryker Frame?

Special bed that allows **horizontal** turning of a spinal cord injury client

❑ What is a Circ-Olectric bed?

Special bed that allows **horizontal** and **vertical** turning of a spinal cord injury client

❑ What instructions are important to teach the client who has a halo vest?

Turn whole body rather than turning head
Wear sheepskin under device
Avoid driving, bath and shower

> ***NCLEX Alert!*** *Place wrench at the client's bedside or taped to the halo vest to be used in an emergency!*

Spinal Nerve Root Compression (Herniated Nucleus Pulposus)

❑ Description	Nucleus pulposus, a jelly-like material in the vertebral disc, swells and herniates → slipped disk → spinal nerve compression
❑ Assessment	Weakness, pain, paralysis, paresthesia, difficulty sitting or walking, **sciatica**
❑ What is sciatica?	Tingling, numbness or leg weakness
❑ What is myelography?	X-ray of the spinal canal using a dye
❑ Interventions	Hot moist packs, Muscle relaxants Steroids, Diskectomy with spinal fusion
❑ What is **laminectomy**?	Removal of the posterior part of the vertebra to remove pressure from the spinal nerve

E. Nervous System Drugs

1. Drugs for Parkinson's Disease (Dopaminergics)

❑ Description	Promotes acetylcholine and dopamine balance to decrease tremors
❑ Drugs	Examples: ▪ carbidopa-levodopa (Sinemet) ▪ levodopa (Larodopa) ▪ bromocriptine (Parlodel) ▪ selegiline hydrochloride (Eldepryl) ▪ amantadine (Symmetrel) ▪ pramipexole (Mirapex) ▪ ropinirole (Requip)
❑ Side effects (Dopaminergics)	Dyskinesia, nausea and vomiting, **orthostatic hypotension**, urinary retention dry mouth, constipation
❑ Interventions	Change positions slowly Do not stop drug use abruptly Avoid alcohol
❑ What should be avoided by clients taking levodopa?	High **Vitamin B_6** and **protein** diet → inhibits drug absorption

2. Anticholinergic drugs

❑ Description	Inhibits acetylcholine → reduced tremors in Parkinson's disease
❑ Drugs	Examples: ▪ benztropine mesylate (Cogentin) ▪ trihexyphenidyl HCl (Artane) ▪ biperiden hydrochloride (Akineton)
❑ Side effects (Anticholinergic effects)	Dry mouth, constipation, urinary retention
❑ Interventions	Monitor bladder and bowel function Avoid smoking, alcohol and caffeine Encourage fluids Ice chips for dry mouth

3. Drugs for Myasthenia Gravis (Anticholinesterase)

❑ Description	Inhibits the breakdown of acetylcholine Treats myasthenia gravis and Alzheimer's disease
❑ Drugs	Examples: ▪ neostigmine (Prostigmin) ▪ pyridostigmine (Mestinon) ▪ galantamine (Reminyl) ▪ rivastigmine (Exelon) ▪ donepezil (Aricept)
❑ Side effects	PARASYMPATHETIC EFFECTS anorexia, nausea, vomiting, salivation, bradycardia, hypotension
❑ Interventions	Take drugs on time especially before meals Monitor for cholinergic or myasthenic crisis

MYASTHENIC CRISIS (undermedication)	CHOLINERGIC CRISIS (overmedication)
Assessment ❑ **Severe muscle weakness** ❑ Severe respiratory distress ❑ Tachycardia ❑ Mydriasis ❑ Dysphagia ❑ Tensilon relieves the weakness	Assessment ❑ **Severe muscle weakness** ❑ Severe respiratory distress ❑ Bradycardia ❑ Miosis ❑ Parasympathetic effects: *abdominal cramps, vomiting, diarrhea, hypotension, wheezing* ❑ Tensilon worsens the weakness
Antidote: Tensilon	Antidote: Atropine sulfate (anticholinergic)

4. Anticonvulsant Drugs

HYDANTOINS	BENZODIAZEPINES	BARBITURATES
Treats tonic-clonic seizures and arrhythmias	Treats absence seizure Promotes muscle relaxation Drug of choice for status epilepticus	Treats tonic-clonic seizures and status epilepticus
Drugs ❑ phenytoin (Dilantin) ❑ fosphenytoin (Cerebryx)	Drugs ❑ diazepam (Valium) ❑ lorazepam (Ativan)	Drugs ❑ phenobarbital (Luminal) ❑ amobarbital (Amytal)
Side effects ❑ **Pink-red or red-brown urine** ❑ **Gingival hyperplasia** ❑ **Sedation**, slurred speech, skin rash, nausea and vomiting, blood dyscrasias	Side effects ❑ Sedation ❑ Drug tolerance and dependence ❑ Hepatotoxicity ❑ Thrombocytopenia ❑ Leukopenia	Side effects ❑ Sedation ❑ Hypotension ❑ Ataxia ❑ CNS depression ❑ Drug tolerance
OXAZOLIDINEDIONES	**SUCCINIMIDES**	**VALPROATES**
Treats absence seizures	Treats absence seizure (petit mal)	Treats tonic-clonic, partial, myoclonic and psychomotor seizures
Drugs ❑ trimethadione (Troxidone)	Drugs ❑ ethosuximide (Zarontin)	Drugs ❑ valproic acid (Depakene)
Side effects ❑ Drowsiness, headache, blood dyscrasia	Side effects ❑ Drowsiness, dizziness, nausea, vomiting, blood dyscrasia	Side effects ❑ Sedation, blood dyscrasia, hepatoxicity
Interventions ❑ Do not stop taking the drug abruptly. ❑ Avoid alcohol and over-the-counter drugs. Alcohol intake may potentiate drowsiness or sedation. ❑ Report sore and fever (indicates infection due to leukopenia). ❑ Report signs of toxicity such as drowsiness, dizziness, disorientation, ataxia, nausea and vomiting. ❑ **Hydantoins**: Avoid taking with antacids and milk (inhibits absorption); Provide frequent **oral care**; Massage the gums; Avoid administration with **tube feedings** (inhibits absorption); Contraindicated in pregnancy (teratogenic)		

Other Anticonvulsants

❑ topiramate (Topamax), carbamazepine (Tegretol), lamotrigine (Lamictal), levetiracetam (Keppra), gabapentin (Neurontin), oxcarbazepine (Trileptal), pregabalin (Lyrica)

5. Osmotic Diuretics

- ❑ Description

  Decreases the ICP and intra-ocular pressure

- ❑ Drugs

  Examples:
  - mannitol (Osmitrol)
  - urea (Ureaphil)

- ❑ Side effects

  Fluid and electrolyte imbalance

- ❑ Interventions

  Monitor urine output

  Monitor for signs of dehydration

Sensory System 13

A. The Sensory System

The Eyes

❑ Three layers of the eye	Sclera, Uvea-Choroid, Retina
❑ Regulates the size of the pupil	Iris
❑ The opening within the iris	Pupil
❑ A transparent layer in front of the eye	Cornea
❑ Center of the retina that gives the best detailed vision	Macula
❑ Inner layer of the eye	Retina
❑ Receptors for night vision	Rods
❑ Receptors for day vision	Cones
❑ Nerve that transmits visual stimulus from the retina to the occipital lobe of the brain	Optic nerve
❑ Watery fluid located in the anterior and posterior chambers of the eye	Aqueous humor
❑ Colorless gelatinous fluid that fills the eyeball behind the lens	Vitreous humor
❑ Angle between the cornea and the iris	Anterior chamber
❑ Angle between the iris and the lens	Posterior chamber
❑ Produces aqueous humor	Ciliary body
❑ Where does the aqueous humor drain?	Trabecular meshwork, Canal of Schlemm
❑ Change in the shape of the lens to adjust vision of objects in various distances	Accommodation

The Ears

❑ Three divisions	Outer ear, middle ear, inner ear
❑ Bones in the middle ear	Malleus, incus, stapes
	Vibrates to transmit sounds
❑ Spiral cavity that contains the Organ of Corti	Cochlea
❑ Fluid-filled tubes in the inner ear	Semicircular canals
❑ Receptor for hearing	Organ of Corti
❑ Nerve for balance and hearing	Vestibulocochlear nerve
❑ What happens when the vestibular nerve is damaged?	Incoordination and vertigo
❑ What happens when the cochlear nerve is damaged?	Deafness

B. Diagnostic Tests

Visual and Extraocular Muscle Function Tests

❑ Test for visual acuity	Snellen eye chart (normal is 20/20)
❑ Test for near vision	Jaeger chart Rosenbaum pocket vision screener
❑ Test for color vision	Ishihara polychromatic plates
❑ Test for eye alignment	Corneal light reflex test
❑ Test for extraocular muscle function	Cover-uncover test
❑ Examination of fundus and interior of the eye	Ophthalmoscopy
❑ Test for intraocular pressure (IOP)	Tonometry
❑ Normal IOP	10 to 21 mm Hg
❑ Test performed in glaucoma and stroke	Visual field examination
❑ Test for macular degeneration	Amsler grid
❑ Magnifies the surface of the eye to detect microscopic injuries and cataracts	Slit-lamp exam
❑ Assesses vascular changes and blood flow through the retinal vessels; Diagnoses diabetes or hypertension	Retinal angiography
❑ What does PERRLA mean during a pupillary exam?	P-upils E-qual, R-ound, and R-eactive to L-ight and A-ccommodation
❑ Assesses eye alignment using light reflection from a penlight	Corneal light reflex test
❑ Assesses for the presence of ocular deviation(strabismus)	Cover-Uncover test

> ***NCLEX Alert!*** *SNELLEN EYE CHART*
>
> *Numerator → distance from chart); Denominator → distance at which the normal eye can read*

Hearing and Balance Tests

1. Rinne Test

❑ Description — Compares air conduction (AC) and bone conduction (BC) hearing

❑ Steps:

1. Strike the tuning fork
2. Place the vibrating tuning fork on the base of the **mastoid bone**
3. Ask the client to tell you when the sound is no longer heard
4. Note the time interval and immediately move the tuning fork to the **front of the ear**
5. Ask the client to tell you when the sound is no longer heard

6. Note the time interval and findings
7. AC 2x longer than BC means ________ — Normal finding
8. BC longer than AC means ________ — Conductive deafness

2. Weber Test

- ❑ Description — Distinguishes between conductive and sensorineural hearing loss
- ❑ Steps:
  1. Strike the tuning fork
  2. Place the vibrating fork on the **middle** of the client's forehead
  3. Ask client if the sound is heard better in one ear or the same in both ears
  4. Sound heard on both ears indicates _______ — Normal finding
  5. Lateralization (heard on one side only) indicates ______ — Abnormal finding
     Loud side → conductive deafness
     Weak side → nerve deafness

> ***NCLEX Alert!*** *Conductive deafness is reversible and sensorineural deafness is permanent!*

Audiometry

- ❑ Description — Tests hearing levels and ability to differentiate between various sound intensities and pitch

Caloric Stimulation Test

- ❑ Description — Detects hearing loss caused by vertigo or brain damage in comatose clients
  Involves cold or warm water ear irrigation
- ❑ What is a normal finding? — Cold water → nystagmus away from irrigated ear
  Warm water → nystagmus towards irrigated ear
- ❑ Severe nystagmus and dizziness means ________ — Meniere's disease
- ❑ Absence of nystagmus means _________ — Brain tumor

Electronystagmography

- ❑ Description — Test for vestibular function that records eye movement (nystagmus) to diagnose the cause of vertigo

Doll's Eye Test

- ❑ Description — Test for brainstem function
- ❑ What is a normal finding? — Rotate head to right → eye turns left
  If absent → brain stem damage

C. Eye Disorders

Glaucoma

OPEN-ANGLE (CHRONIC, SIMPLE)	ANGLE-CLOSURE (ACUTE)
Blockage at the trabecular meshwork and Canal of Schlemm → decreased aqueous humor drainage → increased intraocular pressure → permanent blindness	Sudden **pupil dilation**, darkness, mydriatic drugs → sudden closure of the angle → decreased aqueous humor drainage → increased intraocular pressure → permanent blindness
Assessment ❑ Asymptomatic ❑ Painless ❑ **Tunnel vision** (loss of peripheral vision) ❑ Halos around lights	Assessment ❑ Symptomatic ❑ Painful ❑ Nausea and vomiting, blindness ❑ **Emergency**!

- ❑ Interventions — Miotics to open the angle and promote drainage of aqueous humor
- ❑ What should the client avoid? — **Atropine sulfate**, stress, straining
- ❑ Why should the client avoid atropine? — It causes pupil dilation that increases IOP
- ❑ Is there a cure for this condition? — No, but it can be controlled
- ❑ Surgery — Laser iridectomy, Laser trabeculoplasty

Cataract

- ❑ Description — Cloudy appearance or opacity of the lens
- ❑ Causes — **Aging**, diabetes, steroids, UV light
- ❑ Assessment — **Blurred vision**, halos around lights, faded color vision, increased IOP

- ❑ Interventions

  INTRACAPSULAR EXTRACTION
  - Removal of the lens within capsule
  - Done through cryosurgery

  EXTRACAPSULAR EXTRACTION
  - Removal of the lens except the posterior capsule for lens insertion
  - Done through phacoemulsification

- ❑ What are the effects of cataract glasses?

  Objects appear larger
  Decreased peripheral vision

- ❑ What instructions are important to teach the client?

  Apply eye shield at night to prevent rubbing of the eyes
  Wear sunglasses when in bright light
  Avoid exertion, coughing and straining

> ***NCLEX Alert!*** *The client should report sudden, intense eye pain. It indicates increased intraocular pressure!*

Retinal Detachment

- ❑ Description

  Retina pulls away from supportive layer that provides nutrients and oxygen → blindness

- ❑ Assessment

  Blind spots in vision, **flashes of lights**, **floaters,** veil-like or falling curtain shadow in vision

- ❑ Is this condition painful?

  No, this is painless but an emergency

- ❑ What is best position for this condition?

  Affected eye on dependent position (e.g. left outer side tear → left side)

- ❑ Interventions

  Cryosurgery, Photocoagulation
  Scleral buckling

Macular Degeneration

- ❑ Description

  Deterioration of the central part of retina

- ❑ Causes

  Aging, smoking, heredity

- ❑ Assessment

  Blurred vision, wavy letters, bull's eye vision diminished color perception

- ❑ What is **bull's eye** vision?

  Loss of central vision

- ❑ Interventions

  Laser photocoagulation
  Photodynamic therapy

Refractive Errors

❑ Nearsightedness due to an elongated eyeball; Treated with concave lens	Myopia
❑ Farsightedness due to a short eyeball; Treated with convex lens	Hyperopia
❑ Degenerative changes and loss of lens elasticity	Cataract
❑ Imperfect focusing on the retina due to unequal curvature and shape of the cornea	Astigmatism

D. Ear Disorders

Otitis Media

❑ Description	Infection of the middle ear → pressure on the eardrum → rupture → deafness, labyrinthitis, meningitis
❑ Assessment	Fever, tinnitus, malaise, otorrhea
❑ Interventions	Wear earplugs when swimming Avoid high altitudes Blow nose with mouth open
❑ Surgery	Myringotomy, Myringoplasty
❑ What is the purpose of tympanostomy tubes?	To ventilate and dry the ears

NCLEX Alert! *Tympanostomy tubes will fall spontaneously in 6 months.*

Otosclerosis

❑ Description	Abnormal growth of bone in middle ear → overgrowth of stapes → fixation → conductive deafness
❑ Assessment	Progressive, bilateral deafness tinnitus (ringing in the ears)
❑ What is the result of Rinne Test?	Sound is heard best behind the ear
❑ What is the result of Weber Test?	Lateralization
❑ Surgery	Stapedectomy
❑ What instructions are important to teach after ear surgery?	Take antiemetics for dizziness Move head slowly to prevent dizziness Avoid blowing nose, exertion and flying

NCLEX Alert! *Temporary deafness is expected after stapedectomy due to ear swelling.*

Meniere's Disease (Endolymphatic Hydrops)

❑ Description	Increase in fluid within the labyrinth
❑ Causes	Heredity, allergy, smoking, high salt diet
❑ Assessment	TRIAD SYMPTOMS ▪ V - ertigo ▪ T - innitus ▪ U- nilateral hearing loss
❑ What is a warning symptom before the attack?	Feeling of ear pressure
❑ What is the goal of treatment?	Reduce fluid in ear and promote drainage
❑ Interventions	Bed rest, Low salt diet, Diuretics, meclizine (Antivert), diazepam (Valium), promethazine (Phenergan)
❑ Surgery	Endolymphatic sac decompression Labyrinthectomy (last resort)

E. Eye Drugs

1. Administering Eye Drugs

❑ Steps:

1. Always give eye drops before an ointment	
2. Use gloves (optional if client has eye infection)	
3. Place drug on the lower ___________________ sac	Conjunctival
4. Close the eye gently	
5. Apply _______ over the inner canthus to prevent systemic absorption of drug	Pressure
6. Wait _____ before administering another eye drop on the same eye	3-5 minutes
7. Dropper should not touch the cornea	

2. Drugs for Glaucoma

MIOTICS	ALPHA-ADRENERGIC AGONIST	PROSTAGLANDIN ANALOGS
Constricts the pupil → opens the angle → increased aqueous humor drainage → reduced IOP	Decreases the aqueous humor production → decreased IOP	Increases the outflow of aqueous humor → decreased IOP
Drugs ❑ pilocarpine hydrochloride (Isopto Carpine) ❑ phospholine iodide (Echothiophate)	Drugs ❑ apraclonidine (Iopidine) ❑ brimonidine (Alphagan)	Drugs ❑ bimatoprost (Lumigan) ❑ latanoprost (Xalatan)
Side effects ❑ **Blurred vision** ❑ Poor night vision	Side effects ❑ Blurred vision ❑ Itchy eyes	❑ Blurred vision, eye tearing ❑ Darkening of eye color, eyelid and eyelashes
Interventions ❑ Avoid driving at night ❑ Adequate lighting at night	Interventions ❑ Avoid wearing contact lens after taking drug	Interventions ❑ Avoid wearing contact lens after taking drug
BETA-ADRENERGIC BLOCKERS	**CARBONIC ANHYDRASE INHIBITORS**	**OSMOTIC DRUGS**
Decreases the aqueous humor production → decreased IOP	Decreases the production of carbonic acid → decreased aqueous humor production → decreased IOP	Increases the urinary output → decreased IOP For emergency treatment of glaucoma
Drugs ❑ timolol maleate (Timoptic) ❑ levobetaxolol (Betaxon) ❑ carteolol HCl (Ocupress)	Drugs ❑ dorzolamide (Trusopt) ❑ brinzolamide (Azopt)	Drugs ❑ mannitol (Osmitrol) ❑ glycerin (Osmoglyn)
Side effects ❑ **Bradycardia**, hypotension, bronchospasm	Side effects ❑ Eye burning and stinging, mild eye pain	Side effects ❑ Fluid and electrolyte imbalance
Interventions ❑ Avoid in clients with asthma and COPD ❑ Check HR before giving drug ❑ Monitor for dyspnea	Interventions ❑ Avoid prolonged sun exposure	Interventions ❑ Monitor intake and output

3. Mydriatic-Cycloplegic and Anticholinergic Drugs

- ❑ Description — Causes pupil dilation. Used before eye exams for better examination of deeper structures such as the retina
- ❑ Drugs — Examples:
  - cyclopentolate (Cyclogyl)
  - scopolamine (Isopto Hyoscine)
  - tropicamide (Mydriacil)
  - atropine (Isopto Atropine)
- ❑ Side effects — Hypertension, tachycardia, **photophobia**
- ❑ What are the signs of atropine toxicity? — Tachycardia, urinary retention, dry mouth
- ❑ Interventions — Avoid driving 24 hours after giving drug. Wear sunglasses

4. Drugs for Macular Degeneration

- ❑ Drugs — Examples:
  - bevacinumab (Avastin)
  - pegabtanib (Macugen)
  - ranibizumab (Lucentis)
- ❑ Side effects — Blurred vision, corneal swelling
- ❑ Interventions — Prepare for eye injection procedure

F. Ear Drugs

1. Decongestants and Antihistamines

- ❑ Description — Produces vasoconstriction
- ❑ Drugs — Examples:
  - naphazoline HCl (Allerest)
  - cetirizine (Zyrtec)
  - chlorpheniramine (Chlor-Trimeton)
- ❑ Side effects — **Drowsiness**, dry mucous membranes
- ❑ Interventions — Avoid operating dangerous machinery. Suck on hard candy for dry mouth

> ***NCLEX Alert!*** *INSTILLING EAR MEDICATIONS*
>
> *Adult → Pull the ear back and up*
>
> *Child <3 years-old → Pull the ear back and down*

Urinary System

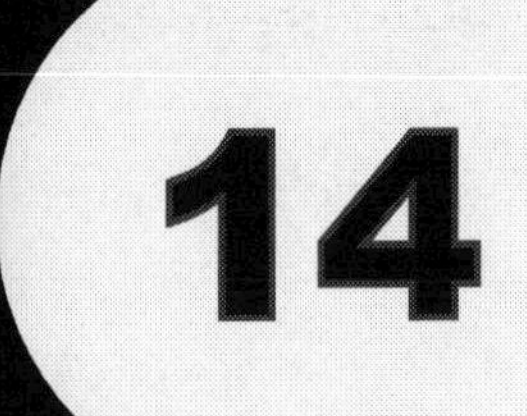

A. The Urinary System

❑ Functions	Filtration and removal of wastes Maintains homeostasis (BP, fluid and electrolytes, pH) Secretes renin and erythropoietin
❑ Structures	Two kidneys Two ureters Urinary bladder Urethra
❑ Functional units of the kidney that form urine	Nephrons
❑ Parts of the nephron	Glomerulus and Bowman's capsule, Loop of Henle, proximal and distal convoluted tubules
❑ What are the normal components of urine?	Glucose, water, urea, creatinine, electrolytes
❑ Is it normal to find RBC and protein in urine?	No
❑ What is the normal urine output?	1,000–1,500 mL per day (30-50 mL/hour)

B. Diagnostic Tests

Intravenous Pyelogram and Retrograde Pyelogram

❑ Description	Excretory urogram or IV urography X-ray to determine obstruction and stones through a series of x-rays
❑ What is the purpose of retrograde pyelogram?	To visualize the ureter and renal pelvis through cystoscopy Guides ureteral stent placement
❑ What is important to remember about this test?	Should be done before any barium or iodine tests
❑ Complication	Urosepsis

Cystoscopy

❑ Description	Visualization of the bladder to identify causes of hematuria, incontinence or retention and to collect urine samples
❑ Interventions	Give sedatives and antispasmodics ATB after the procedure
❑ Complication	Urosepsis

Cystogram

❑ Description	Evaluates abnormalities in bladder structure and filling through the instillation of contrast dye and x-ray
❑ How is this procedure different from voiding cystourethrogram (VCUG)	They are similar but in VCUG the client is instructed to void followed by x-rays

Urodynamic Studies

❑ Description	Determines the cause of decreased urine flow, retention and urinary incontinence
❑ What is uroflowmetry?	Measurement of urinary flow rate
❑ What is cystometrogram?	Assesses bladder tone and capacity through insertion of retention catheter and injection of saline into the bladder

24-Hour Urine Collection

❑ Description	Collection of urine for 24 hours to assess for the presence of substances (e.g. ketosteroids, creatinine clearance)
❑ Steps:	
1. Void and ______ the urine	Discard
2. Mark collection bottle with the time and date the client voided	
3. Collect urine for the entire 24 hours	
4. Last urine is voided at the ________ time the test began; Urine is added to collection.	Same
5. Entire specimen is ____________________	Refrigerated

> ***NCLEX Alert!*** *The procedure should start with an empty bladder. Repeat the test if some 24-hour urine specimens are not taken!*

C. Urinary System Disorders

Acute Glomerulonephritis

❑ Description	Inflammation of the glomeruli → RBC and protein leakage in urine
❑ Causes	Group A beta-hemolytic streptococcus
❑ Assessment	Fever, hematuria, hypertension, **periorbital edema**, anasarca, flank pain Dark, smoky, bloody urine
❑ Diagnostic Tests	↑ ASO titer, ↑ BUN and creatinine
❑ What is the purpose of the Antistreptolysin O (ASO) titer?	To determine recent strep infection
❑ Interventions	Bed rest, Steroids, Diuretics, Penicillin Fluid restriction, Monitor BP Low sodium, low protein diet

Pyelonephritis

❑ Description	Inflammation of the kidney and renal pelvis
❑ Causes	Catheterization, cystoscopy, urinary stasis sexual intercourse, E. coli infection
❑ Assessment	Flank tenderness, chills, fever, frequency, dysuria, burning sensation upon urination
❑ Interventions	Increase fluids, Avoid caffeine and alcohol Trimethoprim sulfamethoxazole (Septra)
❑ Wipe perineum from front to back after voiding	To prevent ascending infection
❑ Encourage intake of acid-forming foods	To inhibit the growth of bacteria

> ***NCLEX Alert!*** *To prevent recurrent UTI, the client should void after each sexual intercourse.*

Kidney and Ureteral Stones

❑ Description	Urolithiasis → trauma → renal colic → hydronephrosis → kidney damage
❑ Causes	Bedrest, dehydration, hyperparathyroidism
❑ What is hydronephrosis?	The kidney swells due to urine backflow
❑ What are the common compositions of stones?	Calcium oxalate or phosphate, uric acid, cysteine, magnesium phosphate

❑ Assessment	Sharp, severe flank pain (**renal colic**), chills, fever, dysuria, nephritis, nausea, vomiting
❑ What is **costovertebral angle tenderness** or Murphy's punch sign?	Pain is elicited when the area of the back overlying the kidney is percussed
❑ Where does the pain radiate?	Suprapubic region and genitalia
❑ Interventions	Narcotics, Antibiotics, Increase fluids, Limit sodium, Limit Vitamin C
❑ Calcium oxalate and phosphate stones	Give thiazide diuretics
❑ Magnesium ammonium phosphate stones	Acidify the urine
❑ Cystine and uric acid stones	Alkalinize the urine
❑ What foods should the client avoid?	Restrict **oxalate-containing** foods such as dark, leafy vegetables, rhubarb, potato chips, french fries, spinach, chocolates, tofu, tea, nuts, wheat bran, beans, berries and draft beer
❑ What is the purpose of an **acid ash diet** for alkaline stones?	To acidify the urine; Foods include meat, poultry, cheese, fish, eggs, grains, cranberries, plums and prune
❑ What is the purpose of an **alkaline ash diet** for acidic stones?	To alkalinize the urine; Foods include fruits and vegetables, except cranberries, prunes and plums
❑ Extracorporeal shock wave lithotripsy (ESWL)	Uses sound waves to destroy stones
❑ Surgery	Percutaneous nephrolithotomy Ureterolithotomy, Pyelolithotomy, Nephrolithotomy, Nephrectomy
❑ What is the purpose of a nephrostomy tube?	Catheter tube is inserted through the skin into the kidney to drain the urine
❑ Is the nephrostomy tube being irrigated?	No, unless ordered by HCP

NCLEX Alert! *A client with renal stones should be encouraged to ambulate to encourage the passage of stones. The client should be instructed to strain the urine to catch the stones. Send the stone to the laboratory in order to determine its composition!*

Polycystic Kidney Disease

❑ Description	Multiple clusters of kidney cysts
❑ What is the greatest risk factor?	Genetic (autosomal dominant transmission)
❑ Assessment	Hypertension, back pain, renal stones
❑ Interventions	Antihypertensive drugs, Epogen Nephrectomy, Renal transplant

Urinary Retention

❑ Due to general anesthesia or atropine	Acute retention
❑ Due to a neurogenic bladder	Chronic retention
❑ Interventions	ACUTE ▪ Immediate catheterization ▪ Urethral dilators CHRONIC ▪ Suprapubic cystostomy ▪ Clean intermittent catheterization (CIC)
❑ What is **Crede's maneuver**?	Gently pressing the bladder to aid voiding

Urinary Incontinence

❑ Incontinence due to disability; has normal urinary function	Functional incontinence
❑ Sudden, strong bladder contractions without warning	Reflex incontinence
❑ Accidental urination when sneezing or coughing	Stress incontinence
❑ Sudden strong urge to void before reaching the toilet	Urge incontinence
❑ Overdistended bladder leads to urine leakage	Overflow incontinence
❑ Interventions	oxybutynin (Ditropan), tolterodine (Detrol) ▪ decreases spastic bladder contractions phenoxybenzamine HCl (Dibenzaline) ▪ relaxes the urinary sphincter betanechol (Urecholine) ▪ contracts the bladder amitriptyline (Elavil) ▪ decreases bladder contractions pseudoephedrine (Sudafed) ▪ decreases stress incontinence
❑ What exercise helps improve urinary function and control?	Kegel Exercise

- Steps in performing Kegel exercise
  1. Sit or stand with legs apart; may also lie down
  2. Contract pelvic floor muscle similar to defecation or stopping the flow of urine
  3. Hold contraction for 3 seconds
  4. Release for 10 seconds, then repeat 4-5 times
  5. Repeat exercise 3 times per day

Cystitis

Description	Inflammation of the urinary bladder
Assessment	Urgency, frequency, dysuria, suprapubic pain, foul-smelling urine
Interventions	TMP-SMZ (Septra, Bactrim) Nitrofurantoin (Macrodantin) Wipe perineum from front to back Void after sexual intercourse Shower instead of bathing in a tub
What should the client avoid?	Soda, alcohol, caffeine, nylon underwear and scented toilet paper

Bladder Stones

Assessment	Hematuria, suprapubic pain, dysuria
Interventions	Low oxalate or low purine diet (based on stone composition) Transurethral cystolitholapaxy

Bladder Cancer

Causes	Smoking, bladder stones, UTI
Assessment	**Painless hematuria**, dysuria, urgency
Diagnostic Tests	Cystoscopy, Biopsy
Interventions	Chemotherapy, Radiation, Intravesical immunotherapy using BCG Topical antineoplastic drug
Surgery	Cystectomy with urinary diversion
Types of urinary diversion methods	Non-continent (Ileal conduit) Continent (creation of Kock Pouch)

D. Renal Failure

- ❑ Sudden and reversible with early treatment — Acute renal failure
- ❑ Chronic, slow, progressive and irreversible — Chronic renal failure
- ❑ Causes

PRERENAL CAUSE	INTRARENAL CAUSE	POST-RENAL CAUSE
Sudden decrease in renal blood flow	Direct injury to the kidneys	Obstruction in the urinary tract
❑ Shock ❑ Dehydration	❑ Nephritis ❑ Nephrotoxicity	❑ Benign prostate hypertrophy ❑ Bladder stones

- ❑ Phases of Acute Renal Failure

INITIATION	OLIGURIC	DIURETIC	RECOVERY
❑ Reduced blood flow ❑ Severely low glomerular filtration rate (GFR)	❑ Oliguria, edema ❑ Hypertension ❑ Azotemia ❑ Increased BUN and creatinine ❑ Hyperkalemia	❑ Usually 10-12 days after oliguric phase ❑ Nephrons recover ❑ Increased urination	❑ Usually occurs within a month ❑ Takes up to 12 months ❑ GFR returns

- ❑ Assessment (Chronic Renal Failure) — ↑ K, ↑ Phosphorus, ↑ Mg, ↑ BUN, ↑ creatinine
  ↓ Na, ↓ Ca
  metabolic acidosis, edema, hypertension, weight gain, anemia, puffy face, dry skin, lethargy, muscle cramps, osteoporosis
- ❑ What is uremic frost? — Crystallized urea deposits on the skin
- ❑ Interventions — IV bicarbonate, Calcium supplements
  Sodium polysterene sulfonate (Kayexalate)
  Low potassium, low sodium, low protein diet, Epogen, Dialysis
- ❑ Why is IV insulin and glucose given? — Decreases the potassium levels by moving potassium inside the cell
- ❑ Why is aluminum hydroxide (Amphojel) given? — Decreases the phosphorus levels

> ***NCLEX Alert!*** *A client with ESRD is placed on a low protein diet but encouraged to maximize intake of complete proteins such as meat, eggs, fish and dairy products.*

Hemodialysis

❑ Lesser risk for thrombosis and infection	Arteriovenous fistula
❑ Synthetic and requires healing time before use	Arteriovenous graft
❑ Check the graft site for redness, warmth and drainage	To determine the presence of infection
❑ Palpate the site for the presence of a thrill	To determine a well-functioning access site
❑ Auscultate for bruit	To determine a well-functioning access site
❑ Observe for ____________________ during dialysis	Disequilibrium syndrome
❑ What is **disequilibrium syndrome**?	Cerebral edema caused by waste removal
❑ What are the signs of disequilibrium syndrome?	Headache, confusion, vomiting, seizures
❑ Management for disequilibrium syndrome	Slow down the dialysis procedure

> ***NCLEX Alert!*** *Avoid pressure, injections and BP taking on the dialysis access site.*

Peritoneal Dialysis

CONTINUOUS AMBULATORY PERITONEAL DIALYSIS	CONTINUOUS CYCLIC PERITONEAL DIALYSIS	INTERMITTENT PERITONEAL DIALYSIS
❑ Instillation: 30-40 minutes ❑ Dwell: 4-10 hours ❑ Drain: 30-40 minutes ❑ Performed several times a day on a continuous basis	❑ Automated machine fills and drain dialysate while client sleeps at night ❑ Allows activities during the day	❑ Whole day or night sessions done 2-3 times a week

❑ Monitor laboratory results especially potassium	To determine presence of hyperkalemia
❑ Obtain pre- and post-dialysis weights	To determine amount of fluid to remove
❑ Is the dialysate being warmed before administration?	Yes
❑ If infusion is slow, move client from side to side	This facilitates infusion to drain
❑ Monitor blood pressure and pulse rate	To determine the presence of hypotension
❑ Clear appearance of drainage means ________	Normal
❑ Cloudy or blood-tinged drainage means ________	Abnormal (indicates infection or trauma)
❑ Complication	Peritonitis
❑ What are the signs of peritonitis?	Fever, nausea, and vomiting, abdominal tenderness, board-like rigid abdomen

E. Urinary System Drugs

1. Fluoroquinolones

- ❑ Description: Antibacterial, Treats UTI
- ❑ Drugs: Examples:
  - levofloxacin (Levaquin)
  - ciprofloxacin (Cipro)
- ❑ Side effects: Nausea, vomiting, and diarrhea
  Dizziness, drowsiness, **tendinitis**
- ❑ Interventions: Report joint pain (tendinitis)

2. Sulfonamides

- ❑ Description: Antibacterial, Treats UTI
- ❑ Drugs: Examples:
  - trimethoprim-sulfamethoxazole (TMP-SMZ) (Bactrim, Septra))
  - sulfamethoxazole, sulfadiazine
- ❑ Side effects: Allergy, blood dyscrasias, **crystalluria**, Stevens-Johnson Syndrome
- ❑ Interventions: Increase fluid intake, Monitor CBC

> ***NCLEX Alert!*** *Stevens-Johnson syndrome is a life-threatening, rare disease affecting the skin and mucous membranes and is usually a reaction to infection or a drug. The reaction starts as flu-like symptoms, followed by the appearance of red or purplish painful rash that later ruptures as blisters.*

3. Urinary Tract Analgesics

- ❑ Description: Decreases pain due to UTI
- ❑ Drugs: Examples:
  - phenazopyridine (Pyridium, Urogesic)
- ❑ Contraindications: Renal or liver disease
- ❑ Side effects: Nausea, headache, dizziness
  Red-orange or brown urine (harmless)
  Staining of contact lens
- ❑ Interventions: Given with ATB

4. Urinary Tract Antiseptics

methenamine (Mandelamine, Urex)

- ❑ Description: Treats chronic UTI
- ❑ Side effects: **Crystalluria**, nausea, diarrhea
- ❑ Interventions: Give after meals and at bedtime
  Keep urine acidic, Increase fluid intake

nalidixic acid (NegGRAM)

❑ Description	Treats UTI Can cause hypertension in children who are <3 months
❑ Side effects	Dizziness, drowsiness, blurring of vision, photosensitivity, nausea, diarrhea
❑ Interventions	Monitor CBC and liver function

nitrofurantoin (Macrodantin, Macrobid)

❑ Description	Antibacterial, Treats UTI
❑ Interventions	Give with meals
❑ Side effects	**Rusty or brown urine** (harmless), anorexia, diarrhea
❑ Interventions	Avoid taking with antacids, Take with food

NCLEX Alert!

You should take note which drugs cause urine to change color! Most of these side effects are harmless!

5. Anticholinergic-Antispasmodic Drugs

❑ Description	Treats overactive bladder and incontinence
❑ Drugs	Examples ▪ solifenacin (Vesicare) ▪ tolterodine (Detrol) ▪ darifenacin (Enablex) ▪ trospium (Sanctura) ▪ oxybutynin chloride (Ditropan)
❑ Side effects	Dry mouth, blurred vision, **constipation**
❑ Interventions	Monitor bowel movements Suck on hard candies for dry mouth

6. Cholinergic Drugs

❑ Description	Treats urinary retention
❑ Drugs	Example: betanechol chloride (Urecholine)
❑ Side effects	Salivation, abdominal cramps, vomiting, **diarrhea**, bronchoconstriction, incontinence
❑ Interventions	Use caution in clients with asthma

Immune System

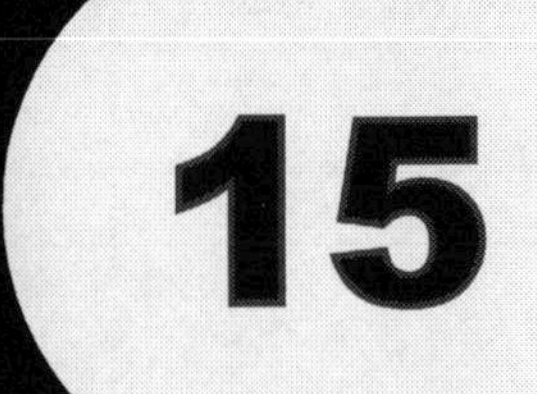

A. Immune System Disorders

Anaphylaxis

❑ Description	Severe sudden allergic reaction → release of histamine by mast cells
❑ Assessment	**Angioedema**, wheezing, itchiness, erythema, hives, stridor, hypotension, anaphylactic shock
❑ Interventions	Maintain a patent airway Elevate legs, Oxygen, IV fluid replacement, Antihistamines, Diphenhydramine, Epinephrine, Steroids

Latex Allergy

❑ Description	Allergy to proteins found in rubber latex → more frequent exposure → more allergy
❑ Exposure modes	Inhaled, Cutaneous, Parenteral route
❑ What products contain latex?	Elastic bandage, stethoscopes, BP cuff, Ambu bag, balloons, feeding tubes, condoms, diaphragms, gloves, syringes, catheters
❑ Risk factors	Multiple surgeries, **spina bifida,** allergy to grapes, potatoes, kiwis, mango, chestnut, avocados, bananas, pineapples, celery, melons, fig, papaya, tomato, apple, hazelnuts, papaya and strawberry
❑ Assessment	Contact dermatitis, redness, vesicles, crusts
❑ Interventions	Use non-latex supplies Wear Medic-Alert bracelet

Multiple Myeloma (Plasma Cell Myeloma)

❑ Description	Cancerous plasma cells infiltrate the bone marrow → pathologic fractures
❑ Assessment	Insidious onset and vague symptoms, bone pain, infection, anemia, bleeding renal failure, hyperuricemia
❑ Diagnostic Tests	**Bence-Jones protein** in urine, hypercalcemia, elevated creatinine
❑ Interventions	Chemotherapy, Analgesics, Steroids, Increase fluids, Weight-bearing exercises, Gentle handling, Protect from infection

Systemic Lupus Erythematosus

❑ Description	Chronic, systemic inflammatory disease → immune antibodies attack connective tissues → inflamed brain, blood vessels, lymph nodes, GI, kidneys and pleura
❑ Causes	Autoimmune, heredity
❑ Risk factors	Stress, medication, **UV light,** pregnancy
❑ Assessment	**Butterfly rash on face,** fever, anorexia, dry, scaly and red rashes, weight loss, malaise, joint pain, **photosensitivity**, red palms, anemia, pericarditis, nephritis
❑ Diagnostic Tests	Positive Antinuclear Antibody Test **(ANA test)** and LE cell testing Increased ESR and +C-reactive protein
❑ What is the goal of treatment?	Relief of symptoms and induce remission
❑ Interventions	Rest periods, Steroids, NSAIDs, Avoid stress and exposure to sunlight Immunosuppressants, Plasmapheresis Prevent infection

Polyarteritis Nodosa

❑ Description	Inflammation of small and medium arteries in the brain and skin (vasculitis)
❑ This condition is similar to____	SLE
❑ Assessment	Fatigue, low-grade fever, bloody stool, weight loss, elevated ESR, renal failure
❑ Interventions	Supportive care, Analgesics, Steroids

Goodpasture's Syndrome

❑ Description	Autoimmune disorder → antibodies attack the kidneys and lungs
❑ Assessment	Dyspnea, oliguria, edema, hypertension
❑ What is the goal of treatment?	Suppress the immune response
❑ Interventions	Steroids, Plasmapheresis

Pemphigus

❑ Description	Rare autoimmune disease
❑ Assessment	Fragile, huge, **painful thin bullae** Wet and crusty lesions
❑ What is Nikolsky's sign?	Separation of the epidermis even with slight rubbing of the skin
❑ What is the goal of treatment?	Suppress the immune system
❑ Interventions	Increase fluid intake, ATBs, Steroids

Lyme Disease

❑ Description	Caused by Borrelia burgdorferi transmitted through a tick bite
❑ Assessment	1. FIRST STAGE ▪ **Bulls-eye rash**, flu-like symptoms 2. SECOND STAGE ▪ Joint pain, nervous, cardiac disease 3. THIRD STAGE ▪ Severe joint pains
❑ Diagnostic Tests	ELISA and Western Blot Test
❑ Interventions	ATBs (Doxycycline, Amoxicillin) Avoid wooded areas, Tick repellant spray Wear long-sleeved dress, long pants, shoes and hats while outside

Chronic Fatigue Syndrome

- ❑ Description — Presence of profound fatigue worsened by exertion and not relieved by rest
- ❑ Cause — Infection, immune-related, stress, neurally mediated **hypotension**
- ❑ Assessment — Severe fatigue **(> 6 months),** non-restful sleep, confusion, anxiety, depression, muscle pain, headaches, IBS
- ❑ Interventions — Rest periods, Cognitive behavioral therapy

Infectious Mononucleosis (Mono/Kissing Disease)

- ❑ Description — Epstein-Barr virus → transmission through saliva → swollen lymph glands
- ❑ Assessment — Fever, sore throat, malaise, swollen tonsils
- ❑ Diagnostic Tests — EBV Test, Monospot Test
- ❑ Interventions — Self-limiting, Rest, Increase fluid intake

B. Acquired Immunodeficiency Syndrome (AIDS)

- ❑ Description — Human Immunodeficiency Virus (HIV) destroys T-cells (CD4) in order to replicate → immunosuppression → infection
- ❑ What is the normal CD4 cell count? — 500-1600 cells/mm3
- ❑ What are the 3 enzymes necessary for HIV replication? — Protease, Invirase, Reverse transcriptase
- ❑ Sources of HIV transmission — Blood, semen, vaginal fluids, breast milk
- ❑ How is HIV transmitted? — Anal or vaginal sex, injecting drugs, perinatal transmission
- ❑ When is the viral load highest? — During early and late infection
- ❑ Is HIV transmitted through saliva, urine or tears? — No
- ❑ Is HIV transmitted by hugging, dry kissing, shaking hands, sharing utensils, coughing or sneezing? — No

- Assessment

STAGE	DESCRIPTION
1. Acute HIV Infection Stage	❑ Acute Retroviral Syndrome (ARS) or Primary HIV Infection stage ❑ Within 2 to 4 weeks after infection ❑ Development of flu-like symptoms ❑ Fever, lymphadenopathy, muscle and joint pains, headache, sore throat, rash ❑ Highly infectious with decreasing CD_4 cell counts as HIV replicates ❑ Client may have produced antibodies against HIV (**seroconversion**)
2. Clinical Latency Stage	❑ Asymptomatic HIV Infection or Chronic HIV Infection stage ❑ May last for 10 years; Client remains infectious
3. AIDS Stage	❑ **CD4 <200 cells/mm3** plus clinical symptoms of opportunistic infections ❑ Cytomegalovirus, Candidiasis, Cachexia, Non-Hodgkin's lymphoma ❑ Herpes simplex, **Pneumocystis carinii** infection ❑ **Kaposi's sarcoma** (skin cancer with red or purple skin patches)

Reference: U.S. Department of Health & Human Services (www.hiv.gov)

- Diagnostic Tests

  HIV Antibody Testing
  (ELISA Test, Western Blot Test)
  Viral load monitoring
  CD4 cell count monitoring
  Polymerase Chain Reaction Test (RNA-PCR)
  Nucleic Acid Amplification Test (NAAT)

- What test confirms a positive ELISA Test?

  Western Blot Test

- How soon can a client get tested for HIV antibody production?

  2 weeks to 6 months (**window period**)
  Newer testing methods can detect HIV infection sooner by looking for the HIV-RNA instead of the antibody

- Interventions

  Highly Active Antiretroviral Therapy (HAART), Reverse isolation for clients with AIDS

- What is a Pre-Exposure Prophylaxis (PrEP) regimen?

  Includes taking a pill daily as a preventive treatment for persons who don't have HIV but are at very high risk for infection

C. Immune System Drugs

1. Immunosuppressants

- ❑ Description — Blocks rejection after organ transplant and treats autoimmune diseases
- ❑ Drugs — Examples:
  - cyclophosphamide (Neosar)
  - cyclosporine (Sandimmune, Gengraf)
  - tacrolimus (Prograf)
  - azathioprine (Imuran)
  - methotrexate (Rheumatrex, Trexall)
- ❑ Side effects — Nephrotoxicity, gastrointestinal upset, hyperlipidemia, neurotoxicity, **neutropenia**, diarrhea, hemorrhagic cystitis, cirrhosis, stomatitis, vomiting, allergy
- ❑ Interventions — Report sore throat and fever
Monitor CBC, Neutropenic precautions

2. Drugs for HIV and AIDS

NON-NUCLEOSIDE REVERSE-TRANSCRIPTASE INHIBITORS (NNRTIs)	NUCLEOSIDE/ NUCLEOTIDE REVERSE TRANSCRIPTASE INHIBITORS (NRTIs)
❑ delavirdine (Rescriptor) ❑ nevirapine (Viramune) ❑ efavirenz (Sustiva) ❑ etravirine (Intelence)	❑ zidovudine (Retrovir, AZT) ❑ tenofovir (Viread) ❑ abacavir (Ziagen) ❑ emtricitabine/tenofovir (Truvada) ❑ efavirenz/emtricitabine/tenofovir (Atripla)
PROTEASE INHIBITORS	**MISCELLANEOUS DRUGS**
❑ fosamprenavir (Lexiva) ❑ saquinavir (Invirase) ❑ indinavir (Crixivan) ❑ lopinavir/ritonavir (Kaletra) ❑ atazanavir (Reyataz) ❑ nelfinavir (Viracept) ❑ tipranavir (Aptivus) ❑ atazanavir/cobicistat (Evotaz) ❑ darunavir/cobicistat (Prezcobix)	Integrase Inhibitor ❑ raltegravir (Isentress) Fusion Inhibitor ❑ enfuvirtide (Fuzeon)

- Common side effects of HIV and AIDS drugs

Nausea
allergic reaction
diabetes mellitus
diarrhea
hepatotoxicity
hyperlipidemia
lactic acidosis
lipodystrophy (fat redistribution)
lipoatrophy (loss of fats in cheeks)
nephritis
neutropenia
osteoporosis
peripheral neuropathy
Stevens-Johnson syndrome

3. Antibiotics/Antimicrobials

CLASS	ANTIBIOTICS	DISEASES	SIDE EFFECTS
Aminoglycosides	tobramycin (Nebcin) amikacin (Amikin) kanamycin (Kantrex) gentamycin, neomycin streptomycin	endocarditis pseudomonas TB	**ototoxicity** **nephrotoxicity**
Cephalosporins	cefaclor (Ceclor) ceftriaxone (Rocephin) cefazolin (Ancef) cefdinir (Omnicef) loracarbef (Lorabid) cefadroxil (Duricef)	meningitis pneumonia peritonitis UTI's	gastric upset nephrotoxicity C. difficile superinfections allergy
Fluoroquinones	ciprofloxacin (Cipro) levofloxacin (Levaquin)	urinary and respiratory infections	headaches dizziness C. difficile bone marrow depression
Lincosamides	clindamycin (Cleocin) lincomycin (Lincocin)	streptococcal and staphylococcal infections	gastric upset bone marrow depression C. difficile
Macrolides	azithromycin (Zithromax) clarithromycin (Biaxin) erythromycin	respiratory and skin infections STD's	C. difficile gastric upset superinfections

CLASS	ANTIBIOTICS	DISEASES	SIDE EFFECTS
Monobactam	aztreonam (Azactam)	gonorrhea pseudomonas pneumonia meningitis	gastric upset hepatoxicity
Penicillins	penicillin G (Bicillin) amoxicillin (Amoxil)	respiratory, skin and urinary infections	**allergy** gastric upset superinfections
Sulfonamides	trimethoprim- sulfamethoxazole (TMP-SMZ; Bactrim, Septra) sulfasalazine sulfisoxazole sulfadiazine	UTI fungal infection inflammatory bowel disease	gastric upset nephrotoxicity hepatoxicity bone marrow depression photosensitivity **crystalluria** allergy
Tetracyclines	minocycline (Minocin) doxycycline (Vibramycin)	acne rosacea respiratory and genital infections	gastric upset **teeth staining** allergy superinfections hepatotoxicity photosensitivity

NCLEX Alert! *Superinfections refer to the occurrence of new infections due to the destruction of normal, protective bacterial flora when taking antibiotics (e.g. oral thrush, C. difficile).*

NCLEX Alert! *Antimicrobial stewardship is a program that promotes the proper use of antimicrobials to decrease bacterial resistance and spread of infections caused by multi-drug resistant organisms. (Association for Professionals in Infection Control and Epidemiology)*

Oncology Nursing

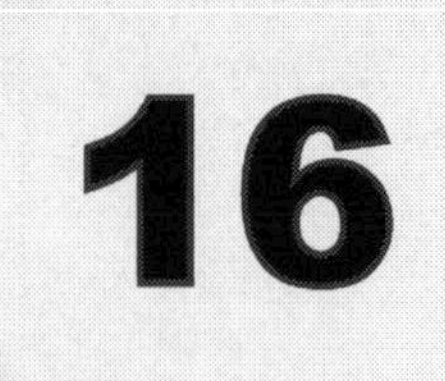

A. Cancer

❑ Slow growing and encapsulated	Benign
❑ Increases in size and causes pressure on organs	Benign
❑ Usually freely movable	Benign
❑ Metastasizes via the bloodstream and lymphatic system	Malignant
❑ Refers to the extent of spread and size of tumor	Staging
❑ TNM (tumor, node, metastasis) classification method	Staging
❑ Refers to the cellular appearance of cancer	Grading
❑ Risk factors for cancer	Smoking, Radiation, UV light, Hepa B virus, HPV, Epstein-Barr virus, H. Pylori, Obesity, Hereditary, Aging, Immunosuppression, Nitrate preservatives

Breast Self-Examination

❑ Steps:	
1. Perform breast self-examination ______ days after menstruation	3-5
2. Choose a specific ____ of the month if client is a post-menopausal female	Day
3. Use pads of fingers on shower	
4. Visually inspect breasts with mirror	
5. Lie down and palpate for breast mass including axillary area	

Testicular Self-Examination

❑ Steps:	
1. Choose a specific ______ of the month	Day
2. Best done after a warm shower or bath	Warmth relaxes the scrotum for easy exam
3. Lift and roll each testicle	
4. Feel for lump and mass and observe for changes in size shape and consistency of the testicles	

Warning Signs of Cancer

❑ What does CAUTION means in cancer?	C - hange in bowel or bladder habits A - sore that does not heal U - nusual bleeding or discharge T - hickening or lump in the breast, testicles, or elsewhere I - ndigestion or difficulty swallowing O - bvious change in the size, color, shape, or thickness of a wart, mole, or mouth sore N - agging cough or hoarseness

B. Cancer Therapies

Surgery

❑ Prevents cancer especially for those with known family history (e.g. presence of $BRCA_1$ in breast cancer)	Prophylactic
❑ Destructs the tumor using radio-frequency	Ablative
❑ Decreases pain to enhance quality of life	Palliative

Chemotherapy

❑ Description	Destroys both cancer and normal cells Systemic effect on skin, hair, GI, sperms, and blood cells
❑ Side effects	Alopecia, nausea and vomiting, mucositis, immunosuppression, anemia, thrombocytopenia, **hyperuricemia**
❑ Is the hair loss permanent?	No

> ***NCLEX Alert!*** *Side effects of chemotherapeutic drugs are serious so make sure you remember them!*

Radiation Therapy

EXTERNAL BEAM RADIATION	BRACHYTHERAPY
❑ External radiation rays focused into tumor ❑ Client does not emit radiation ❑ Radiation precautions **not** required	❑ Direct contact with a tumor for a period of time ❑ Client emits radiation and a danger to others ❑ Requires radiation precautions

Question	Answer
❑ Side effects	Skin irritation, alopecia, fatigue
❑ Guidelines for external radiation therapy	Wash area with mild soap and water Do not erase markings Avoid exposure to the sun
❑ What are the 3 principles of radiation precautions?	TIME – 15-minute exposure period only DISTANCE – 6 feet away from client SHIELDING – Use lead shield
❑ Interventions for sealed radiation source	Provide private room and bathroom Place caution sign on door Place flat on bed to prevent dislodgment Use dosimeter badge to monitor exposure Rotate nursing staff who cares for client Restrict visitors <16 years-old Pregnant staff not allowed to care for client Save linens and dressings until implant is removed
❑ What should you do when the radiation implant is accidentally dislodged?	Use **long-handled forceps** to pick up dislodged implant Place implant in lead container Report incident to radiation department

Bone Marrow Transplantation

Question	Answer
❑ Description	Used for treatment of leukemia, lymphoma, myeloma and aplastic anemia Given with high doses of chemotherapy
❑ Types	Autologous (stem cells from self) Allogenic (stem cells from another person)
❑ Is this procedure given through central line transfusion?	Yes

C. Chemotherapy or Antineoplastic Drugs

Question	Answer
❑ General side effects	Neutropenia, alopecia, anemia, anorexia cardiotoxicity, diarrhea, mucositis, nausea and vomiting, sterility, thrombocytopenia

Interventions for Chemotherapy Drug Side Effects

Side Effect	Intervention
❑ Neutropenia	Avoid crowds, ill visitors, fresh flowers and raw foods Monitor CBC and differential counts Monitor for fever and sore throat
❑ Thrombocytopenia	Bleeding precautions Use a soft toothbrush and electric razor
❑ Cardiotoxicity	Monitor ejection fraction (EF%)
❑ Mucositis	Avoid strong mouthwash
❑ Hyperuricemia	Give allopurinol (Zyloprim)
❑ Sterility	Discuss options for sperm banking
❑ Alopecia	Purchase a wig before treatment to match the original hair
Chemotherapy Administration Safety Considerations	Ensure good air flow in the room Avoid preparing the drug when pregnant Assess for extravasation and phlebitis

Chemotherapy Drugs

ALKYLATING DRUGS		ANTITUMOR ATB DRUGS
NITROGEN MUSTARDS ❑ chlorambucil (Leukeran) ❑ mechlorethamine (Mustargen) ❑ melphalan (Alkeran) ❑ cyclophosphamide (Neosar) NITROSOUREAS ❑ streptozocin (Zanosar) ❑ carmustine (BiCNU, Gliadel)	ALKYLATING-LIKE DRUGS ❑ carboplatin (Paraplatin) ❑ busulfan (Myleran) ❑ cisplatin (Platinol)	ANTHRACYCLINES ❑ daunorubicin ❑ mitomycin-C ❑ actinomycin-D ❑ bleomycin doxorubicin (Adriamycin®)
ANTIMETABOLITE DRUGS	**ANTIMITOTIC DRUGS**	**TOPOISOMERASE INHIBITORS**
❑ 5-fluorouracil (5-FU) ❑ hydroxyurea ❑ methotrexate ❑ pemetrexed (Alimta) ❑ 6-mercaptopurine (6-MP) ❑ cytarabine (Ara-C)	❑ taxanes: paclitaxel (Taxol) and docetaxel (Taxotere) ❑ estramustine (Emcyt) ❑ vinca alkaloids: vinblastine (Velban), vincristine (Oncovin)	TOPOISOMERASE I INHIBITORS ❑ topotecan (Hycamtin, Potactasol) TOPOISOMERASE II INHIBITORS ❑ teniposide (Vumon) ❑ etoposide (VP-16, Toposar)

1. Hormonal Drugs

Estrogens

❑ Description	Treats advanced breast, endometrial and prostate cancer
❑ Drugs	Examples: ▪ estramustine (Emcyt)
❑ Side effects	Breast tenderness (males), leg swelling, nausea, diarrhea, decreased libido

Antiestrogens

❑ Description	Treats breast cancer
❑ Drugs	Examples: ▪ tamoxifen citrate (Nolvadex, Soltamox) ▪ anastrozole (Arimidex) ▪ raloxifine (Evista) ▪ exemestane (Aromasin) ▪ letrozole (Femara)
❑ Side effects	Gastric upset, blurred vision, dizziness

Progestins

❑ Description	Treats advanced breast and endometrial cancer Megestrol is also used for anorexia
❑ Drugs	Examples: ▪ megestrol acetate (Megace) ▪ medroxyprogesterone (Depo-Provera)
❑ Side effects	Nausea, diarrhea, vaginal bleeding, weight gain

Antiandrogens

❑ Description	Treats prostate cancer
❑ Drugs	Examples: ▪ bicalutamide (Casodex) ▪ goserelin acetate (Zoladex) ▪ flutamide (Eulexin) ▪ triptorelin (Trelstar)
❑ Side effects	**Decreased libido**, impotence, diarrhea, feeling of warmth

Other Hormonal Antagonists and Enzymes

- ❑ Description — Asparaginase treats acute lymphocytic leukemia
  Leuprolide treats prostate cancer in men and endometriosis in women
- ❑ Drugs — Examples:
  - leuprolide acetate (Lupron)
  - asparaginase (Elspar)

> ***NCLEX Alert!*** *HORMONAL DRUGS CAN CAUSE SEXUAL ALTERATIONS*
> *Androgens → decreased menstruation, hirsutism and virilization effect in women*
> *Estrogens → decreased libido, gynecomastia and feminization effect in men*

2. Immunomodulatory Drugs (Biologic Response Modifiers)

- ❑ Description — Stimulates the immune system to identify and destroy cancer cells
- ❑ Drugs — Examples:
  - interferon alfa-2a (Roferon-A)
  - aldesleukin (Proleukin, Interleukin-2)

3. Monoclonal Antibodies

- ❑ Description — Synthetic antibody made in laboratory to mimic the action of the immune system
- ❑ Drugs — Examples:
  - rituximab (Rituxan)
  - trastuzumab (Herceptin)
  - alemtuzumab (Campath)

4. Cell Stimulating Drugs (Colony-Stimulating Factors)

- ❑ Description — Stimulates the production of blood cells

GRANULOCYTE STIMULATING FACTOR	ERYTHROPOIESIS STIMULATING FACTOR	THROMBOPOIESIS STIMULATING FACTOR
Increases the WBC count	Increases the RBC count	Increases the platelet count
Drugs ❑ pegfilgrastim (Neulasta) ❑ filgrastrim (Neupogen) ❑ sargramostim (Leukine)	Drugs ❑ epoetin alfa (Epogen) ❑ darbepoetin alfa (Aranesp)	Drugs ❑ oprelvekin (Interleukin-11, Neumega) ❑ romiplostim (Nplate) ❑ eltrombopag (Promacta)

Reproductive System

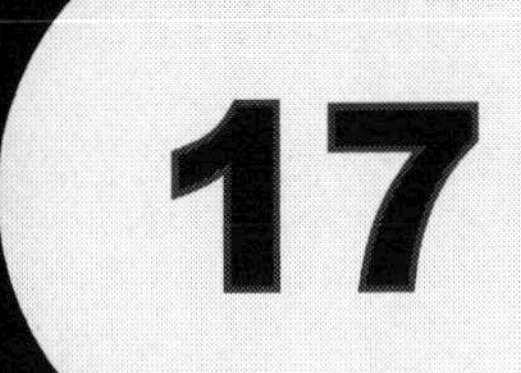

A. The Reproductive System

The Female Reproductive System

❑ External structures	Mons pubis, vulva, labia majora and minora, clitoris, Bartholin glands or bulbourethral glands, fourchette, hymen
❑ Internal structures	Vagina, uterus, fallopian tubes, ovaries
❑ Monthly release of an ovum	Ovulation
❑ Hormone responsible for the development of follicle	Follicle-Stimulating Hormone (FSH)
❑ Hormone that stimulates rupture of the follicle (ovulation)	Luteinizing Hormone (LH)
❑ Secretes progesterone after ovulation	Corpus luteum
❑ Implantation occurs ___ days after fertilization	7
❑ Ovulation occurs ___ weeks before menstruation	2
❑ Promotes breast development	Estrogen
❑ Promotes milk production	Prolactin
❑ Hormone that maintains pregnancy	Progesterone
❑ Promotes the development of secondary female sex characteristics	Estrogen and Progesterone
❑ Promotes milk ejection and uterine contractions	Oxytocin

The Male Reproductive System

❑ External structures	Penis, scrotum, prepuce
❑ Internal structures	Testes, epididymis, ductus deferens, spermatic cord
❑ Accessory structures	Seminal vesicles, prostate gland, bulbourethral glands
❑ Hormone that promotes development of secondary male sex characteristics	Testosterone
❑ What does the prostate gland secrete?	Alkaline substance to protect the sperm from the acidity of the vagina

B. Diagnostic Tests

Breast Self-Examination

❑ Done at age _____ years and older	20
❑ Perform ____ days after end of menstruation	3-5

Mammography

❑ Done at ____ years of age or prior depending on history; every 1-2 years after	40

> ***NCLEX Alert!*** *The client should avoid using deodorant with aluminum hydroxide or talc under the arms or breasts before mammography. These will make the images harder to read due to the presence of artifacts.*

Papanicolaou (Pap) Test

❑ Performed ___ weeks after the first day of last menstrual period (LMP)	2
❑ Initial Pap Test should start at ____ years of age	21
❑ Females aged 21 to 29, should have a Pap test every ___ years	3
❑ What instructions are important to teach the client?	Avoid sex, douching and vaginal foams

HPV DNA Testing

❑ Done at ____ years of age or older	30
❑ Testing is not recommended before the age of 30	
❑ Performed with the Pap test every ___ years	5

Laparoscopy

❑ Description	Examination of the abdomen and involves small incisions below the umbilicus
❑ What gas is injected into the abdomen?	Carbon dioxide

Hysterosalpingogram

❑ Description	X-ray of the uterus and fallopian tubes

Abdominal Ultrasound

❑ Description	Drink 1 quart of water before the test Client should not void before procedure

C. Female Reproductive System Disorders

Menopause

❑ Description	Ovaries stop functioning → decreased estrogen and progesterone → cessation of menstruation
❑ Assessment	Menstrual irregularities, **hot flashes**, insomnia, vaginal dryness, dyspareunia, decreased libido, night sweats, alopecia, breast and uterine atrophy, **osteoporosis**, **cardiovascular disease, stroke**, depression
❑ Interventions	Hormonal Replacement Therapy (HRT) Low-dose androgens, Antidepressants alendronate (Fosamax), raloxifene (Evista)

Premature Ovarian Failure

❑ Description	Ovaries stop releasing hormones at age <40 years → infertility
❑ Assessment	Menstrual irregularities, menopause
❑ Interventions	Manage symptoms of menopause

Pelvic Inflammatory Disease (PID)

❑ Description	Infection of the uterus, fallopian tubes, and ovaries
❑ Causes	STDs (gonorrhea, chlamydia)
❑ Assessment	Foul-smelling discharge, pelvic pain, fever,
❑ Interventions	Bed rest, ATBs, Contact isolation

Endometriosis

❑ Description	Endometrial cells develop outside uterus Disappears with menopause
❑ Assessment	**Dysmenorrhea**, menorrhagia, abdominal, pelvic or vaginal pain, dyspareunia, infertility
❑ Diagnostic Tests	Ultrasound reveals **"chocolate cysts"**
❑ Interventions	Estrogen-progestin contraceptive
❑ Surgery	Cauterization, Ablation, Panhysterectomy

Pelvic Organ Prolapse

- ❑ Description — Pelvic organ drops and presses on vagina
- ❑ Types — CYSTOCELE - bladder
  RECTOCELE - rectum
  ENTEROCELE - intestines
  UTERINE PROLAPSE – uterus
- ❑ Causes — **Childbirth**, obesity, constipation, cancer
- ❑ Assessment — **Stress incontinence**, cystitis, back pain,
- ❑ Interventions — Pessary device insertion, Kegel exercise
- ❑ What is a pessary? — A device inserted into the vagina to support the uterus
- ❑ Surgery — Anterior or posterior colporrhaphy
  Vaginal hysterectomy

> ***NCLEX Alert!*** *Clients with pelvic organ prolapse are at risk for cervical cancer!*

Vaginal Fistulas

- ❑ Description — An abnormal connection between the vagina and bladder or rectum
- ❑ Types — RECTOVAGINAL – rectum and vagina
  URETHROVAGINAL – urethra and vagina
  VESICOVAGINAL – bladder and vagina
- ❑ Causes — **Childbirth**, cancer, radiation, surgery
- ❑ Assessment — Leaking of urine or stool from vagina
  Malodorous, foul-smelling discharge
- ❑ Interventions — Skin care, Emotional support

Uterine Displacement

- ❑ Description — Uterus deviates from normal position
- ❑ Types — RETROVERSION – backward tilting
  ANTEVERSION – forward tilting
  RETROFLEXION– bending towards rectum

- ❑ Assessment — **Dysmenorrhea**, backache, painful sex
- ❑ Interventions — Surgery, Pessary insertion
- ❑ Why should the client assume a knee-chest position several times a day? — To reposition the retroverted uterus

Uterine Leiomyoma (Myoma or Fibroid Tumors)

- ❑ Description — Benign tumor growth in the uterus
- ❑ Cause — Estrogen
- ❑ Assessment — Disappears with menopause; Menorrhagia, dysmenorrhea, pressure
- ❑ Interventions — Dilatation and curettage, Myomectomy

Endometrial and Cervical Cancer

- ❑ Risk factors

ENDOMETRIAL CANCER	CERVICAL CANCER
❑ Nulliparity	❑ Multiple sexual partners
❑ Early menarche, late menopause	❑ Sexually active at an early age
❑ >50 years of age taking estrogens or HRT	❑ HPV infection
❑ Obesity, Diabetes mellitus	❑ Smoking

- ❑ Assessment — **Vaginal bleeding**, pelvic pain, dyspareunia, cachexia, weakness
- ❑ Interventions — Chemotherapy, Radiation, Hysterectomy
- ❑ How can cervical cancer be prevented? — Gardasil vaccination (9-26 years-old); Children receive shots at 11-12 years-old

Ovarian Cancer

- ❑ Risk factors — Family history, breast cancer, nulliparous
- ❑ Assessment — **Vague lower abdominal pain**, bloating, change in bowel habits, urinary frequency, urgency, mass felt during exam
- ❑ Interventions — Chemotherapy, Radiation, Prophylactic bilateral oophorectomy, Total hysterectomy
- ❑ How can ovarian cancer be prevented? — Pregnancy, breastfeeding, contraceptives

Toxic Shock Syndrome

- ❑ Description — Fatal sepsis caused by staphylococcus
- ❑ Causes — **Use of superabsorbent tampons**, internal contraceptives, open wounds
- ❑ Assessment — High fever, chills, nausea, vomiting
- ❑ Interventions — ATBs, IVF replacement, dopamine (Intropin)

Cancer of the Breast

- ❑ Risk factors — Female >30 age, family history radiation, alcohol, nulliparous, obesity, early menarche, late menopause, late age of pregnancy
- ❑ What are $BRCA_1$ or $BRCA_2$? — Genes linked to breast cancer
- ❑ Assessment — Painless mass, fixed or movable lesion, **"peau de orange"** appearance, asymmetry of the breast size, bloody discharge from nipples, dimpling of breast skin, retraction or inversion of nipple, enlarged axillary lymph nodes
- ❑ What is sentinel lymph node mapping? — Method to determine if the breast cancer cells have spread to adjacent lymph nodes in the axillary region
- ❑ Drugs for Breast Cancer

ANTI-ESTROGEN DRUGS	AROMATASE INHIBITORS	ANTIPROGESTIN	IMMUNE TARGETED THERAPY
Treats estrogen-sensitive breast cancer Blocks the effects of estrogen	Decreases estrogen levels	Treats progesterone-dependent cancer	Monoclonal antibody that stops the growth of cancer
❑ tamoxifen (Nolvadex)	❑ anastrazole (Arimidex) ❑ letrozole (Femara) ❑ exemestane (Aromasin)	❑ mifepristone (RU486)	❑ transtuzumab (Herceptin)

❑ Surgery

SIMPLE/TOTAL MASTECTOMY	MODIFIED RADICAL MASTECTOMY	RADICAL MASTECTOMY
Removal of the breast with no lymph node dissection	Removal of the breast, some lymph nodes, lining over the pectoralis minor and chest muscles	Removal of the breast, axillary lymph nodes and minor and major pectoralis muscles

❑ Interventions after radical mastectomy with removal of axillary lymph nodes

Elevate arm on surgical side to reduce lymphedema
Avoid BP taking, injections and arm abduction on surgical side
Encourage deep breathing and coughing
Splint the incision during activity
Manage negative-pressure drains

D. Male Reproductive System Disorders

Benign Prostatic Hyperplasia (BPH)

❑ Description

Increase in prostate size due to aging
→ obstruction of the urethra
→ weak urinary stream and cystitis

❑ Assessment

Remember FUN!

- F – requency of urination
- U – rgency of urination
- N – octuria

❑ Diagnostic Test

Digital Rectal Exam (DRE)

❑ Interventions

terazosin (Hytrin)

- Relaxes the muscles in the prostate and treats urinary symptoms

finasteride (Proscar, Propecia)

- Androgen hormone inhibitor

❑ Surgery

Transurethral Resection of Prostate (TURP)
Suprapapubic Prostatectomy
Perineal Prostatectomy

❑ Complications

Hemorrhage, thrombosis, infection

- ❑ What is the purpose of the **three-way Foley catheter** after TURP surgery?

  To irrigate the bladder and remove clots
  Discontinued after 24 hours if no clots are present
  Monitor for **hyponatremia** due to the use of hypotonic irrigating solution

- ❑ Why is it important to maintain the patency of the three-way Foley catheter?

  Bladder distention and spasms can cause bleeding

- ❑ What instructions are important to teach the client after prostate surgery?

  Avoid straining and heavy lifting
  Perform Kegel exercises to treat urinary incontinence

> ***NCLEX Alert!*** *Transurethral resection of the prostate (TURP) can cause retrograde ejaculation and urinary incontinence. Perineal prostatectomy can cause permanent erectile dysfunction.*

Cancer of the Prostate

- ❑ Causes

  Increased **testosterone**, High fat diet

- ❑ Assessment

  Urinary frequency, nocturia, dysuria

- ❑ Diagnostic Tests

  Digital rectal exam (DRE)
  Prostate specific antigen (PSA) level

- ❑ Interventions

  Radiation, Chemotherapy
  Suprapubic or radical prostatectomy

- ❑ Why is bilateral orchiectomy performed?

  To stop the production of testosterone which enhances the growth of cancer

- ❑ When is prostate cancer screening recommended?

  At age 50 years-old or earlier if high-risk
  Tests include DRE and PSA level

Erectile Dysfunction (Impotence)

- ❑ Types

  Physiological and psychogenic

- ❑ Causes

  Diabetes mellitus, spinal cord injury, decreased testosterone, depression

- ❑ Diagnostic Tests

  NOCTURNAL PENILE TUMESCENCE TEST

- Involves application of an elastic device around the penis during sleep
- Absence of spontaneous erections during sleep indicates that the cause of erectile dysfunction is organic or physiologic in nature

❑ Interventions

Oral phosphodiesterase type 5 inhibitors (PDE5)

- sildenafil (Viagra)
- avanafil (Stendra)
- vardenafil (Levitra)
- tadalafil (Cialis)

❑ When is the best time to take PDE5 inhibitors?

30 minutes-1 hour before sexual activity

❑ What are the side effects of PDE5 inhibitors?

Hypotension, mild headache, flushing

Maternity Nursing

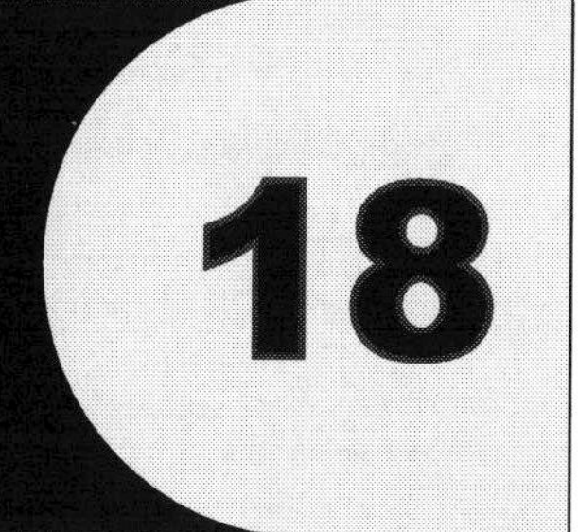

A. Female Reproductive System

Female Pelvis

❑ Normal, round; Favorable for delivery	Gynecoid
❑ Heart-shaped; Favorable for delivery	Android
❑ Oval-shaped; Normal or narrow	Anthropoid
❑ Flat and narrow; Not favorable for delivery due to short antero-posterior diameters	Platypelloid

Menstrual Cycle

❑ What are the 3 phases of the menstrual cycle?	Proliferative, secretory, menstrual phase
❑ Average regular menstrual cycle is ____ days	28
❑ Menstrual phase lasts for ____ days	3-5
❑ Ovulation occurs ____ days before menstruation	14

Hormones

❑ Stimulates the maturation and development of the ovum	Follicle-stimulating hormones (FSH)
❑ Stimulates endometrial growth and proliferation	Estrogen
❑ What hormone is high before ovulation?	Estrogen
❑ Promotes ovulation	Luteinizing hormones (LH)
❑ What hormone remains high after ovulation and prepares the uterus after fertilization?	Progesterone
❑ What structure secretes estrogen and progesterone after ovulation?	Corpus luteum

Fertilization

❑ Sperm lifespan	3-5 days
❑ Ovum lifespan	12-24 hours
❑ Fertilization occurs in the ____ of the fallopian tube	Outer third
❑ A fertilized ovum is called a ____________	Zygote
❑ A zygote has ____ chromosomes	46 (23 from each parent)

❑ XY: _______ and XX: _______	Male, Female
❑ What determines the sex of the fetus?	Sperm cell carries X or Y chromosome that fuses with the egg cell's X chromosome

Implantation

❑ Fertilized ovum (zygote) travels to the _______	Uterus
❑ Implantation occurs approximately after ____ days after fertilization	7-10
❑ Zygote becomes a morula then becomes a _______	Blastocyst
❑ A blastocyst secretes _______	Human chorionic gonadotropin (hCG)
❑ The presence of hCG is the basis for a positive _______	Pregnancy test (6 days after fertilization)

Major Milestones in Fetal Development

❑ **Development of embryo**	3rd - 8th Week
❑ Formation of the brain and spinal cord	Week 4
❑ Closure of neural tube structure	Week 8
❑ **Development of fetus**	9th Week – Birth
❑ Heart rate detectable with a Doppler device	Week 10
❑ Kidneys secrete urine	Week 12
❑ Lanugo covers the entire body	Week 20
❑ Fetal heart tones heard with a fetoscope	Week 16
❑ **Period of viability**	Week 20
❑ What is viability?	Fetus is able to survive when delivered
❑ Vernix caseosa, alveoli and surfactant production	Week 24
❑ Lungs are fully developed	Week 28
❑ Testes descend into the scrotum	Week 28

Amniotic Fluid

❑ Functions	Acts as a cushion, Protection from infection
❑ Does the fetus swallow amniotic fluid?	Yes
❑ Normal amount: _________ mL	800-1200
❑ Oligohydramnios = ________	<500 mL of amniotic fluid
❑ Polyhydramnios = ________	>1000 mL of amniotic fluid

Placenta

❑ Functions	Fetal nourishment, Excretion (e.g. urine)
❑ Fully developed at _________	Week 12
❑ Umbilical cord has ___ arteries and ___ vein	2, 1

Fetal Circulation Bypass Structures

❑ Diverts blood from the liver as it returns from the placenta	Ductus venosus
❑ Directs blood from the right to the left atrium, bypassing the lungs	Foramen ovale
❑ Diverts blood from the pulmonary artery into the aorta, bypassing the lungs	Ductus arteriosus
❑ Do these fetal structures close after birth?	Yes

B. Prenatal Assessment and Diagnostic Tests

❑ Approximately how long is a normal pregnancy?	280 days or 40 weeks

FIRST TRIMESTER	SECOND TRIMESTER	THIRD TRIMESTER
Week 1-13	Week 14-26	Week 27-40

Naegele's Rule

❑ Description	Estimates Expected Date of Delivery (EDD) Applies to a regular 28-day menstrual cycle

FORMULA: -3 +7 +1

1. Obtain the first day of the last menstrual period (LMP) (Ex. October 9, 2013)
2. Subtract 3 months (July 9, 2013)
3. Add 7 days (July 16, 2013)
4. Change the year = EDD of July 16, 2014

You should note which months have 30 days (September, April, June and November) or 31 days; February is always 28 days

Example: LMP of November 28, 2017 = EDD of September 4, 2018

NCLEX Alert! *Year is not changed when pregnancy ends in same year!*

Terminologies

❑ Pregnancy	Gravida
❑ Never been pregnant	Nulligravida
❑ First pregnancy	Primigravida
❑ Having more than one pregnancy	Multigravida
❑ Number of pregnancy that reached viability	Parity
❑ Never had pregnancy that reached viability	Nullipara
❑ First pregnancy that reached viability	Primipara
❑ Having pregnancies that reached viability periods	Multipara

NCLEX Alert! *Parity does not refer to the number of live births. Rather, it refers to the number of pregnancies that reached the period of viability – which is at 20 weeks.*

GTPAL System

❑ Description	An acronym used by clinicians to determine a client's obstetrical history
❑ GTPAL means ________	G- ravidity T - erm births (after 37th week) P - reterm births (before 37th week) A – bortions L - ive births
❑ Example: Elizabeth is 26 weeks pregnant. Her previous three pregnancies ended in a live birth at 38 weeks. She also had a pregnancy that terminated at 10 weeks.	Answer: G-5, T-3, P-0, A-1, L-3

Signs of Pregnancy

PRESUMPTIVE SIGNS	PROBABLE SIGNS	POSITIVE SIGNS
❑ Amenorrhea ❑ Nausea and vomiting ❑ Urinary frequency ❑ Increased breast size ❑ Quickening ❑ Fatigue ❑ Discoloration of vaginal membranes	❑ Goodell's sign ❑ Hegar's sign ❑ Chadwick's sign ❑ Ballottement ❑ Braxton-Hick's contractions ❑ Uterine enlargement ❑ + Pregnancy test	❑ Fetal outline on x-ray or ultrasound ❑ Fetal movements felt on palpation ❑ Presence of FHR → Doppler 10-12 weeks → Fetoscope 20 weeks

❑ What is quickening?	Mother feels the first fetal movement (around 16-20 weeks) Occurs earlier for multiparous women
❑ What is Goodell's sign?	Softening of the cervix
❑ What is Chadwick's sign?	Bluish discoloration of the cervix, vagina, and labia due to increased vascularization
❑ What is Hegar's sign?	Softening of the lower uterine segment
❑ What is ballottement?	Manual vaginal exam elicits **rebound impact** of floating fetus when pushing upward against the uterine wall
❑ What is Braxton-Hick's contractions?	Infrequent and irregular uterine contractions where the uterus contracts for 30 to 60 seconds then stops
❑ Braxton-Hick's contractions begin around the ____ trimester but are commonly experienced on ____ trimester	2nd 3rd

Diagnostic Tests During Pregnancy

❑ Confirms gestational age and Expected Date of Delivery; Done during 18 and 20 weeks but may have one before 12 weeks to confirm due date	Ultrasound
❑ Evaluates fetal well-being; Assesses the fetal heart rate, movements, breathing, muscle tone and amniotic fluid index through ultrasound and non-stress test	Biophysical Profile
❑ Detect hepatitis B infection	Hepatitis B Surface Antigen Testing
❑ Detects gonorrhea, syphilis, herpes and chlamydia	Venereal Diseases (STDs) Testing
❑ Detects bacteria which can infect the mother's uterus, urinary tract and also harm the fetus during birth; Specimen is taken from the vagina and rectum	Group B Streptococcus Testing
❑ Test done for women who have TB symptoms or are at high risk for TB; If positive, chest x-ray is done after 20 weeks gestation when fetal organs are fully developed	Mantoux Skin Test
❑ Detects rubella antibody	Rubella Testing

> ***NCLEX Alert!*** *Hepatitis B vaccine may be given during pregnancy.*

❑ Detects infections that can harm the fetus	Toxoplasmosis, Rubella, Cytomegalovirus, Herpes Simplex and HIV (TORCH) Panel
❑ Detects if mother is a sickle cell carrier	Sickle Cell Screening
❑ Detects gestational diabetes mellitus; Performed between 26 to 28 weeks	Glucose Tolerance Test
❑ Mother monitors fetal movements; Instruct mother to report **<10 kicks** in a consecutive 2-hour period; Performed starting week 28	Kick Counts
❑ Assesses fetal well-being and FHR in response to fetal movement; Performed after 28 weeks gestation	Non-Stress Testing
❑ Assesses placental function and oxygenation and fetal well-being during stress of contractions through the IV administration of oxytocin; Done during 34 or more weeks pregnant	Contraction Stress Testing
❑ Examines blood from the fetal umbilical cord to detect genetic abnormalities	Umbilical Cord Sampling (cordocentesis)
❑ Detects genetic disorders; Obtains sample of chorionic villi through needle aspiration	Chorionic Villi Sampling
❑ Detects genetic disorders and assesses fetal **lung maturity** (**L/S ratio: 2:1**); Done during 15 and 20 weeks of pregnancy, if recommended; After week 32 of pregnancy if risk of pre-term delivery	Amniocentesis
❑ Detects **neural tube** defects (spina bifida) and Down Syndrome; Done between 15 and 20 weeks	Alpha-Fetoprotein (AFP) Test
❑ Determines presence of amniotic fluid in the vaginal secretions; BLUE COLOR → amniotic fluid	Nitrazine Paper Test
❑ Specimen collected from cervix and visualized through microscope; FERNLIKE PATTERN → amniotic fluid	Fern Test

NCLEX Alert! *Rubella vaccine is never given during pregnancy. A woman should also not get pregnant 1-3 months after receiving a rubella vaccination. The live virus vaccine can harm the developing fetus!*

Contraction Stress Test

- ❑ Uterus is stimulated to contract by administering ________ or stimulating the ________ — Oxytocin, nipple
- ❑ Negative result (normal) — Absence of late or variable decelerations
- ❑ Positive result (abnormal) — Presence of late decelerations with more than 50% of the contractions

Non-Stress Test

- ❑ Mother will be instructed to press a button every time she experiences fetal ________________. — Movement
- ❑ "Reactive" indicates a ________________. — Normal result or healthy fetus
- ❑ Normal result — 2 or more FHR accelerations in 20 minutes; At least 15 beats above baseline FHR; Lasting at least 15 seconds

Measuring Fundal Height

- ❑ 14-16 weeks — Fundus is above the symphysis pubis
- ❑ 20-22 weeks — Fundus is at the level of umbilicus
- ❑ 36 weeks — Fundus is at the xiphoid process

Leopold's Maneuver

- ❑ Description — Palpation for determining presentations and fetal heart sounds
- ❑ How are fetal positions determined in Leopold's maneuver? — Head (movable, round, hard)
  Back (firm, smooth surface)
  Buttocks (irregular, soft surface)
  Hands, feet, elbows and knees (small irregularities)
- ❑ Steps in Leopold's maneuver —
  FIRST MANEUVER
  - determines the presenting part

  SECOND MANEUVER
  - determines the fetal back

  THIRD MANEUVER
  - determines engagement

  FOURTH MANEUVER
  - determines fetal attitude and descent

External Version

- ❑ Description — Procedure to change an abnormal presentation (e.g. breech, transverse) into a vertex presentation
- ❑ When is this procedure usually done? — Between 36 and 38 weeks to prevent preterm birth
- ❑ What are the contraindications of this procedure? — Cephalopelvic disproportion, placenta previa, active herpes, multiple pregnancies

Danger Signs of Pregnancy

- ❑ What are the dangers signs of pregnancy? —
  Severe, persistent vomiting
  blurred vision or dizziness
  chills with fever over 38°C (100.4°F)
  decreased or absent fetal movements
  dyspnea
  dysuria or oliguria
  edema of the feet and hands
  epigastric or abdominal pain
  severe, persistent headache
  sudden vaginal fluid discharge
  vaginal bleeding

C. Prenatal Period

Normal Changes During Pregnancy

- ❑ What are the normal changes during pregnancy? —
  Blood volume increases by 50%
  dyspnea due to enlarging uterus
  water and sodium retention
  formation of mucus plug
  urinary frequency ($1^{st}/3^{rd}$ trimesters)
  vascular spider nevi on face, neck or chest
  darkened areolae
  chloasma gravidarum (mask of pregnancy)
  linea nigra (dark line across the abdomen)
  striae gravidarum (stretch marks)
  Chadwick's Sign
- ❑ What is physiologic anemia? — Decreased concentration of hemoglobin due to **hemodilution** that results from increase in maternal blood volume

❑ What is the initial emotional reaction to pregnancy?	Ambivalence due to fear of the unknown and anticipated role and body image changes

Interventions for Discomforts of Pregnancy

Discomfort	Intervention
❑ Nausea and vomiting	Eat dry crackers upon awakening
❑ Urinary frequency	Perform Kegel's exercises
❑ Increased vaginal discharge	Wear absorbent cotton underwear
❑ Ankle edema	Elevate feet, Avoid prolonged standing
❑ Leg cramps	Increase calcium intake, Dorsiflex the foot
❑ Hemorrhoids	Perform warm sitz bath
❑ Back pain	Perform **pelvic rocking** exercise
❑ Constipation	Eat high-fiber foods, Increase fluid intake
❑ Syncope	Change positions slowly Avoid lying in supine position Elevate legs

Nutritional Needs During Pregnancy

❑ What is the normal weight gain during pregnancy?	25-35 lbs. Gains 3 lbs. for the first trimester; then 1 lb per week thereafter
❑ How many extra calories are needed during pregnancy?	300 calories per day
❑ How many extra calories are needed during lactation?	300-500 per day
❑ How many milligrams of folic acid is needed to prevent spina bifida?	0.4 mg per day
❑ How many milligrams of calcium is needed?	1000 mg per day
❑ Is alcohol intake safe during pregnancy?	No, it can cause fetal alcohol syndrome

Prenatal Visit Schedules

❑ Weeks 4 to 28	1 prenatal visit a month
❑ Weeks 28 to 36	1 prenatal visit every 2 weeks
❑ Weeks 36 to 40	1 prenatal visit every week

D. Complications of Pregnancy

Abortion

❑ Description	Pregnancy terminates before period of viability (20 weeks)
❑ Passage of some fetal tissues	Incomplete abortion
❑ Failure to expel a dead fetus	Missed abortion
❑ 3 or more abortions in pregnancies	Recurrent abortion
❑ Cervix is closed with intermittent, slight bleeding	Threatened abortion
❑ Cervix dilates with increased bleeding and cramps; Delivery is unavoidable	Inevitable abortion
❑ Expulsion of all products of conception	Complete abortion
❑ Interventions	Bed rest, Dilation and curettage, Count perineal pads, RhoGAM given as needed

Gestational Diabetes

❑ Description	Maternal hyperglycemia → fetus receives more glucose and produces insulin
❑ Risk factors	Age >35, multiple pregnancies, obesity genetics
❑ When does this condition occur?	2nd /3rd trimester
❑ When is glucose screening performed?	24-28 weeks of pregnancy
❑ What are the insulin needs during pregnancy?	1st trimester → ↓ insulin needs 2nd and 3rd trimesters → ↑ insulin needs After delivery → ↓ insulin needs
❑ What are the risks associated with this condition?	**Fetal macrosomia**, **hypoglycemia**, hyperbilirubinemia, congenital anomalies respiratory distress syndrome
❑ Assessment	3 P's (polyuria polydipsia, polyphagia) weight loss, UTI, fungal infections, polyhydramnios, glycosuria, ketonuria
❑ Interventions	Diet, Insulin, Exercise
❑ Complications	Hypertension, pre-eclampsia
❑ What problems should be monitored post-partum?	Maternal and fetal hypoglycemia

❑ What are the chances of getting diabetes after gestational diabetes?	Lifetime risk exists for the development of Type 2 diabetes

Ectopic Pregnancy

❑ Description	Implantation of a zygote in fallopian tube
❑ Assessment	Vaginal bleeding, missed menstrual period abdominal pain and cramping
❑ Report severe and referred shoulder pain	Indicates rupture of the fallopian tube
❑ Interventions	Monitor bleeding, Laparotomy, Laparoscopic surgery, Give RhoGAM
❑ Why is Methotrexate (chemotherapy agent) given?	To hinder the growth of the embryo

Disseminated Intravascular Coagulation (DIC)

❑ Description	Excessive bleeding and clotting leads to severe depletion of clotting factors and platelets → bleeding and vascular blockage
❑ Risk factors	**Abruptio placentae**, sepsis, fetal death
❑ Assessment	Bruising, petechiae, purpura, hematuria
❑ Diagnostic Tests	Prolonged PT, PTT and clotting time
❑ Interventions	Treat the cause, Blood transfusion, IVF

Fetal Death in Utero

❑ Assessment	Absence of FHR or fetal movements, lack of increase in fundal height
❑ Complication	Sepsis, DIC
❑ Interventions	Labor induction and delivery

Hepatitis B

❑ Complications	Premature birth, low birth weight
❑ Transmission	Blood, vaginal secretions, breastmilk, transplacental transmission
❑ Interventions	Limit vaginal exams Suction newborn immediately after birth
❑ Can a mother with hepatitis B breastfeed the infant?	Yes, infants born to Hepa B infected mothers should receive a HBV immune globulin for protection but it is not necessary to delay the breastfeeding

HIV and AIDS

❑ When is the greatest risk of transmission?	During delivery due to possible exposure of fetus to maternal blood
❑ Interventions	Avoid invasive procedures in pregnancy May have cesarean delivery Suction newborn immediately after birth HIV drug given to newborn for 4-6 weeks
❑ Is breastfeeding restricted?	Yes, HIV can be transmitted in breast milk

> ***NCLEX Alert!*** *Not all newborns will be infected with HIV but they acquire the maternal anti-HIV antibodies and may show an HIV positive result after birth.*

Hematoma

❑ Causes	Prolonged labor, Forceps delivery
❑ Assessment	Severe perineal pain, edema, ecchymosis, difficult urination, maternal shock
❑ Is blood loss evident?	Blood loss may not be visible
❑ Interventions	Apply ice, Analgesics, Monitor for shock

Hydatidiform Mole (Gestational Trophoblastic Disease)

❑ Description	Noncancerous tumor → trophoblasts develop into abnormal grapelike clusters and not into fetus → choriocarcinoma
❑ Assessment	Absence of fetal heart rate Bright red or dark brown vaginal bleeding Fundal height higher than expected
❑ Diagnostic Test	"**Snowstorm**" pattern on ultrasound, abnormally **elevated hCG** levels
❑ Interventions	Dilation and curettage Vacuum aspiration Check tissue for cancer Monitor hCG levels for 1 year
❑ Why is birth control needed until 1-year follow-up?	Pregnancy will alter the result of the hCG levels which identifies success of treatment

Incompetent Cervix

❑ Description	Premature dilation of a weakened cervix → spontaneous abortions
❑ Assessment	Vaginal bleeding, back pain
❑ Interventions	Bed rest, Tocolytic drugs **Cervical cerclage** done at 10-14 weeks Restrict sexual intercourse
❑ What is cervical cerclage procedure?	Stitching the cervix to keep it closed

> ***NCLEX Alert!*** *Cervical cerclage is removed at 37 weeks of pregnancy or when preterm labor occurs!*

Hyperemesis Gravidarum

❑ Description	Severe nausea and vomiting in pregnancy
❑ Assessment	Persistent nausea and vomiting Morning sickness, weight loss, dehydration
❑ Interventions	Antiemetics, IV fluid replacement

Multiple Gestation

❑ Fraternal (dizygotic)	Two eggs fertilized by two sperm cells
❑ Identical (monozygotic)	One egg fertilized by one sperm cell but later on divides into two fetuses
❑ Complications	Premature labor, abortion, polyhydramnios post-partum hemorrhage, intrauterine growth retardation (IUGR)
❑ Assessment	Increased fundal height with enlarged uterus, multiple FHR's, severe weight gain
❑ Interventions	Cesarean delivery Monitor for uterine atony

> ***NCLEX Alert!*** *Multiple gestation increases the mother's risk of developing post-partum hemorrhage due to uterine atony!*

Pregnancy-Induced Hypertension (PIH)

GESTATIONAL HYPERTENSION	GESTATIONAL PROTEINURIA	PREECLAMPSIA	ECLAMPSIA
Mild hypertension only	Proteinuria after 20 weeks gestation	**Hypertension**, **edema**, **proteinuria** after 20 weeks gestation	Seizures + HELLP Syndrome

- ❑ Risk factors — Multiple gestation, primigravida, diabetes mellitus, hypertension, age <19 or > 40 years-old
- ❑ Complications — Abruptio placentae; Fetal death; Thrombocytopenia; Disseminated Intravascular Coagulation
- ❑ What is the cure for this condition? — Birth is the only cure

> ***NCLEX Alert!*** *Severe headache and epigastric pain indicate the occurrence of an impending seizure!*

❑ Interventions

MILD PRE-ECLAMPSIA	SEVERE PRE-ECLAMPSIA	ECLAMPSIA
❑ Frequent neurochecks ❑ Monitor blood pressure ❑ Bed rest ❑ Left side-lying position ❑ High protein, high carbohydrate diet ❑ Avoid added salt diet ❑ Antihypertensive drugs ❑ Monitor intake and output ❑ IV fluid replacement ❑ Assess for HELLP syndrome	❑ Monitor for signs of magnesium sulfate toxicity ▪ CNS depression ▪ decreased respiration ▪ oliguria, hypotension ▪ sweating, flushing ▪ absence of deep tendon reflexes (DTR) ❑ Antihypertensives ❑ Bed rest ❑ Induction of labor	❑ Seizure precautions ❑ Anticonvulsants ❑ O_2 by face mask 10 L/minute ❑ Left side-lying position ❑ Monitor fetal heart rate ❑ Delivery of fetus

> ***NCLEX Alert!*** *HELLP (Hemolysis, Elevated Liver Enzymes and Low Platelet Count) syndrome is a fatal complication secondary to severe preeclampsia. Symptoms include: RUQ pain, blurry vision, nausea, vomiting, headaches, nosebleeds, edema, weight gain and seizures.*

Infections During Pregnancy

❑ Presence of rash and influenza-like symptoms	Toxoplasmosis
❑ Treated with folic acid, sulfadiazine and antimalarial drug	Toxoplasmosis
❑ Avoid handling or cleaning **cat litter**	Toxoplasmosis
❑ Avoid consumption of raw eggs, uncooked meat and unpasteurized milk	Toxoplasmosis
❑ Wash fruits and vegetables thoroughly	Toxoplasmosis
❑ Harmful to fetus on 1st trimester	Rubella
❑ Do not give vaccine if allergic to eggs and neomycin	Rubella
❑ Avoid pregnancy 1-3 months after vaccination	Rubella
❑ Complications include low birth weight, mental retardation and loss of vision	Cytomegalovirus
❑ Cesarean delivery is required only for **active** lesions	Genital herpes
❑ Causes sepsis and neurological complications	Group B Streptococcus (GBS)
❑ Administer penicillin during labor and birth	Group B Streptococcus (GBS)
❑ Respiratory isolation required, Breastfeeding is allowed if non-infectious	Tuberculosis

E. The Process of Labor and Delivery

FETAL PRESENTATION	FETAL LIE	FETAL STATION	FETAL POSITION
Refers to the fetal part that enters the pelvis	Refers to the relationship of the fetus to the mother's spine	Refers to measurement as to how far the fetal head has descended into the maternal pelvis	Refers to the relationship of a fetal structural landmark to the mother's pelvis
Types 1. Cephalic 2. Shoulder 3. Breech (frank, full, footling) ❑ *Meconium-staining is normal for breech presentation*	Types 1. Longitudinal (cephalic or breech) 2. Transverse ❑ *Shoulder presentation will require cesarean delivery*	❑ "Station 0" means fetal presenting part is at the level of the ischial spine (engaged) ❑ "Minus or plus station" means fetal presenting part is below (plus) or above (negative) the ischial spine	❑ Best position → Left Occiput Anterior (LOA) ❑ Right Occiput Posterior (LOP, ROP) positions are longer and more painful labor because the fetal head presses on the mother's sacrum (back labor)

- ❑ Mechanisms of Labor — Engagement, Descent, Flexion, Internal Rotation, Extension, Restitution, External Rotation, Expulsion

- ❑ Signs of Impending Labor — Lightening
  Appearance of bloody show
  Sudden burst of energy
  Increased Braxton-Hicks contractions
  Spontaneous rupture of membranes

- ❑ What is lightening? — Fetus drops into the lower pelvis of the mother; Causes relief from dyspnea

True versus False Labor

TRUE LABOR	FALSE LABOR
❑ Regular contractions with increasing intensity	❑ Irregular contractions with unchanged intensity
❑ Intervals become shorter	❑ Intervals remain long
❑ Pain worsens with walking	❑ Pain stops with walking
❑ Contractions felt in back and lower abdomen	❑ Contractions usually in lower abdomen
❑ Progressive cervical dilatation, effacement or descent	❑ Lack of cervical dilatation, effacement or descent
❑ Fetal engagement and descent	❑ Lack of fetal engagement and descent

Breathing Techniques

- ❑ Description — Promotes relaxation
  Maximizes oxygenation
  Decreases pain experience during labor

- ❑ Cleansing Breath — Contraction starts and finishes with a deep, relaxing inspiration and expiration to provide more oxygen to the fetus

- ❑ Slow-Paced Breathing — A slow-deep breathing in a relaxed manner
- ❑ Modified-Paced Breathing — Faster than slow-paced breathing
- ❑ Pattern-Paced Breathing — A pant-blow technique
- ❑ Short Puffs — Breathing when urge to push is strong

- What will happen if the mother is breathing too fast?

  It can result into exhaustion and loss of carbon dioxide; Respiratory alkalosis occurs as manifested by dizziness, numbness and tingling sensations

- How is respiratory alkalosis prevented?

  Have the mother breathe into cupped hands or paper bag to retain CO_2.

Fetal Monitoring

- Description

  Displays FHR and uterine contraction tracings to monitor quality of uterine activity such as frequency and duration

- Normal Fetal Heart Rate (FHR)

  120-160 beats per minute

Reassuring (Normal) Fetal Heart Rate Patterns

VARIABILITY	ACCELERATIONS	EARLY DECELERATIONS
❑ Fluctuations in the baseline FHR	❑ Caused by fetal movement or stimulation ❑ FHR increases 15 beats above the baseline for 15 seconds	❑ Caused by **fetal head compression** ❑ FHR decreases and returns to the baseline FHR **by the end** of contraction ❑ FHR tracing "mirrors" the contractions tracing

Non-Reassuring (Abnormal) Fetal Heart Rate Patterns

ABSENT OR DECREASED VARIABILITY	BRADYCARDIA/ TACHYCARDIA	LATE DECELERATIONS	VARIABLE DECELERATIONS
❑ Lack of fluctuations in the baseline FHR ❑ Caused by fetal hypoxemia or acidosis	❑ FHR <120 or >160 beats per minute	❑ Caused by **uteroplacental insufficiency** ❑ Begins after the start of the contraction and returns to the baseline **after** contraction	❑ Caused by **umbilical cord compression** ❑ No uniform pattern ❑ Falls and rises suddenly ❑ FHR tracing shows V or W shaped waves

Fetal Heart Rate Pattern Tracings

ACCELERATIONS **(Reassuring)** ▪ Caused by fetal movement or stimulation ▪ FHR increases 15 beats above the baseline for 15 seconds	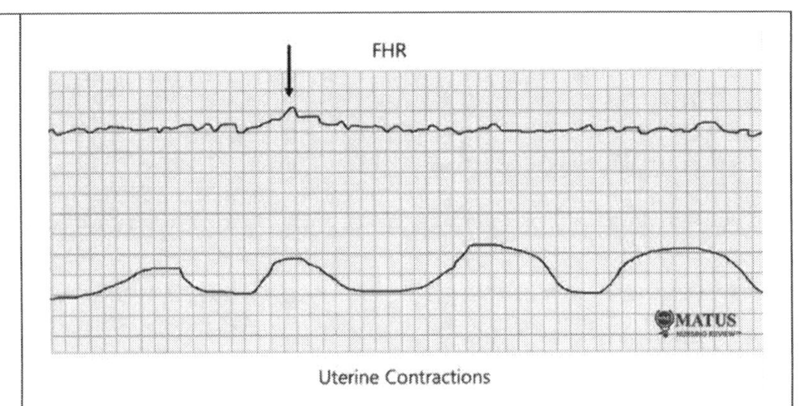
EARLY DECELERATION **(Reassuring)** ▪ Caused by **fetal head compression** ▪ FHR decreases and returns to the baseline FHR **by the end** of contraction ▪ FHR tracing "mirrors" the contractions tracing	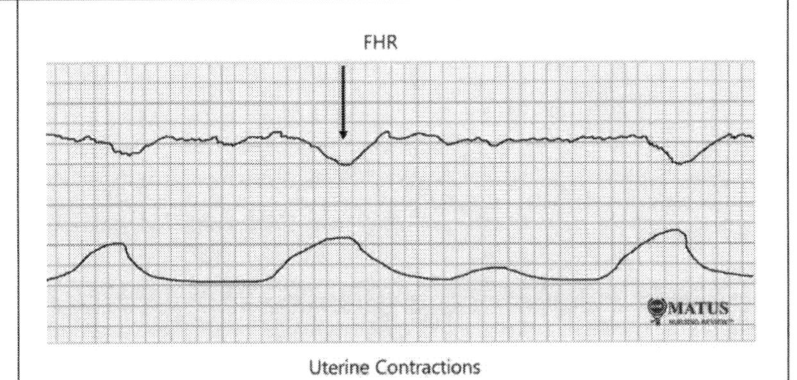
LATE DECELERATION **(Non-Reassuring)** ▪ Caused by **uteroplacental insufficiency** ▪ Begins after the start of the contraction and returns to the baseline **after** contraction	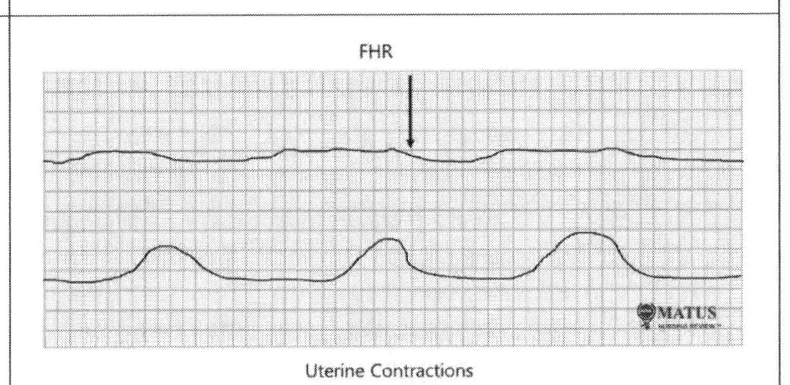
VARIABLE DECELERATION **(Non-Reassuring)** ▪ Caused by **umbilical cord compression** ▪ No uniform pattern; Falls and rises suddenly ▪ FHR tracing shows V or W shaped waves	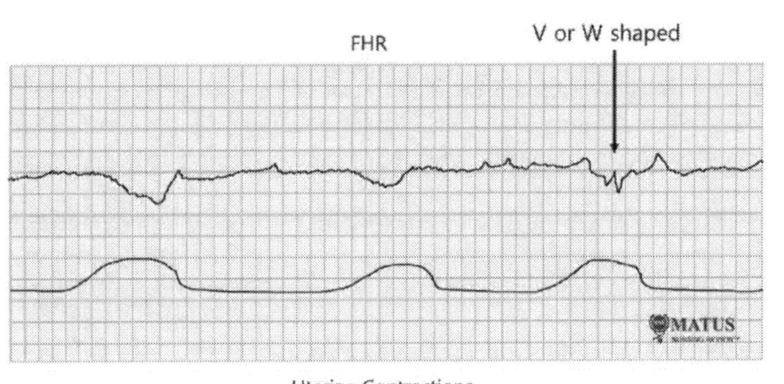

❑ Nursing Actions for Non-Reassuring FHR Patterns

Determine the cause of abnormal tracing
Stop the oxytocin infusion
Change mother's position to left side
Provide O_2 by face mask
Prepare for emergency cesarean section

Stages of Labor

STAGE 1	Onset of uterine contractions to cervical dilation
STAGE 2	Delivery of fetus
STAGE 3	Delivery of placenta
STAGE 4	First 4 hours after delivery

First Stage of Labor - Three Phases of Labor

LATENT	ACTIVE	TRANSITIONAL
❑ Cervical dilation: 1-4 cm	❑ Cervical dilation: 5-7 cm	❑ Cervical dilation 8-10 cm
❑ Uterine contractions *Frequency - every 15-30 mins.* *Duration - 15-30 seconds* *Intensity - mild*	❑ Uterine contractions *Frequency - every 3-5 mins.* *Duration - 30-60 seconds* *Intensity - moderate*	❑ Uterine contractions *Frequency - every 2-3 mins* *Duration - 45-90 seconds* *Intensity - strong*
Interventions ❑ Monitor FHR, contractions and cervical dilation ❑ Provide fluids or ice chips ❑ Assist to void ❑ Reinforce breathing technique	Interventions ❑ Monitor FHR, contractions and cervical dilation ❑ Assist in breathing techniques ❑ Provide back rubs, massage or sacral pressure to reduce pain	Interventions ❑ Monitor FHR, contractions and cervical dilation ❑ Promote rest between contractions ❑ Assist to void

NCLEX Alert! *After rupture of membranes, immediately assess the FHR and color of the amniotic fluid to assess for fetal distress!*

❑ Report meconium-stained amniotic fluid

This indicates fetal distress; Hypoxia causes a vagal reaction relaxing the anal sphincter

❑ Why should the mother avoid pushing when the cervix is not yet fully dilated?

Exhaustion and fetal hypoxia will occur

Second Stage of Labor

❑ Assess FHR, contractions and vital signs every ___ minutes	5
❑ Signs of imminent fetal delivery	Fetal head appears, perineal bulging

Third Stage of Labor

❑ Placental expulsion occurs how many minutes after birth?	5 minutes
❑ Schultze mechanism	Delivery of shiny side of placenta
❑ Duncan mechanism	Delivery of dirty side of placenta
❑ What are the 4 signs of placental separation?	1. Uterus assumes globular shape (Calkin's sign) 2. Uterus rises upward 3. Sudden gush of blood from vagina 4. Lengthening of umbilical cord

Fourth Stage of Labor

❑ Where is the fundus immediately after delivery?	At the midline and halfway between the symphysis pubis and umbilicus; Within 12 hours, it is 1 cm above the umbilicus; It then descends 1 cm every 24 hours
❑ Interventions	Monitor vital signs Massage uterus if boggy Provide warmth Apply ice packs to the perineum
❑ What will happen if the uterus remains boggy and soft?	Maternal hemorrhage
❑ What will happen if the bladder becomes distended?	Bladder distention can hinder uterine contractions which leads to bleeding
❑ What is a sign of bladder distention after birth?	Fundus is deviated from the midline

Procedures During Labor and Delivery

Anesthesia

❑ Blocks pain in the perineal area during episiotomy	Local anesthesia, pudendal block
❑ Decreases perineal and uterine pain; does not cause headache	Epidural anesthesia
❑ Causes urinary retention and hypotension	Epidural anesthesia
❑ Causes maternal **hypotension** and spinal **headache**; Mother should lie flat for 12 hours; IV fluid is given to replace leaked CSF	Spinal or subarachnoid block

Amniotomy

- ❑ Description — Rupturing of membranes to stimulate labor
  Fetus should be at "0" or a plus station
- ❑ What are the risks of this procedure? — Maternal sepsis, cord prolapse

Induction

- ❑ Description — Initiation of contractions to stimulate labor
  Uses oxytocin (Pitocin) IV infusion

> ***NCLEX Alert!*** *MONITOR FOR HYPERTONIC UTERINE CONTRACTIONS*
> *Frequency < than 2 minutes, Duration > than 90 seconds → Stop oxytocin infusion!*

Bishop Score

- ❑ Description — Assesses and predicts the readiness of the cervix for labor induction
  Includes five factors given a score of 0-3
  Score of >6 → readiness for induction
- ❑ What are the 5 factors being scored in Bishop scoring? — Cervical dilation, effacement, position, consistency, fetal station

Episiotomy

- ❑ Description — Surgical incision of the perineum to enlarge the passageway for fetal delivery
- ❑ Interventions — Apply ice pack for first 24 hour, Sitz baths
- ❑ How do you assess the episiotomy? — Remember REEDA!
  - R - edness
  - E - cchymosis
  - E - rythema
  - D - ischarge
  - A - pproximation

Vacuum Extraction

- ❑ Description — Application of a vacuum pump during vaginal delivery to assist fetal birth
- ❑ What are the risks of this procedure? — **Chignon**, cephalhematoma
- ❑ What is a chignon? — Temporary swelling of the fetal head due to vacuum extraction

Forceps Delivery

- ❑ Description — Forceps is applied on the baby's head to facilitate fetal delivery
- ❑ What is the risk of this procedure? — Facial nerve damage

Cesarean Delivery

- ❑ Indications — Cephalopelvic disproportion; Active maternal herpes virus infection; Pregnancy-Induced hypertension
- ❑ Normal blood loss for cesarean section — <1000 mL for first 24 hours after birth

F. Complications During Labor and Delivery

ABRUPTIO PLACENTAE	PLACENTA PREVIA
Premature separation of placenta usually occurring after 20 weeks of pregnancy	Low implantation of the placenta with symptoms appearing on 3rd trimester
Causes: **hypertension**, trauma, multiple pregnancy	Causes: **multiparity**, multiple pregnancy
Assessment ❑ Dark, red vaginal bleeding ❑ Painful abdomen with board-like rigidity ❑ Maternal hypotension ❑ Fetal distress	Assessment ❑ Bright-red vaginal bleeding ❑ Painless, soft abdomen ❑ Fundal height higher than normal ❑ Maternal hypotension and fetal distress
Interventions ❑ Monitor bleeding ❑ Bed rest ❑ Monitor for DIC ❑ Fetal delivery	Interventions ❑ Monitor bleeding ❑ Bed rest ❑ Avoid vaginal exam to minimize bleeding ❑ Arrange **double set-up** for vaginal exam ❑ Tocolytic medications

Precipitous Labor and Delivery (Express Delivery)

- ❑ Description — Unusually rapid labor less than 2-3 hours from onset of labor contractions
  → sudden expulsion of fetus
  → vaginal lacerations and fetal trauma
- ❑ Causes — Strong contractions, large pelvic canal

- Assessment — Rapid cervical dilation, strong uterine contractions, hemorrhage
- Interventions — Prepare precipitous tray (scissors, hemostats, gloves, cord clamp)
  Pant between contractions
  Apply pressure to fetal head
  Deliver between contractions

Premature Rupture of Membranes

- Description — Amniotic membrane ruptures before onset of labor → chorioamnionitis
- Assessment — Positive nitrazine test
  Vaginal secretions → yellow color
  Amniotic fluid → blue color
- Interventions — Avoid vaginal exam, Monitor for fever

Amniotic Fluid Embolism

- Description — Fetal particles enter maternal circulation → pulmonary embolism
- Assessment — Sudden chest pain, dyspnea, heart failure, pulmonary edema
- Interventions — O_2 at 10 L/min. by face mask, CPR, Intubation, Emergency cesarean section

Dystocia

- Description — Painful, difficult and prolonged labor
- Hypotonic contractions — Short, weak contractions
- Hypertonic contractions — Painful, uncoordinated contractions
- Causes — Fetal macrosomia, abnormal presentation
- Assessment — Severe uterine pain, non-progressive labor, abnormal contraction pattern
- Interventions — Monitor FHR and uterine contractions
  Prophylactic ATBs to prevent sepsis

> ***NCLEX Alert!*** *Prolonged rupture of membranes and labor process increases the risk of maternal infection. Monitor for fever and change in vital signs.*

Preterm Labor

❑ Description	Labor before 37th week of pregnancy
❑ Risk factors	Primigravida, multiple pregnancy
❑ Assessment	Painful or painless uterine contractions, rupture of amniotic membranes, pelvic pressure, low dull backache, abdominal cramping
❑ Interventions	Bed rest, Left side-lying position Tocolytic drugs (e.g. magnesium sulfate)

Supine Hypotension (Vena Cava Syndrome)

❑ Description	Enlarged uterus presses on vena cava → decreased venous return → hypoxia
❑ Assessment	Dizziness, tachycardia, pallor, clammy skin
❑ Interventions	Avoid supine position Place client on left side-lying position

Prolapsed Umbilical Cord

❑ Description	Umbilical cord drops through the cervix → cord compression → fetal distress
❑ Causes	**Premature rupture of membranes**, breech presentation, multiple pregnancy, multiparity, polyhydramnios
❑ Types	OVERT (visible) and OCCULT (hidden)
❑ Assessment	Sensation that "something is slipping", abnormal FHR, palpable cord, variable deceleration or bradycardia
❑ Interventions	Apply pressure on the presenting part Place on Trendelenburg, left lateral or knee-chest position with head down O_2 at 10 L/min. by face mask Prepare for emergency cesarean section

G. The Postpartum Period

Maternal Physiological Changes

Lochia

❑ Rubra	Bright red (1-3 days)
❑ Serosa	Pale pinkish to brownish (3-10 days)
❑ Alba	White yellow (10-14) Has menstrual-like odor, Weigh pads, Report excessive amount and change in color of lochia

Menstruation

❑ When does menstruation return?	Within 1-2 months (non-breastfeeding) Within 3-6 months (breastfeeding)

> ***NCLEX Alert!***
> *Breastfeeding is not a reliable form of contraception. The mother may ovulate without menstruating!*

Involution

❑ Description	Uterus returns to pre-pregnancy state Breastfeeding promotes involution
❑ Fundal height decreases about ____ fingerbreadth /___ cm per day	1, 1
❑ Fundus is nonpalpable on the _____ day	10th
❑ What should you do if the uterus remains flaccid?	Massage until firm

Rubin's Postpartum Phases of Emotional Adjustment

TAKING-IN PHASE (FIRST 3 DAYS)	TAKING-HOLD PHASE (3-10 DAYS)	LETTING-GO PHASE (5th WEEK)
❑ Preoccupied with own needs for food, fluids and sleep ❑ Shares labor experience	❑ Receptive to mothering role ❑ Best time to teach ❑ Provide reassurance	❑ Gives up previous lifestyles to accommodate the newborn and embrace reality

Interventions During Post-Partum Period

❑ Assessment	Height, tone, and location of fundus Bowel and voiding status Color, amount and odor of the lochia Emotional bonding, Pain level Perineum for swelling or bruising
❑ What is Kangaroo Care after birth?	Method of holding a newborn and involves skin-to-skin contact to promote bonding and stabilize fetal well-being
❑ What is postpartum blues?	A normal, transient feeling of sadness after birth due to maternal hormonal changes

> ***NCLEX Alert!*** *Remember "BUBBLE HE" in Post-Partum Assessment*
>
> *B – reast, U – terus, B – owels, B – ladder, L – ochia, E – pisiotomy, H – oman's sign, E – motion/Bonding*

Breastfeeding

❑ What is proper latching during breastfeeding?	The mother's nipple reaches the soft palate of the newborn, thus preventing pain when breastfeeding and cracking of nipples
❑ Why does breastfeeding cause abdominal cramps?	Oxytocin is released which causes the uterus to contract to prevent bleeding
❑ Why are hormonal contraceptives not allowed?	Hinders milk supply; Use progestins only
❑ How long can breastmilk be frozen?	3 months in a freezer kept at 0°F (–18°C)
❑ What is demand feeding?	Feeding when the newborn shows hunger
❑ Management for breast engorgement	Wear support bra, **Ice packs** after feeding, **Warm packs** before breastfeeding
❑ Management for cracked nipples	Ensure proper latching technique Expose nipples to air after breastfeeding Change positions during breastfeeding

Hemorrhage

❑ Causes	**Retained placental fragments**, uterine atony, vaginal lacerations
❑ Types	EARLY: First 24 hours after delivery LATE: More than 24 hours after delivery

❑ Amount	Vaginal delivery: >**500 mL** blood loss Cesarean delivery: >**1000 mL** blood loss
❑ Interventions	Massage the fundus, Give Pitocin, Check pooled blood by turning client

Subinvolution

❑ Description	Uterus fails to return to pre-pregnant state
❑ Assessment	Pain on uterine palpation, uterus larger than expected, increased vaginal bleeding
❑ Interventions	Monitor the fundus, Give methergine

Mastitis

❑ Description	A painful infection of the breast
❑ Interventions	Proper breastfeeding techniques Manual expression of breastmilk Warm or cold application, ATB's
❑ Is breastfeeding allowed?	Yes, if there is no abscess

H. Care of the Newborn

Care After Birth

❑ Interventions	Suction mouth and nares Dry and wrap in blankets Place a cap on head to prevent cold stress Inject IM Vitamin K Apply ID Bracelets Erythromycin eye ointment
❑ Vital Signs	HR: 100-160 beats/minute (100 – sleeping; 160 – crying) RR: 30-60 breaths/minute, irregular (average: 40 breaths/minute) BP: approximately 75/55 mmHg Temperature: 97.6-99° F (axillary)
❑ Assess the umbilical cord	Remember AVA! 2 arteries, 1 vein

Apgar Scoring System

	SIGN	2	1	0
A	Activity (muscle tone)	Active	Arms and legs flexed	Absent
P	Pulse	> 100 bpm	< 100 bpm	Absent
G	Grimace (reflex irritability)	Sneezes, coughs	Grimaces	No response
A	Appearance (skin color)	Pink over entire body	Pink except extremities	Cyanotic or pale all over
R	Respirations	Good, crying	Slow, irregular	Absent

- ❑ Assess Apgar score ___ minute and ___ minutes after birth — 1, 5
- ❑ Results — 8-10 - normal; 4-7 - stimulate by rubbing the back; 0-3 - requires emergency resuscitation

Physical Examination and Care of the Newborn

- ❑ Diamond-shaped; Closes between 12-18 months — Anterior fontanel
- ❑ Triangle-shaped; Closes at 2-3 months — Posterior fontanel
- ❑ Milky secretion from breast due to maternal hormones — Witch's Milk
- ❑ Color change in which one half of the body blanches and the other half turns red; May indicate severe infection or cardiac defect — Harlequin sign
- ❑ Stool that is pale yellow to light brown in color — Breastfed stool
- ❑ Looser, greenish brown stool passed on the 2nd or 3rd day of life — Transitional stool
- ❑ Signs of respiratory distress in newborn — Nasal flaring, grunting, chest retractions, apnea >15 seconds
- ❑ Cheese-like white substance coating the skin — Vernix caseosa
- ❑ Fine, thin, downy hair — Lanugo
- ❑ Tiny, flat, yellow or white spots on the nose and chin — Milia
- ❑ White cysts on hard palate — Epstein's pearls
- ❑ Blood-tinged mucoid vaginal discharge — Pseudomenstruation
- ❑ Thick, white mucus on genitalia — Smegma
- ❑ Dimple in the lower back with a tuft of hair — Indicates spina bifida
- ❑ Asymmetry of the head; disappears in 72 hours — Molding (due to pressure on head)
- ❑ Temporary collection of blood that **CROSSES** over the suture line — Caput succedaneum
- ❑ Temporary edema that does **NOT CROSS** the suture line — Cephalhematoma
- ❑ Cross-eyed — Indicates strabismus; normal at birth
- ❑ Use ATB ointment, water and soap — Umbilical cord care
- ❑ Use petroleum jelly gauze — Circumcision care

Skin Discolorations

❑ Jaundice present **within** the first 24 hours after birth	Pathologic jaundice; abnormal
❑ Jaundice appears on the second or third day of life.	Physiologic jaundice; normal
❑ Flat, pink spots on skin on eyelids or nape due to the dilation of blood vessels	Port-wine stain
❑ Red or purple marks often on the face	Telangiectatic nevi (stork bites)
❑ Accumulation of blood vessels forming a lump under the skin	Strawberry mark/hemangioma
❑ Blue-gray pigmentation usually on the sacral area common among African or Asian ethnicities	Mongolian spots

Reflexes of the Newborn

❑ Infant makes sucking movements when the area around the mouth is gently touched	Sucking reflex
❑ Stroking the side of the infant's cheek is followed by turning of the head and sucking movements with mouth	Rooting reflex
❑ Suddenly lowering the infant is followed by throwing out of arms and legs while extending the neck	Moro or startling reflex
❑ Infant turns head to the left while left arm will extend with right arm raised above the head	Tonic neck or fencing reflex
❑ When the sole of the foot is stroked, the big toe bends back and the other toes fan out	Babinski reflex
❑ Infant grasps the examiner's finger tightly when the palm is stroked	Grasping reflex
❑ Holding the infant with toes touching the floor is followed by attempts to walk in place	Stepping or walking reflex
❑ Holding the infant facing downward then suddenly being swooshed down is followed by arm extension	Parachute reflex

I. Disorders of the Newborn

Large for Gestational Age

❑ Description	Neonate plotted at or above the 90th percentile on the growth curve
❑ Assessment	Hypoglycemia, respiratory distress
❑ Interventions	Assess for signs of respiratory distress Check for birth trauma or injury Monitor for signs of hypoglycemia Monitor for infection

Small for Gestational Age

- ❑ Description — A neonate plotted at or below the 10th percentile on the growth curve
- ❑ Assessment — **Hypoglycemia**, ruddy appearance, low or high body temperature
- ❑ Interventions — Provide warmth, Monitor for infection; Monitor for signs of hypoglycemia

Preterm Newborn

- ❑ Description — Fetus born before 37 weeks → immaturity of organ structures
- ❑ Assessment — Apnea, abundant lanugo, jaundice, subnormal body temperature, limbs more extended, poor suck and swallow reflexes, minimal creases, undescended testes
- ❑ Interventions — Keep warm, Nutrition by tube feeding; Monitor for infection and hypoglycemia

Retinopathy of Prematurity

- ❑ Description — Abnormal development of retinal blood vessels in premature infants → scarring → blindness
- ❑ Causes — Prematurity, **prolonged O_2 treatment**
- ❑ Assessment — **Leukokoria**, vitreous hemorrhage, myopia, strabismus, cataracts, blindness
- ❑ Interventions — Laser surgery, cryosurgery

Respiratory Distress Syndrome

- ❑ Description — Lack of surfactant due to prematurity → hypoxia and respiratory acidosis
- ❑ Assessment — Tachypnea, apnea, flaring nostrils, grunting
- ❑ Interventions — Assess respiration; Check for retinal damage due to oxygen; Surfactant replacement through ET

Bronchopulmonary Dysplasia

- ❑ Description — Affects infants who are premature, had long-term mechanical ventilation and oxygen administration → lung damage
- ❑ Assessment — Tachypnea, chest retractions, nasal flaring
- ❑ Interventions — Assess airway, Surfactant, Diuretics, Bronchodilators, Steroids

Necrotizing Enterocolitis

- ❑ Description — Premature newborn → bacteria → intestinal inflammation and infection
- ❑ Assessment — Increased abdominal girth, abdominal bloating tenderness, bloody stools, vomiting, diarrhea, decreased or absent bowel sounds
- ❑ Interventions — NPO, Gastric decompression ATBs, IVF, Surgery

Hyperbilirubinemia

- ❑ Description — Bilirubin levels more than 12 mg/dL
- ❑ Assessment — Jaundice, poor sucking reflex
- ❑ How do you check jaundice in an infant? — Gently press the forehead or nose → skin appears yellow
- ❑ What is the goal of treatment? — Prevent brain damage (**kernicterus**)
- ❑ Interventions — Phototherapy, Cover genital area Apply eye shields, Provide fluids Reposition frequently
- ❑ What is **bronze baby skin syndrome**? — Dark grey-brown pigmentation of skin, and urine following phototherapy

Erythroblastosis Fetalis

- ❑ Description — Rh negative (-) mother with Rh positive (+) fetus → maternal production of anti-Rh antibodies → hemolysis of fetal RBCs
- ❑ When is maternal exposure to Rh (+) fetal RBC's most likely to occur? — Exposure occurs during amniocentesis, delivery and abortion

❑ Is there a danger of erythroblastosis fetalis in an Rh (-) fetus?	No, it only occurs when the fetus is Rh (+) and the mother is Rh (-)
❑ Assessment	Pathologic jaundice within 24 hours after birth, anemia, edema
❑ Interventions	Rho (D) immune globulin (RhoGAM) injection to mother at 28 weeks gestation and within 72 hours after delivery
❑ What is the action of RhoGAM?	RhoGAM destroys Rh (+) blood that entered the mother's circulation
❑ What is exchange transfusion?	Infant blood is replaced with Rh (-) blood

NCLEX Alert! *It's plain simple! During an Rh negative mother's first pregnancy with an Rh positive fetus, complications will not occur because the fetus is often delivered before the mother becomes exposed to fetal RBCs and produces anti-Rh antibodies. If RhoGAM is not given during the first pregnancy as a prophylaxis treatment and the mother later becomes pregnant with another Rh positive fetus, the formed maternal antibodies will cross the placenta and destroy the fetal red blood cells.*

Fetal Alcohol Syndrome

❑ Assessment	Abnormal facial characteristics, small head, smooth ridge between upper lip and nose, thin upper lip, low nasal bridge, abnormal palmar creases, wide-set eyes
❑ Interventions	Monitor for respiratory distress and hypoglycemia

The Newborn with Addiction

❑ Assessment	Tremors, hypertonicity, irritability, high-pitched cry, sneezing, fever, diaphoresis, convulsion
❑ Interventions	Seizure precautions, IV fluid replacement

J. Maternity Drugs

1. Uterine Stimulants

- ❑ Description — Stimulates uterine contraction; Promotes milk ejection
- ❑ Drug — Example: oxytocin (Pitocin)
- ❑ Side effects — Hypertension, **water intoxication**
- ❑ Interventions — Monitor BP, uterine contractions and FHR
- ❑ What should you do when hypertonic contractions are present? — Stop Pitocin, turn mother to side and give oxygen

2. Ergot Alkaloids

- ❑ Description — Stimulates uterine contractions
- ❑ Drug — Example:
  - methylergonovine (Methergine)
- ❑ Side effects — **Hypertension**, uterine cramping
- ❑ Interventions — Monitor BP and uterine contractions

3. Tocolytics

- ❑ Description — Inhibits uterine contractions to stop preterm labor

DRUGS	SIDE EFFECTS
magnesium sulfate	Hypermagnesemia, hypotension, bradycardia, flushing, sweating
nifedipine (Adalat)	Tachycardia, hypotension, lightheadedness, nausea
terbutaline (Brethine)	Tachycardia, hypotension, chest pain
ritodrine (Yutopar)	Tachycardia, hypotension, arrhythmias
indomethacin (Indocin)	Gastric upset, nausea, vomiting, diarrhea, stomach pain, heartburn, rash

NCLEX Alert! *REMEMBER 3 R'S FOR SIGNS OF MAGNESIUM SULFATE TOXICITY*

R - espirations <12/min
R - enal (urine) output <100 mL/4 hours
R - eflexes: absence of deep tendon reflexes

The normal level of magnesium sulfate is 4-7.5 mEq/L or 5-8 mg/dL
Antidote: Calcium gluconate

4. Betamethasone and Dexamethasone

❑ Description	Promotes production of lung surfactant to accelerate fetal lung maturity in preterm labor
❑ Side effects	Maternal infection, hyperglycemia
❑ Interventions	Monitor for hyperglycemia and infection

5. Lung Surfactants

❑ Description	Replaces pulmonary surfactant to prevent respiratory distress syndrome
❑ Drugs	Intratracheal Route ▪ beractant (Survanta) ▪ calfactant (Infasurf)
❑ Side effects	Transient bradycardia, hypotension
❑ Interventions	Monitor BP and HR

6. Prostaglandins (Cervidil)

❑ Description	Ripens and dilates the cervix Applied vaginally to induce labor Left in place for 12 hours
❑ Drugs	Example: dinoprostone (Cervidil, Prepidil)
❑ Side effects	Stomach pain, nausea, diarrhea
❑ Interventions	Mother should maintain side-lying position

7. Rho (D) Immune Globulin (RhoGAM)

❑ Description	Prevents isoimmunization in Rh (-) mothers exposed to Rh (+) fetal RBC's
❑ What is isoimmunization or sensitization?	Maternal production of anti-Rh antibodies
❑ What tests identify the presence of anti-Rh antibodies?	1. INDIRECT COOMB'S TEST ▪ Blood sample taken from the pregnant woman during prenatal testing 2. DIRECT COOMB'S TEST ▪ Blood sample taken from the newborn's cord to check for the presence of anti-Rh antibodies attached to red blood cells

> ***NCLEX Alert!*** *RhoGAM is not useful if the mother has already been sensitized or has produced antibodies against the Rh antigen!*

Pediatric Nursing

19

A. Growth and Development

Age Groups

❑ 1-12 months	Infant
❑ 1-3 years	Toddler
❑ 3-5 years	Preschool
❑ 6-12 years	School-Age
❑ 12-18 years	Adolescent

Erikson's Psychosocial Theory of Development

❑ Trust versus mistrust	Infant
❑ Autonomy versus shame/doubt	Toddler
❑ Initiative versus guilt	Preschool
❑ Industry versus inferiority	School-Age
❑ Identity versus confusion	Adolescent

Denver II Developmental Screening Test

❑ Description	Assesses the child's developmental skills from 0-6 years of age
❑ Is this an IQ test?	No, this is a test to determine if the child is able to perform skills expected at his age
❑ What are the types of skills being assessed?	Personal-social, speech, fine and gross motor abilities

Teeth Development

❑ When do the first teeth erupt?	At 6 months (lower central incisors)
❑ When do the permanent teeth erupt?	At 6 years-old (molars)
❑ What drug stains the teeth and should be avoided during pregnancy and in children below 8 years old?	Tetracycline
❑ What should you do if a tooth is accidentally avulsed?	Place avulsed tooth in a glass of milk
❑ How can bottle mouth caries syndrome be prevented?	Substitute milk with water Avoid sweet liquids

Types of Play

PLAY	DESCRIPTION	AGE GROUP
Solitary Play	Child plays alone with toys different from others	Infancy to toddlerhood
Parallel Play	Child plays the same activity, playing next to each other, but **does not interact** or do the same game	Toddlerhood
Associative Play	Children participate in the same activities **without** formal interaction or goal; May share toys and imitate others but play independently from each other such as children riding bicycles in the park.	Toddlerhood to preschool
Cooperative Play	Children are working together or against each other **with** formal interaction and a goal	Preschool
Competitive Play	Children participate and understand the importance of rules in games or sports such as basketball and soccer	School-age

The Infant

- ❑ What is the average infant birth weight? — 2.7 – 4.1kg (6 to 9 pounds)
- ❑ Infant loses ______ of weight at 4 days of age — 5-10 % (normal physiologic weight loss)
- ❑ Infant birth weight doubles in _________ and triples in _________ — 6 months, 1 year
- ❑ Why is the infant at risk for ear infections? — Eustachian tubes are shorter and straighter
- ❑ Why are solid foods introduced at 6 months? — Infant has developed ability to swallow
- ❑ What is the preferred first solid food? — Rice cereal
- ❑ Why are single-ingredient foods introduced initially? — To detect food allergy
- ❑ What is weaning? — Gradual replacement of breastmilk or formula with other fluids or foods
- ❑ Can whole milk be given before one year? — No, it may cause allergy or anemia
- ❑ How can parents prevent accidental poisoning? — Lock poisonous items, Use safety latches for cabinets, Never call a drug as "candy"
- ❑ How can parents prevent accidental child drowning? — Use alarms, Fence pools, Never leave child unattended, Wear life jacket

> ***NCLEX Alert!*** *For car safety, use semi-reclined rear-facing infant seat until at least 2 years old or until reaching the manufacturer's stated weight and height maximums (American Pediatric Association).*

The Toddler

❑ Characteristic traits and milestones	Independence, negativism, self-feeding, curiosity, ritualism
❑ Has vocabulary of 900 words	3 years-old
❑ How should parents handle negativism?	Eliminate restrictions, Offer the child reasonable choices, Use distraction
❑ How should parents manage temper tantrums?	Stay calm, Ignore the behavior as long as the child is safe, Enforce a time-out
❑ Preferred toys and plays	Water play, finger painting, dancing to music, push/pull toys

The Preschooler

❑ Characteristic traits and milestones	Control of bladder and bowel functions, magical thinking, egocentric
❑ How should parents handle sibling rivalry?	Allow child to help with care of new sibling Spend special time with older child
❑ Major fears	Fear of mutilation and intrusive procedures Feels responsible when something bad happens due to egocentrism
❑ Are imaginary playmates normal?	Yes, due to magical thinking
❑ Preferred toys and plays	Construction assembly sets, crayons, housekeeping sets, alphabet or number games, books, puzzles, clay

The School-Age Child

❑ Characteristic traits and milestones	Desires knowledge and achievements
❑ Identifies with the parent of the ______ sex	Same
❑ Prefers friends of the ______ sex	Same
❑ Preferred toys and plays	Collecting items and playing games
❑ Is hero worship normal at this age?	Yes

The Adolescent

❑ Characteristic traits and milestones	Independence, Making a career choice
❑ Major concerns	Change in body image, Peer pressure
❑ Periods of puberty	Girls (8-14 years-old); Boys (9-16 years-old)

> ***NCLEX Alert!*** *The leading cause of childhood mortality are accidents or unintentional injuries!*

Approaches to Hospitalization

❑ Stages of Separation Anxiety

PROTEST	DESPAIR	DENIAL/DETACHMENT
❑ Agitated ❑ Screams ❑ Fights caregivers	❑ Withdrawn ❑ Sad ❑ Quiet ❑ Lonely	❑ Appears adjusted ❑ Interested in others ❑ Ignores parents during visits

❑ Interventions during childhood hospitalization

- Allow sucking and cuddling (infant)
- Maintain home rituals
- Bring favorite objects
- Accept and support regression
- Allow the child to handle equipment
- Avoid intrusive procedures (preschool)
- Allow child to contact friends
- Show body diagrams and visual aids
- Offer choices and participation in care

Common Pediatric Milestones – *Take note of these!*

❑ Lifts head slightly when placed on stomach	1 month
❑ Smiles	2 months
❑ Posterior fontanels close	2-3 months
❑ Anterior fontanels close	18-24 months
❑ Supports head steadily	3 months
❑ Turns from back to side	4 months
❑ Rooting, Moro and tonic neck reflexes disappear	4 months
❑ Sits with support	6 months
❑ Pulls to a sitting position	6 months
❑ Two lower teeth appear	6 months
❑ Plays pat-a-cake	7 months
❑ Transfers object from one hand to another	8 months
❑ Sits steadily alone	8-9 months

❑ Understands "no"	9 months
❑ Creeps	9 months
❑ Fears strangers	9 months
❑ Imitates sounds such as "baba' for bye-bye	9 months
❑ Plays peek-a-boo	10 months
❑ Separation anxiety peaks	10 months
❑ Pulls to a standing position in the playpen	10 months
❑ Able to pick up small objects (pincer action)	11 months
❑ Speaks first word	11 months
❑ Stands alone and can sit from standing position	11 months
❑ Understands simple directions	11 months
❑ Drinks from a cup but spills	11 months
❑ Walks with one hand held	12 months
❑ Runs	2 years
❑ Speaks short sentences; Has vocabulary of 300 words	2 years
❑ Speaks five or six sentences	4 years
❑ Ties shoelaces	4 years
❑ Speaks using complete sentences	5 years

B. Neurological Disorders

Spina Bifida

❑ Description	Deficiency of folic acid → spinal vertebrae fail to close in utero
❑ Types	OCCULTA – hidden; with hair tuft on back MENINGOCELE – sac with CSF only MENINGOMYELOCELE – sac has CSF and nerves
❑ Assessment	Paralysis, muscle weakness, bladder and bowel problem, bedwetting, increased ICP, **hydrocephalus**
❑ Diagnostic Test	Increased **alpha fetoprotein** (AFP)
❑ Interventions	Apply **moist sterile dressings** over the sac Bladder or bowel training, Crutches, Braces Intermittent self-catheterization Prone position with abduction of legs or side-lying position

❑ Why is the child at risk for developing latex allergy?	Due to frequent exposure during surgeries and catheterizations

> ***NCLEX Alert!*** *HOW MUCH FOLIC ACID IS NEEDED DURING PREGNANCY TO PREVENT SPINA BIFIDA?*
> *Prevention: 0.4 mg (400 mcg); To prevent recurrence: 4 mg (4000 mcg)*

Hydrocephalus

❑ Description	Accumulation of cerebrospinal fluid
❑ Causes	Tumor, spina bifida
❑ Assessment	Bulging fontanel, high-pitched cry, vomiting, sunset eyes, increased ICP
❑ Interventions	Monitor for increased ICP Ventriculoperitoneal shunting
❑ What is the most common complication of shunting?	Infection
❑ Position after shunt insertion procedure	Flat to prevent sudden drainage of CSF
❑ Monitor for lethargy and vomiting	Indicates increased ICP

> ***NCLEX Alert!*** *Ventriculoperitoneal shunt is revised as the child grows!*

Reye's Syndrome

❑ Description	Causes liver and brain damage
❑ Causes	**Aspirin**, viral infection (chickenpox or flu)
❑ Assessment	Cerebral swelling, increased ICP, diarrhea, confusion, seizure, hepatic encephalopathy
❑ Interventions	Avoid aspirin, Monitor for increased ICP

> ***NCLEX Alert!*** *Give acetaminophen only to prevent Reye's syndrome in children.*

Meningitis

❑ Description	Inflammation of the meninges
❑ Causes	Respiratory infection, otitis media
❑ What are the causative organisms?	Bacterial meningococcus, H. Influenza
❑ Assessment	Increased ICP, nuchal rigidity (stiff neck), headache, fever, high-pitched cry, opisthotonus, photophobia, positive Kernig's and Brudzinski's sign
❑ Diagnostic Tests	Spinal tap with CSF culture

- ❑ Interventions — Monitor for increased ICP, ATBs
  Quiet room, Dim the lights
  Droplet precaution
- ❑ How long is respiratory isolation required? — 24 hours after starting antibiotics

> ***NCLEX Alert!*** *Rifampicin is used for prophylaxis or prevention of meningitis if exposure is suspected.*

Down Syndrome/Trisomy 21

- ❑ Description — Chromosome 21 disorder that leads to mental retardation
- ❑ Cause — Advanced maternal age
- ❑ Assessment — Close-set upward slanting eyes, palmar simian crease, brachycephaly, **low set ears**, round face, flat nose
- ❑ What is a palmar simian crease? — Single line across the palm of the hand
- ❑ Interventions — Maximize potentials, Physical therapy

Cerebral Palsy

- ❑ Description — Disturbances in movement due to brain damage
- ❑ Causes — Traumatic birth, brain anoxia
- ❑ Assessment — **Spastic gait**, muscle rigidity, learning disability, delayed speech or motor skills
- ❑ Does this condition become worse over time? — No, it is a non-progressive disorder
- ❑ Interventions — Maximize potentials, Muscle relaxants
  Physical and occupational therapy

Autism

- ❑ Description — Neurological disorder → impaired communication and social interaction
- ❑ Assessment — Inappropriate social interaction, poor eye contact, compulsive acts, tantrums, repetitive actions and words, attachment to objects, unaware of other's feelings
- ❑ Interventions — Maintain consistency, Promote safety
  Family therapy, Supportive treatment

> ***NCLEX Alert!*** *Asperger's syndrome is a lesser form of autism where affected children show impaired social interactions, little emotions and several persistent, repetitive behaviors.*

Attention-Deficit Hyperactivity Disorder (ADHD)

❑ Description	Brain disorder characterized by hyperactivity, impulsivity and attention difficulty
❑ Assessment	Inattention, impulsivity, learning disability, short attention span, reading difficulty
❑ Interventions	STIMULANTS ▪ methylphenidate (Ritalin) ▪ dextroamphetamine (Dexedrine) ▪ amphetamine/dextroamphetamine (Adderall) NON-STIMULANTS ▪ atomoxetine (Strattera) ▪ clonidine (Kapvay)
❑ Why are cerebral stimulants given for this condition?	They have a paradoxical, relaxing effect on children

Child Abuse

❑ Types	Physical, emotional abuse and neglect
❑ Serious brain injury when shaking an infant	Shaken Baby Syndrome (SBS)
❑ What is the hallmark sign of Shaken Baby Syndrome?	Presence of retinal hemorrhages
❑ Mental health problem in which a caregiver fabricates or intentionally inflicts the illness in a child	Munchausen Syndrome by Proxy
❑ Assessment	Neglected medical and nutritional needs Frequent emergency room visits
❑ Interventions	Protect child from further harm Report a **suspected** child abuse situation

C. Eye, Ear and Throat Disorders

Retinoblastoma

❑ Description	A malignant retinal tumor
❑ Assessment	Yellowish-white reflex in pupil (**cat's eye reflex**), blindness, eye swelling
❑ Interventions	Enucleation, Laser coagulation

Amblyopia (Lazy Eye)

- ❑ Description — Poor vision in one eye leads to the brain favoring the stronger eye
- ❑ Causes — Strabismus, astigmatism, cataracts
- ❑ Assessment — Squinting, poor depth perception
- ❑ Interventions — Patch the **"good"** eye

Otitis Media

- ❑ Description — Infection of the middle ear → pressure → rupture of eardrum → deafness
- ❑ Causes — Defective eustachian tubes, formula feeding, passive smoking
- ❑ Assessment — Pulls ear, rolls head side to side, irritability
- ❑ Interventions — ATB, Avoid high altitudes, Wear ear plugs when swimming, Myringotomy
- ❑ What is the purpose of myringotomy? — To drain the pus and decrease pressure
- ❑ What is the purpose of tympanoplasty tubes? — To ventilate the ear

> ***NCLEX Alert!*** *Tympanoplasty or ventilation tubes fall out spontaneously in 6 months!*

Tonsillitis

- ❑ Description — Infection of the tonsils
- ❑ Assessment — Ear pain, fever, dysphagia, dyspnea
- ❑ Interventions — ATB, Salt water gargles, Tonsillectomy
- ❑ What must be checked before tonsillectomy? — Loose teeth, especially in school-age child
- ❑ Interventions after tonsillectomy — Report frequent swallowing
  Prone or side-lying position
  Clear, cool drinks, No red or purple fluids
  Avoid milk, soda, straw, fork, clearing throat, coughing and forceful blowing of nose

D. Respiratory Disorders

Laryngotracheobronchitis (Viral Croup)

- ❑ Description — Inflammation of the larynx and trachea → laryngeal obstruction → hypoxia
- ❑ Assessment — Brassy, barking cough, dyspnea, **stridor**, crowing sound, wheezing

- ❑ Interventions — Expose child to steam in a hot shower
  Humidified oxygen
  Cool mist tent (croupette)
  Epinephrine, Steroids

Epiglottitis (Bacterial Croup)

- ❑ Description — Infection → laryngeal swelling → severe respiratory distress
- ❑ Assessment — Severe dyspnea, high fever, drooling, tripod positioning (leans forward), froglike sound, inspiratory stridor
- ❑ Interventions — Cool mist humidification, Oxygen
  IV fluid replacement, Tracheostomy, Intubation, ATB
- ❑ Is throat examination allowed? — No, it can trigger laryngeal spasms
- ❑ What immunization is given to prevent this condition? — Haemophilus influenzae type B vaccination

Respiratory Syncytial Virus (RSV) Disease (Bronchiolitis)

- ❑ Description — A viral infection causes pneumonia
- ❑ Transmission — Droplet, direct contact
- ❑ Assessment — Runny nose, cough, fever, wheezing
- ❑ Interventions — Wear mask, gloves and gown
  Ribavirin (Virazole) in mist tent
- ❑ Can a pregnant health care worker care for a child receiving ribavirin treatment? — No, ribavirin exposure is harmful to fetus
- ❑ What should be avoided during aerosol administration of ribavirin? — Staff should avoid wearing contact lens; Wear goggles if contact lenses are worn
- ❑ Why is Respiratory Syncytial Virus Immune Globulin (RespiGam) given? — To enhance immunity against RSV

Sudden Infant Death Syndrome (SIDS, Crib Death, Cot Death)

- ❑ Description — Unexplained death of an infant (<1 year)
- ❑ Causes — Brainstem defect, prematurity, prone or side-lying position in sleep
- ❑ Interventions — Place infant in **supine** position, Use a firm mattress, Remove blankets and toys in crib

E. Cardiovascular Disorders

Congenital Heart Disease

ACYANOTIC HEART DEFECTS	CYANOTIC HEART DEFECTS
Left to right shunting → increased pulmonary blood flow → no cyanosis	Right to left shunting → decreased pulmonary blood flow → cyanosis
❑ Ventricular septal defect ❑ Atrial septal defect ❑ Patent ductus arteriosus (PDA) ❑ Coarctation of the aorta (has higher BP in upper extremities)	TETRALOGY OF FALLOT 1. *Pulmonary stenosis* 2. *Right ventricular hypertrophy* 3. *Ventricular septal defect* 4. *Overriding of the aorta*

- ❑ Assessment — Finger clubbing, dyspnea, **polycythemia**
- ❑ What should you do when the child has an attack of hypercyanotic (Tet) spells? — Place child in **squatting** or knee-chest position
- ❑ Surgery — BLALOCK-TAUSSIG PROCEDURE
  - Connects the subclavian or carotid artery with the pulmonary artery to increase blood flow to the lungs
- ❑ Why is Prostaglandin E1 given? — To open the ductus arteriosus and enhance pulmonary blood flow

Rheumatic Fever

- ❑ Description — Group A streptococcus throat infection → inflammation of connective tissues (e.g. joints, heart, blood vessels, skin)

JONES CRITERIA	
2 major or 1 major + 2 minor (plus history of strep throat) = Rheumatic Fever	
Major Signs	**Minor Signs**
❑ Carditis ❑ Polyarthritis ❑ Rash ❑ Subcutaneous nodules ❑ Chorea	❑ Low-grade fever ❑ Increased ESR and WBC ❑ + C-reactive protein ❑ + Antistreptolysin O (ASO) titer ❑ Prolonged PR interval

- ❑ Interventions — ATB (penicillin), Bed rest, Aspirin
- ❑ Give prophylactic antibiotics before invasive procedures — To prevent bacterial endocarditis

Kawasaki Disease (Mucocutaneous Lymph Node Syndrome)

❑ Description	Inflammation of blood vessels → thrombosis and aneurysms
❑ Assessment	High fever, rashes, **strawberry tongue,** desquamation (peeling) of skin, diarrhea
❑ Interventions	NSAIDs, Blood transfusion, Aspirin Anticoagulants, IV immune globulin IV fluid replacement, Monitor for bleeding

F. Gastrointestinal Disorders

Cleft Lip and Cleft Palate

❑ Description	Splits in the palate or lip
❑ Causes	Heredity, smoking, diabetes mellitus
❑ Complications of cleft palate	Dental decay, speech disorder, stuttering, frequent respiratory infections
❑ When is cheiloplasty usually performed?	Cleft lip (3-4 months of age) Cleft palate (before 18 months of age)
❑ Position after cleft lip repair	Supine or side-lying position
❑ Position after cleft palate repair	Prone or side-lying position
❑ Interventions after cleft lip or palate repair	Apply elbow or jacket restraints Apply Logan lip traction bow Avoid use of pacifiers Use Asepto rubber tipped syringe
❑ What is the ESSR feeding method?	E – nlarge the nipple opening S - timulate the sucking reflex S - wallow fluid appropriately R - est between feedings

> ***NCLEX Alert!*** *Frequently burp the infant with cleft lip or palate!*

Esophageal Atresia and Tracheoesophageal Fistula

❑ Description	Esophagus ends in a blind pouch rather than connecting to the stomach May also be connected to the trachea
❑ Assessment	3 C's – **Coughing, Choking, Cyanosis** drooling, abdominal distention, dyspnea, **polyhydramnios** during pregnancy

- Interventions: Place on NPO; Prevent aspiration pneumonia
- Surgery: Esophageal anastomosis

Celiac Disease (Gluten Enteropathy or Sprue)

- Description: Hypersensitivity to gluten → intestinal inflammation → damage of the microvilli → malabsorption of nutrients
- Assessment: **Intolerance to BROW** (Barley, Rye, Oats, Wheat) bloating, diarrhea, steatorrhea, failure to thrive, abdominal distention, atrophy of the buttocks
- Interventions: Gluten-free diet, Monitor weight

> ***NCLEX Alert!*** *Corn and rice can be used as substitutes to BROW.*

Pyloric Stenosis

- Description: Thickening and narrowing of the pyloric sphincter → foods can't leave the stomach
- Assessment: **Projectile vomiting** after feeding, palpable olive-shaped mass in the RUQ, **non-bile stained vomitus**, visible peristaltic waves, dehydration
- Interventions: Thickened feedings, Burp frequently; Place on right side after feedings; Pyloromyotomy; Resume feedings with glucose water

Hirschsprung's Disease (Aganglionic Megacolon)

- Description: Missing nerve cells in the colon → poor peristalsis → blockage of large intestine
- Assessment: Failure to pass meconium, abdominal swelling, constipation, ribbon-like stools, **bile-stained vomitus**, explosive stools

- Interventions — Stool softeners, Rectal irrigations
- Surgery — Bowel resection and anastomosis with temporary colostomy

Imperforate Anus

- Description — Anal opening is missing or closed
- Assessment — Failure to pass meconium within 48 hours; Inability to insert rectal thermometer
- Interventions — NPO, Emergency surgery with temporary colostomy

Intussusception

- Description — Telescoping of the intestine → intestinal obstruction → peritonitis
- Assessment — Excessive crying, bile-stained vomitus, **sausage-shaped** mass in RUQ of abdomen **red currant-jelly** (bloody) stools
- Interventions — NGT insertion for decompression; IV fluid replacement; Barium enema (treatment of choice)

Lead Poisoning (Plumbism)

- Description — Poisoning caused by accumulation of lead due to eating of paint chips, lead toys, unwashed fruits and herbal or folk remedies
- Assessment — Development delay, anorexia, irritability, anemia, seizures
- Diagnostic Tests — Blood lead level test, Bone x-ray
- Interventions — CHELATING AGENTS
  - calcium disodium edetate (CaEDTA)
  - dimercaprol (BAL)
  - dimercaptosuccinic acid (DMSA)
- What are chelating agents? — Agents that excrete lead through the kidneys

G. Endocrine Disorders

Acute Glomerulonephritis

❑ Description	Group A beta-hemolytic streptococcus infection → inflammation of nephrons → leakage of RBC's and protein in urine
❑ Assessment	**Gross hematuria** smoky brown, pink or cola colored urine, periorbital edema, fever, increased BUN and creatinine, hyperkalemia, hypertension
❑ Interventions	Antihypertensive drugs, Steroids Monitor blood pressure

Phenylketonuria (PKU)

❑ Description	Lacks phenylalanine hydroxylase → decreased tyrosine (an amino acid) and increased phenylalanine → mental retardation
❑ Transmission	Autosomal recessive
❑ Assessment	Mental retardation, musty urine odor, hypopigmentation of skin color, blue eyes, atopic dermatitis
❑ Diagnostic Test	Guthrie blood test (heel prick) → 48-72 hours after birth
❑ Is PKU screening mandatory for all newborns?	Yes
❑ What is important to remember before performing a Guthrie blood test?	Ensure that the newborn has ingested protein to prevent a false negative result
❑ Interventions	Low phenylalanine, low protein diet Restrict aspartame, milk, meat and cheese Special PKU formula
❑ Are the diet restrictions for life?	Yes

Genital Anomalies

❑ Hypospadias	Meatus on the underside of the penis
❑ Epispadias	Meatus is on the upper aspect of the penis
❑ Interventions	Surgery before 10th month of age
❑ Why is circumcision not performed after birth?	Foreskin will be used to repair the defect

Nephrotic Syndrome

❑ Description	Loss of large amounts of protein in urine
❑ Assessment	Gross albuminuria, periorbital edema, puffy eyes, anasarca, weight gain
❑ Interventions	Diuretics, Steroids, Low sodium diet Provide meticulous skin care

H. Musculoskeletal Disorders

Duchenne Muscle Dystrophy

❑ Description	Absence of dystrophin (protein that prevents muscle damage) → progressive muscle degeneration
❑ Transmission	X-linked recessive transmission
❑ Who are usually affected?	Males; Females are carriers
❑ Assessment	Delayed motor development, waddling gait, big calves, muscle weakness, falls, cardiac and respiratory failure
❑ What is Gower's maneuver?	Child uses the hands to stand from squatting position
❑ Diagnostic Tests	Muscle biopsy, Increased creatine kinase
❑ Interventions	Supportive treatment, Rehab therapies

Clubfoot (Talipes)

❑ Description	Foot is improperly positioned and faces sideways or upwards
❑ Interventions	Stretching, Casting, Surgery
❑ What is a Dennis-Browne Splint?	A device attached to the bottom of the child's shoes to keep the feet in position

Scoliosis

❑ Description	Sideways curvature of the spine
❑ Assessment	Back pain, muscle spasms, prominent scapula, uneven shoulder height, hip appears lower, uneven arm length
❑ Interventions	Exercise Spinal fusion with Harrington rods insertion
❑ What is a Milwaukee brace?	A device worn 23 hours per day over a clothing to stop the spinal changes

Legg-Calve Perthes Disease/Coxa Plana

❑ Description	Avascular necrosis of the femoral head
❑ Assessment	Gradual worsening of limping, stiffness in the affected hip, limited range of motion
❑ Interventions	Limit weight-bearing Bed rest, Traction, Hip joint replacement

Congenital Hip Dysplasia (Developmental Hip Dysplasia)

❑ Description	Abnormal hip joint development → unstable hip in the acetabulum → dislocation
❑ Assessment	Limited abduction of the leg on the affected side, asymmetric gluteal folds
❑ What is Galleazi's sign?	Difference in knee height
❑ What is Ortolani's sign?	Click is heard when affected leg is **abducted**
❑ What is Barlow's test?	Dislocation is felt when hip is **adducted**
❑ Interventions	Pavlik harness or Frejka splint, Triple diaper (applied to abduct the legs) Surgery followed by hip spica cast

I. Hematological Disorders

Thalassemia

❑ Description	Genetic blood disorder → abnormal, fragile hemoglobin → anemia
❑ Who are usually affected?	Mediterranean descent
❑ Types	Thalassemia minor and major (Cooley's)
❑ Assessment	Facial bone deformities, pallor, fever, jaundice, fatigue, bronze skin, **hemosiderosis**, protrusion of teeth
❑ Interventions	Blood transfusion, Bone marrow transplant
❑ What is the antidote for iron toxicity?	deferoxamine mesylate (Desferal)

Sickle-Cell Anemia

❑ Description	Abnormal hemoglobin S becomes crescent-shaped → anemia, thrombosis → vaso-occlusive crisis
❑ Transmission	Autosomal recessive
❑ Who are usually affected?	African-Americans
❑ Assessment	Anemia, joint pain, fatigue, fever
❑ What is a Sickledex Test?	Screening test to detect abnormal Hgb S
❑ Interventions	Remember HOP! H - ydration O - xygenation P - ain management

> ***NCLEX Alert!*** *A child with sickle-cell anemia should avoid hypoxia, dehydration, infection and high altitudes to prevent sickling.*

Hemophilia

❑ Description	Deficiency in clotting factors → bleeding
❑ Transmission	X-linked recessive trait
❑ Who are usually affected?	Males; female are carriers
❑ Types	Hemophilia A (Factor VIII deficiency) Hemophilia B (Factor IX deficiency)
❑ Assessment	**Hemarthrosis**, anemia, hematuria
❑ Interventions	Clotting factor replacement
❑ What should the child avoid?	Contact sports to prevent trauma

J. Oncological Disorders

Wilm's Tumor (Nephroblastoma)

❑ Description	A malignant kidney tumor
❑ Assessment	Abdominal mass, hypertension, hematuria, loss of appetite
❑ Interventions	Surgery, Radiation, Chemotherapy

> ***NCLEX Alert!*** *Do not palpate the abdomen to prevent breaking the tumor capsule and cause metastasis.*

Leukemia

❑ Description	Increased production of immature WBC's → anemia, infection, bleeding
❑ Most common type	Acute lymphocytic leukemia
❑ Assessment	Fever, pallor, petechiae, fatigue, infection
❑ Diagnostic Test	Bone marrow biopsy
❑ What is the site for bone marrow biopsy?	Iliac crest
❑ Interventions	Chemotherapy, Bone marrow transplant Reverse isolation

K. Communicable Diseases

Rubeola (Measles)

❑ Transmission	Airborne, contact
❑ Incubation period	10-14 days after exposure
❑ Period of infectivity	4 days before and 4 days after rash appears
❑ Assessment	Fever, runny nose, red, inflamed eyes
❑ Where do the rashes start to appear?	Behind the ear and spreads to the body
❑ What are the 3C's of measles?	**Cough, Coryza, Conjunctivitis**
❑ What are Koplik spots?	Clustered, white lesions on the palate
❑ Interventions	Analgesics, Droplet precautions

Rubella (German Measles)

❑ Transmission	Airborne
❑ Incubation period	14-21 days after exposure
❑ Period of infectivity	1-5 days after appearance of rash
❑ Assessment	Low-grade fever, sore throat

❑ Where do the rashes start to appear?	Face and spreads to the body
❑ Interventions	Analgesics, Isolate from pregnant woman

Chickenpox (Varicella)

❑ Transmission	Airborne, contact
❑ Incubation period	10-21 days after exposure
❑ Period of infectivity	1-2 days before the rash appears until blisters have formed scabs (5-7 days)
❑ Assessment	Red spots turn to blisters and scabs
❑ Where do the rashes start to appear?	Trunk and spreads over the body
❑ Interventions	Isolate until vesicles have dried

Diphtheria

❑ Transmission	Droplet
❑ Incubation period	2-5 days after exposure
❑ Period of infectivity	As long as the bacilli are present on lesions
❑ Assessment	Thick, gray membranes on the pharynx and throat, dyspnea, sore throat, fever, swollen lymph glands
❑ Interventions	ATBs, Diphtheria anti-toxin

Scarlet Fever

❑ Description	Caused by Group A beta-hemolytic strep
❑ Transmission	Droplet
❑ Assessment	Fever, sore throat, **strawberry tongue,** bright red rash starts on the face and spreads over the body
❑ What is Pastia's sign?	Red creases at the bend of the elbow
❑ Interventions	Droplet precautions, ATBs

Erythema Infectiosum (Fifth Disease)

❑ Description	A viral infection
❑ Assessment	Facial rash (**slapped face**), fever
❑ Interventions	Analgesics

Rocky Mountain Spotted Fever

❑ Description	Caused by Rickettsia rickettsia
❑ Transmission	Bite of an infected tick
❑ Assessment	Fever, headache, rash, muscle pain
❑ Interventions	ATB (doxycycline)

Enterobiasis (Pinworm)

- Description — Caused by pinworm *Enterobius vermicularis*
- Transmission — Fecal-oral
- Assessment — Intense itching around the anus
- Interventions — Tape test in the morning before defecation; Antihelminthic drugs (mebendazole)

Pediculosis

- Types
  - Pediculosis capitis (head)
  - Pediculosis corporis (body)
  - Pediculosis pubis ("crabs")
- Interventions
  - Permethrin shampoo with retreatment
  - Remove nits using a fine-tooth combed
  - Laundry linens or articles in hot water
- Who should be treated? — All infected persons (household members and close contacts) must be treated at the same time

L. Recommended Schedule of Immunization (Birth Through 6 Years)

<table>
<tr><th>BIRTH</th><th>1 month</th><th>2 month</th><th>4 months</th><th>6 months</th><th>12 months</th><th>15 months</th><th>18 months</th><th>19-23 months</th><th>2-3 years</th><th>4-6 years</th></tr>
<tr><td></td><td></td><td></td><td></td><td></td><td></td><td></td><td></td><td></td><td></td><td></td></tr>
<tr><td>Hepa B</td><td colspan="2">Hepa B</td><td></td><td colspan="4">Hepa B</td><td></td><td></td><td></td></tr>
<tr><td></td><td></td><td>RV</td><td>RV</td><td>RV</td><td></td><td></td><td></td><td></td><td></td><td></td></tr>
<tr><td></td><td></td><td>DTaP</td><td>DTaP</td><td>DTap</td><td></td><td colspan="2">DTaP</td><td></td><td></td><td>DTaP</td></tr>
<tr><td></td><td></td><td>Hib</td><td>Hib</td><td>Hib</td><td colspan="2">Hib</td><td></td><td></td><td></td><td></td></tr>
<tr><td></td><td></td><td>PCV13</td><td>PCV13</td><td>PCV13</td><td colspan="2">PCV13</td><td></td><td></td><td></td><td></td></tr>
<tr><td></td><td></td><td>IPV</td><td>IPV</td><td colspan="4">IPV</td><td></td><td></td><td>IPV</td></tr>
<tr><td></td><td></td><td></td><td></td><td colspan="7">Influenza (Yearly)</td></tr>
<tr><td></td><td></td><td></td><td></td><td></td><td colspan="2">MMR</td><td></td><td></td><td></td><td>MMR</td></tr>
<tr><td></td><td></td><td></td><td></td><td></td><td colspan="2">Varicella</td><td></td><td></td><td></td><td>Varicella</td></tr>
<tr><td></td><td></td><td></td><td></td><td></td><td colspan="4">Hepa A</td><td></td><td></td></tr>
</table>

Shaded boxes indicate that the vaccine can be given during shown age range

Reference: CDC, 2018 Recommended Schedule of Immunization (Birth Through 6 Years)

Check the CDC website (www.cdc.gov) for updates on immunization schedules for children

Legend:

- ❑ RV - Rotavirus
- ❑ DTaP - Diphtheria, Tetanus, Pertussis
- ❑ Hib - Haemophilus influenzae type B
- ❑ PCV13 - Pneumococcus
- ❑ MMR - Measles, Mumps, Rubella
- ❑ Varicella - Chickenpox

<table>
<tr><th colspan="4">TYPES OF IMMUNITY</th></tr>
<tr><th colspan="2">Naturally Acquired</th><th colspan="2">Artificially Acquired</th></tr>
<tr><td>Active</td><td>Passive</td><td>Active</td><td>Passive</td></tr>
<tr><td>❑ Development of antibodies due to exposure to a disease (antigen)
❑ Long-term protection
❑ e.g. measles, chickenpox</td><td>❑ Newborn receives antibodies from the mother through the placenta or breast milk
❑ e.g. IgG from mother</td><td>❑ Development of antibodies through the injection of live, attenuated vaccines
❑ e.g. Hepa B, Flu vaccines</td><td>❑ Ready-made antibodies (immunoglobulins) are injected to provide immediate protection
❑ e.g. Hepa B immune globulin</td></tr>
</table>

M. Genetic Transmission of Diseases

TRANSMISSION	DESCRIPTION	EXAMPLES
Autosomal Recessive	❑ **Two affected genes** (one from each parent) are required to cause disease in a child ❑ If both parents are carriers (having the affected gene but no symptoms), they have a 25% chance of having a child with disease and a 50% chance of a having a child who is a carrier	❑ Cystic fibrosis ❑ Sickle cell disease ❑ Phenylketonuria ❑ Thalassemia ❑ Tay-Sachs disease
Autosomal Dominant	❑ Only **one affected gene** from a parent is required to cause disease in a child ❑ A carrier mother has a 50% chance of having a son and daughter with the disease ❑ An affected father has a 100% chance of having daughters who will be affected	❑ Polycystic kidney disease ❑ Huntington's chorea ❑ Marfan syndrome ❑ Hyperlipidemia ❑ Neurofibromatosis ❑ Osteogenesis imperfecta
X-Linked Recessive	❑ **Males develop the disease**; Females are the carriers as the father cannot transmit the gene to the children ❑ A carrier mother has a 50% chance of having a son with the disease and 50% chance of having a daughter that is a carrier	❑ Hemophilia ❑ Duchenne muscular dystrophy ❑ Fabry disease
X-Linked Dominant	❑ Both males and females can be affected, but more fatal in males ❑ A carrier mother has a 50% chance of having a child with the disease ❑ An affected father has a 100% chance of having daughters who have the disease (father cannot transmit the gene to his sons)	❑ Fragile X syndrome

NCLEX Alert! *You have to remember the types of genetic transmission for inherited childhood diseases!*

N. Pediatric Dosage and Calculation

- ❑ Most drugs are in what form? — Liquid or suspension
- ❑ Preferred subcutaneous injection sites — Upper arm, abdomen and anterior thigh
- ❑ Preferred intramuscular injection site for infants — Vastus laterals
- ❑ Are special administration sets used? — Yes, microdrip sets are used

Calculation of Medication by Body Weight

- ❑ Calculating Daily Dosage — mg/kg/day or mg/lb/day
  Ex. 2 mg x 10 kg = 20 mg/day
- ❑ Calculating Per Dose — Divide the total daily dosage by the number of doses (frequency) to be administered in one day = per dose
  Ex. 20 mg/day divided by 2 doses (e.g. BID) = 10 mg per dose

Example:

1. A 55-pound child is to receive digoxin (Lanoxin). The daily dosage is 0.15 mg/kg daily to be given every 12 hours. On hand is Lanoxin elixir 0.5 mg/mL. How many mL should the nurse give?

Steps:

55 lbs. = 25 kg

0.15 mg x 25 kg = 3.75 mg daily safe dose

3.75 mg divided by 2 (every 12 hours) = 1.875 mg per dose

$$\frac{1.875\text{ mg}}{0.5\text{ mg}} \times 1\text{ ml} = 3.75\text{ mL (answer)}$$

Pediatric Formula (Per Dose)

1. CLARK'S RULE

$$\text{Child's dose} = \frac{\text{Weight (in pounds)}}{150} \times \text{adult dose}$$

2. FRIED'S RULE

$$\text{Child's dose} = \frac{\text{Age (in months)}}{150} \times \text{adult dose}$$

3. YOUNG'S RULE

$$\text{Child's dose} = \frac{\text{Age (in years)}}{\text{Age (in years)} + 12} \times \text{adult dose}$$

Example:

1. A 54-lb 8-year-old child is prescribed doxycycline (Vibramycin). The adult dose for this drug is 100 mg. Calculate the pediatric (per) dose using Clark's and Young's Rule.

$$\frac{54}{150} \times 100 = 36 \text{ mg (Clark's Rule)}$$

$$\frac{8}{8 + 12} \times 100 = 40 \text{ mg (Young's Rule)}$$

Mental Health Nursing 20

A. Basic Concepts

- ❑ Principles of the Nurse-Client Relationship

  Acceptance
  Client-centered
  Consistency
  Empathy
  Genuineness
  Goal-directed
  Holistic approach
  Individualized care
  Non-judgmental approach
  Problem-solving
  Professional relationship
  Trust

- ❑ What is the meaning of empathy?

  The nurse's ability to understand the client's emotions and experience

- ❑ Why is consistency important in a nurse-client relationship?

  Consistency promotes the client's development of trust towards the nurse, which is essential to ensure client participation and success in treatment

Phases of the Nurse-Client Relationship

PRE-INTERACTION PHASE	ORIENTATION PHASE	WORKING PHASE	TERMINATION/ SEPARATION PHASE
❑ Nurse should be aware of values and biases that can affect the nurse-client relationship (self-awareness)	❑ Define rules and goals ❑ Establish rapport, trust and contract	❑ Problem identification and solving	❑ Evaluate goals met ❑ Asses for signs of separation anxiety

Therapeutic Communication

THERAPEUTIC	NON-THERAPEUTIC
❑ Active listening	❑ Agreeing or disagreeing with client
❑ Asking questions with broad openings	❑ Arguing or giving disapproval
❑ Clarifying understanding	❑ Asking using the word, *"Why?"*
❑ Encouraging verbalization	❑ Belittling the client's problem
❑ Making neutral, non-judgmental responses	❑ Blaming the client
❑ Offering self when needed	❑ Challenging the client's perceptions and thoughts
❑ Presenting reality	❑ Shifting the topic of conversation to another
❑ Reflecting	❑ Giving false reassurances
❑ Restating	❑ Imposing personal values
❑ Setting alternatives for problem-solving	❑ Not listening
❑ Sharing perceptions or observations	❑ Providing advice
❑ Showing empathy	❑ Using cliché' statements
❑ Using open-ended questions	
❑ Using silence	

Therapeutic versus Non-Therapeutic Communication Techniques

1. Nurse: "Your doctor is the best one we have." — Non-Therapeutic, a defensive response
2. Nurse: "Why do you feel that way?" — Non-Therapeutic, elicits defensive response
3. Nurse: "Tell me about that." — Therapeutic, encourages verbalization
4. Nurse: "You are not the Princess of England!" — Non-Therapeutic, arguing with the client
5. Nurse: "Don't worry everything will be okay!" — Non-Therapeutic, this is false reassurance
6. Nurse: "I'm sorry, you were saying something?" — Non-Therapeutic, the nurse is not listening
7. Nurse: "The policy is one cigarette for each client." — Therapeutic, maintains consistency
8. Nurse: "I think you should....." — Non-Therapeutic, giving advice
9. Nurse: "Waiting for the results of your biopsy is hard." — Therapeutic, conveys empathy
10. Nurse: "Let's discuss other options." — Therapeutic, helps set alternatives
11. Nurse: "Can you tell me why you want to leave your wife?" — Therapeutic, encourages verbalization
12. Nurse: "That is interesting. Please go on." — Therapeutic, encourages verbalization
13. Nurse: "That's not serious compared to other clients." — Non-Therapeutic, belittling the problem
14. Nurse: "How did you eat your meal if your arms are missing? — Non-Therapeutic, challenging the client
15. Nurse: "I don't believe you." — Non-Therapeutic, arguing with the client
16. Nurse: "I can tell this must be very difficult for you." — Therapeutic, conveys empathy
17. Nurse: "This is not a moral thing to do." — Non-Therapeutic, imposes own beliefs
18. Client: "My brother always teases me."
    Nurse: "That's not good, but let's talk about your condition." — Non-Therapeutic, changing the topic

Defense Mechanisms

- ❑ What are the reasons for using defense mechanisms? — To decrease anxiety and protect the ego
- ❑ When do defense mechanisms become abnormal? — When they are used excessively

DEFENSE MECHANISM	DESCRIPTION
Displacement	Redirecting feelings toward another powerless person or object
Dissociation	Blocking off or separation of traumatic events from awareness or memory
Fixation	Failure of emotional milestones to advance (e.g. thumb sucking)
Identification	Unconscious action to imitate an admired person
Introjection	Unconscious adoption of traits or values of a person
Compensation	Attempt to excel in one area to overcome a weakness
Conversion	Physical symptoms occur due to unresolved emotional conflicts or issues
Denial	Consciously blocking anxiety-provoking thoughts or situations
Projection	Attributing thoughts, feelings and traits to another person
Rationalization	Making feelings and behaviors acceptable by justification (sour graping)
Intellectualization	Avoids emotions by focusing on facts, logic and excessive reasoning
Reaction formation	Displaying behaviors opposite to what one really feels or thinks
Regression	Act of returning to an earlier stage of development
Repression	Unconscious blocking of unacceptable thoughts
Suppression	Conscious forgetting of unacceptable thoughts
Splitting	Tendency to perceive others either as only totally good or totally bad
Sublimation	Replacement of unacceptable impulses with socially acceptable alternatives
Symbolization	Using an idea, object or symbol to represent an event or another object
Undoing	Behavior that is opposite of a previous unacceptable or destructive behavior

Examples of Defense Mechanisms

1. A blind man learns to sing very well — Compensation
2. A man becomes blind after witnessing a murder — Conversion
3. A woman who has breast cancer tells her children that her biopsy results must be wrong — Denial
4. An athlete slams the door after losing a game — Displacement

5. A girl who was raped was found walking alone. When examined in the ER, she cannot remember what happened	Dissociation
6. A girl dresses and walks like Kim Kardashian	Identification
7. A man claimed to be Saint Joseph, grew a beard and started wearing similar clothing everyday	Introjection
8. A girl who was not invited to a party tells her friend, *"I wanted to go but I have a date anyway."*	Rationalization
9. A man diagnosed with terminal illness spends the whole night researching on the prognosis of his disease	Intellectualization
10. An unfaithful wife accuses her husband of infidelity	Projection
11. A girl who loathes her classmate acts cordial towards him	Reaction formation
12. A 40-year-old man behaves like a 16-year-old on a first date	Regression
13. A woman who hit her husband during a fight cannot remember the event after a week	Repression
14. A student refuses to discuss questions after a finals exam	Suppression
15. A boy who has angry feelings re-channels them by joining the debate team	Sublimation
16. A girl sends chocolates to her mother after an argument	Undoing
17. A girl considers her boyfriend as the worst devil despite the good things he did before their argument	Splitting

Diagnostic and Statistical Manual of Mental Health Disorders

- Description — A reference that lists descriptions, symptoms and other criteria in order to diagnose mental disorders; Provides a uniform language for clinicians during care (*American Psychiatric Association*)

Behavior Modification Therapy

- Description — A therapeutic approach that aims to change an undesirable behavior with favorable ones through positive or negative reinforcement

Family Therapy

- Description — Based on a principle that a problem in one family member affects the whole dynamics of the family; Aims to restore harmony in the family by addressing specific issues and expectations

Milieu Therapy

- Description — Providing changes in the environment to effect behavioral change
  Clients are empowered to take responsibilities and participate in activities

Cognitive Therapy

- Description — Thoughts affect behaviors and feelings
  Treats disorders such as anxiety, panic and depression by changing ways of thinking

Group Therapy

- Description — Members are encouraged to work on achieving effective coping skills and goals
  Applied to rape and substance abuse
  Problem-solving and coping are promoted by peers providing feedback and support

B. Mental Health Disorders

Anxiety

- Description — Subjective experience of apprehension, worry or threat to self-esteem
- Levels of anxiety

MILD	MODERATE	SEVERE	PANIC
❑ Motivating ❑ Enhances concentration	❑ Focuses on immediate situation ❑ Selective inattention ❑ Able to follow directions	❑ Significant narrowing of the perceptual field ❑ Problem solving not possible ❑ Symptoms appear	❑ Severe feeling of dread ❑ Cannot communicate ❑ Escape is the focus

Post-Traumatic Stress Disorder (PTSD)

- Description — Failure to recover after a traumatic event
- Assessment — Recurrent **flashbacks** or nightmares, hypervigilance, anxiety, depression, insomnia, hostility, **suicide attempts**

- ❑ Interventions — Review the traumatic event
  Support groups
  Systematic desensitization
  Antidepressant medications

Panic Disorder

- ❑ Description — Sudden, severe fear with no known cause
- ❑ Assessment — Palpitations, weakness, syncope, choking feeling, dyspnea, chest pain numbness, hyperventilation, "*feeling that something bad is about to happen*"
- ❑ Interventions — Do not leave the client during attack
  Change unhealthy thoughts
  Antianxiety medications

Generalized Anxiety Disorder

- ❑ Description — Persistent worry → physical symptoms and inability to perform ADL's
- ❑ Assessment — Constant worrying, muscle spasm, insomnia
- ❑ Interventions — Stress management, Mindfulness therapy
  Cognitive-behavioral therapy
  Antianxiety and antidepressant medications

Obsessive-Compulsive Disorder

- ❑ Description — Constant intrusive thoughts (obsession) and behaviors (compulsion) usually focusing on germs or arranging items
  Ritualistic acts decrease the anxiety
- ❑ Interventions — Ensure physical needs are provided (e.g. skin care due to handwashing)
  Do **not** interrupt the ritualistic behavior
  Antianxiety and antidepressant medications

Phobias

- ❑ Description — Severe, irrational fears and avoidance of feared situations or objects
- ❑ Interventions — Identify the cause of anxiety
  Relaxation techniques
  Verbalize feelings about the feared object
- ❑ What is desensitization therapy? — Gradual exposure to feared object

- Types of Phobias

PHOBIA	DESCRIPTION
Acrophobia	Fear of heights
Agoraphobia	Fear of open or crowded spaces
Arachnophobia	Fear of spiders
Astraphobia	Fear of thunder and lightning
Claustrophobia	Fear of closed spaces
Gerascophobia	Fear of growing old
Hematophobia	Fear of blood
Monophobia	Fear of being alone
Mysophobia	Fear of germs
Nyctophobia	Fear of darkness or night
Ophidiophobia	Fear of snakes
Pyrophobia	Fear of fire
Thanatophobia	Fear of death
Xenophobia	Fear of people or strangers
Zoophobia	Fear of animals

Dissociative Disorder

- Description: Breakdown in memory, awareness, emotion, identity or perception due to a traumatic experience

- Interventions: Cognitive behavioral therapy
  Antidepressant and antianxiety medications

Types of Dissociative Disorders

DISSOCIATIVE IDENTITY DISORDER (formerly called Multiple Personality Disorder)	DISSOCIATIVE AMNESIA
Existence of two or more distinct personalities	Blocks out information due to a stressful event
Assessment ❑ Inability to remember the personalities ❑ Stress triggers transition to another personality ❑ Dissociation serves to decrease anxiety	Assessment ❑ LOCALIZED: unable to remember an event ❑ SELECTIVE: recalls some aspects of the events ❑ GENERALIZED: total loss of identity and memory
DISSOCIATIVE FUGUE	**DEPERSONALIZATION/ DEREALIZATION DISORDER**
Assumes a new identity and unexpectedly travels into new places for weeks or months	Perception of self from outside the body or things around are not real
Assessment ❑ Sudden loss of identity ❑ Client is unable to recall what happened	Assessment ❑ Feelings of detachment from one's body or mind (depersonalization) ❑ Feelings of detachment from environment which seems unreal (derealization)

Somatoform Disorders

❑ Description

Persistent symptoms such as pain without apparent physical cause
Client is not faking (**malingering**) the symptoms

❑ Interventions

Determine the source of anxiety
Rule out the physical cause of illness
Symptoms are **real** for the client
Cognitive behavioral therapy
Antianxiety medications

❑ What is the difference between **primary** and **secondary** gain?

Primary and secondary gains are motivators for sick roles. Primary gain refers to a **decrease in anxiety** and secondary gain refers to benefits such as increased attention or relief from responsibility.

Types of Somatoform Disorders

CONVERSION DISORDER	ILLNESS ANXIETY DISORDER (formerly Hypochondriasis)	SOMATIZATION DISORDER
A physical symptom occurs due to a psychological conflict	Severe preoccupation with a serious, undiagnosed disease	Persistent physical complaints with no obvious cause
Assessment ❑ Complaints of deafness, blindness or paralysis ❑ "*la belle indifference*" - client does not worry about the symptoms	Assessment ❑ Frequent bodily complaints ❑ Overuse of home treatments ❑ "doctor shopping "	Assessment ❑ Complaints of recurring pain or fatigue ❑ Denial of emotional conflict

Bipolar Disorder (Manic-Depressive Illness)

- ❑ Description — Episodes of mood swings with unusual shifts between depression and mania

MANIA	DEPRESSION
❑ High-level energy	❑ Low-level energy
❑ Easily gets angry	❑ Psychomotor retardation
❑ Inappropriate dress	❑ Internalizing hostility
❑ Sexually promiscuous	❑ Difficulty making decisions
❑ Easy distractibility	❑ Low self-esteem
❑ **Flight of ideas**	❑ Suicidal thoughts
❑ **Delusions of grandeur**	❑ **Anhedonia**
❑ Insomnia	❑ Insomnia
❑ Restlessness	❑ Social isolation

- ❑ Interventions (Manic Phase)
  - Prevent exhaustion and death
  - Promote rest and sleep periods
  - Orient to reality
  - Do not argue with client
  - Limit group activities
  - Assign a private room if possible
  - Avoid competitive activities
  - Distract from grandiose delusions
  - Set limits and maintain consistency
  - Provide **high-calorie finger** foods

Reduce environmental stimuli
Provide physical outlets for high energy
Lithium carbonate, Sedatives

Major Depression

- ❑ Description — Constant depressed mood and loss of interest → impaired activities of daily living
- ❑ Assessment — Poor decision-making skills, bodily complaints, lack of concentration, lack of sexual interest, powerlessness, suicidal thoughts
- ❑ What is rumination? — Repetitively going over a thought
- ❑ What is anhedonia? — Lack of pleasure in enjoyable activities
- ❑ Interventions — Provide simple, repetitive activities
  Avoid a cheerful attitude
  Ask client directly, "*Have you thought of hurting yourself?*"
  Monitor at irregular intervals
  One-on-one supervision
  Create a suicide contract
- ❑ Electroconvulsive Therapy (ECT) — Treats severe depression
- ❑ What are the side effects of ECT? — Short-term memory loss and confusion

Suicidal Behavior

- ❑ Risk factors — History of suicidal attempts, severe depression, personality disorders, family history, adolescent, substance abuse, elderly clients, dementia
- ❑ What are the signs of a possible suicide attempt? — Giving away prized or personal possessions
  Statements about death or hopelessness
  Negative statements about self

Changing a will or life insurance policy
Questions on ways to kill self
Canceling social activities
Isolation from friends or family

NCLEX Alert! *A sudden improvement in mood or calmness indicate that the client has the potential to implement plans of committing suicide!*

Schizophrenia

- ❑ Description — Disturbed thought, mood and affect

- ❑ Combination of schizophrenia and mood disorder symptoms — Schizoaffective Disorder
- ❑ Severe social withdrawal, Disorganized behavior and speech — Disorganized Schizophrenia
- ❑ Immobility, **Waxy flexibility**, Repetitive behavior — Catatonic Schizophrenia
- ❑ Delusion of persecution, Mistrust — Paranoid Schizophrenia
- ❑ Shows signs of schizophrenia but doesn't meet any type — Undifferentiated Schizophrenia
- ❑ Previous diagnosis with no major symptoms — Residual Schizophrenia

- ❑ Assessment of Schizophrenia
    - Linking of words with similar sounds: *"I'll fly in the sky!"* — Clang association or rhyming
    - Repeating the speech of a person — Echolalia
    - Repeating the movements of a person — Echopraxia
    - Rigid positioning of the body for a length of time — Catatonic stupor
    - Constant agitation and excitation — Catatonic excitement
    - Maintains the same limb position for a long time — Waxy flexibility
    - Absence of energy — Anertia
    - No facial expression; Affect is incongruent with the situation — Flat or inappropriate affect
    - Conflicting attitudes and emotions — Ambivalence
    - A newly coined word or expression — Neologism
    - Responses do not relate to the questions — Loose associations
    - Stops speaking suddenly without explanation — Thought blocking
    - Answering with excessive, unnecessary details — Circumstantiality
    - Filling a memory gap with fantasy — Confabulation
    - Jumps from one topic to another — Flight of ideas
    - Unintelligible mixtures of words with no meaning — Word salad
    - Obsessive repetition of same words — Verbigeration or perseveration
    - Absence of speech — Mutism
    - Doing only what is instructed to avoid responsibility — Overcompliance

- False perception **without** any stimulus *(e.g. seeing spiders on the wall)* — Hallucination
- False perception with stimulus *(e.g. seeing spiders instead of coins)* — Illusion
- A fixed, false belief — Delusion
- False belief of being superior and powerful — Delusion of grandeur
- False belief of being harmed by people — Delusion of persecution
- Belief that events are related to one's own situation — Ideas of reference
- Hallucinations and delusion — Positive symptoms of schizophrenia
- Lack of emotion, social isolation, flat affect — Negative symptoms of schizophrenia

❑ Interventions

Address physical needs
Set limits on disruptive behaviors
Maintain a neutral approach
Orient to reality
Canned foods for paranoid schizophrenia

❑ What are the interventions for a client who is actively having hallucinations?

Ask directly about the hallucination such as *"Do you hear strange voices?"*
Present reality or your own perception
Say, *"I know you are hearing voices but I cannot hear them."*
Never agree or disagree with hallucinations
Do not touch the client

> ***NCLEX Alert!*** *Auditory hallucinations pose safety concern to a client especially when command hallucinations tell the client to perform dangerous actions.*

Personality Disorders

❑ Description — Inflexible and abnormal pattern of behavior → impaired social relationships

❑ Can stress make this condition worse? — Yes

❑ Do people with personality disorders lack insight? — Yes

❑ Are they in touch with reality? — Yes

CLUSTER A (ECCENTRIC) PERSONALITY DISORDERS	
Schizoid	Social detachment, solitary, aloof, cold
Paranoid	Suspicious, hostile, aloof
Schizotypal	Unusual ideas, magical thinking, eccentric

CLUSTER B (OVEREMOTIONAL) PERSONALITY DISORDERS	
Narcissistic	Need for self-importance, recognition for accomplishments, undermines others
Histrionic	Extremely dramatic, attention-seeking, overly-expressive behavior
Antisocial	Irresponsible behavior, guiltless, manipulative, shameless
Borderline	*"Walking on eggshells"*, unstable mood, unpredictable, poor self-image, emptiness, fear of abandonment, dependent, self-destructive behavior, splitting, uses guilt tripping, *"I hate you but don't leave me!"*

CLUSTER C (ANXIOUS) PERSONALITY DISORDERS	
Avoidant	Social isolation, feeling of inferiority, sensitivity to rejection
Obsessive-Compulsive	Perfectionism, engages in ritualistic behavior
Dependent	Poor self-confidence and self-esteem, cannot make decisions

- ❑ Interventions — Protect from self-destructive behaviors
  Maintain consistency
  Set limits on inappropriate behavior

Dementia

- ❑ Description — Not a specific disease but refers to disorders that cause impairment in memory, judgment, language and motor skills
- ❑ Most common type — Alzheimer's Disease
- ❑ Assessment — Remember 5 A's!
  1. AGNOSIA
     - Inability to recognize objects or people
  2. AMNESIA
     - Memory loss
  3. APHASIA
     - Inability to express through speech
  4. ANOMIA
     - Inability to recall names of objects
  5. APRAXIA
     - Difficulty in performing simple tasks
- ❑ What are the late symptoms of dementia? — Personality changes, **wandering**, hallucination, paranoia, **sundowning**

❑ What is sundowning (late-day confusion)?	Confusion becomes worse in late afternoon
❑ What are the 3 R's when caring for clients with dementia?	Repetition, Reinforcement, Reorientation
❑ Interventions	Provide **structured** routines Bring familiar objects from home Identify self always, Call client by name Place a calendar and clock Use familiar objects Encourage client to reminisce Assess **cause** of agitated behavior

Delirium versus Dementia

❑ Sudden change in mental state that is treatable	Delirium
❑ Gradual, progressive, chronic and irreversible	Dementia
❑ Caused by substance abuse, metabolic imbalance, liver failure, infection or congestive heart failure	Delirium
❑ Caused by neurological degeneration	Dementia

Eating Disorders

Anorexia Nervosa

❑ Description	Disturbed self-image and perception → starvation and weight loss
❑ Assessment	Weight loss, denial of hunger, self-induced vomiting and enemas, excessive exercising, perfectionist personality, scaly, dry skin, lanugo on extremities, amenorrhea, electrolyte and hormonal imbalance

Bulimia Nervosa

❑ Description	Eating large amounts of food → guilt and depression → self-induced vomiting
❑ Assessment	**Binge-purge** syndrome overuse emetic, enemas, and amphetamines, **dental decay**
❑ Interventions for Eating Disorders	Remain non-judgmental Antidepressants Behavior modification

- What intervention is important before, during and after meals? — Supervise the client to prevent self-induced vomiting

Substance Abuse Disorders

Alcohol Abuse

- Risk Factors — Genetics, low-self-esteem, depression
- Assessment — Slurred speech, uncoordinated movements, decreased inhibition, black-outs
- What is the screening test for alcoholism? — CAGE screening questionnaire
- What is **Wernicke's-Korsakoff psychosis**? — **Thiamine** or vitamin B_1 deficiency caused by alcoholism; Characterized by ataxia, **memory loss** and nystagmus
- What is confabulation? — Making up stories to fill in memory gaps

Alcohol Withdrawal

- Description — Develops hours after stopping alcohol
- Assessment — Anxiety, vomiting, tremors
- What is **delirium tremens**? — Life-threatening form of alcohol withdrawal characterized by confusion, hallucinations and seizures
- Interventions — Be non-judgmental, Provide quiet room Sedatives, Seizure precaution

Disulfiram Therapy

- Description — A form of aversion therapy to eliminate addictive behavior to alcohol
- What will happen If the client drinks alcohol? — Severe unpleasant reactions such as hypotension, tachycardia, flushing, sweating, throbbing headache, syncope, nausea and vomiting, dyspnea
- What instructions are important to teach the client? — Avoid substances containing alcohol such as perfumes, cough medicines, vinegar, mouthwashes, aftershave lotions, glues, thinners, spirits and fermented foods

> ***NCLEX Alert!*** *Avoid alcohol 12 hours before start of dose and until 14 days after disulfiram cessation.*

Drug Dependency

Controlled Substances Schedules

	CRITERIA	PRESCRIPTION	EXAMPLES
Schedule 1	Highest potential for abuse or dependency; No accepted use		*heroin, LSD, marijuana*
Schedule 2	Prescriptions with high potential for abuse or dependency; Some accepted medical use	Written prescriptions required with no refills	*hydromorphone, oxycodone, morphine*
Schedule 3	Intermediate potential for dependency or abuse	Written/oral prescription no longer than 6 months	*hydrocodone, dihydrocodeine*
Schedule 4	Less abuse or dependency risk	Written/oral prescription no longer than 6 months	*diazepam, lorazepam*
Schedule 5	Small potential for dependency or abuse; widespread use	Multiple refills or OTC	*buprenorphine, diphenoxylate/atropine*

Reference: US Drug Enforcement Administration (DEA)

	CNS DEPRESSANTS	CNS STIMULANTS
Substances	❑ Alcohol, barbiturates, benzodiazepines, opioids	❑ Ecstasy ("Molly"), amphetamines, cocaine, crack
Signs of Intoxication	❑ Hypotension, drowsiness, unsteady gait, bradypnea, amnesia	❑ Euphoria, **dilated pupils**, insomnia, hypertension, tachycardia, paranoia
Signs of Overdose	❑ Respiratory depression, coma	❑ Fever, seizures, cardiac arrest, coma

Opioids

❑ Drugs

Examples:

- Heroine, morphine, meperidine (Demerol), codeine, methadone, hydromorphone (Dilaudid), fentanyl (Sublimaze)

❑ Signs of intoxication

Decreased respiration, lethargy, euphoria, confusion, slurred speech, hypotension, **constricted pupils**

❑ Signs of withdrawal

Yawning, insomnia, **runny nose**

Hallucinogens

❑ Substance	Lysergic acid diethylamide (LSD), psilocybin (mushrooms), phencyclidine (PCP)
❑ Signs of intoxication	Anxiety, blank stare, hallucinations, paranoia, slurred speech, **dilated pupils**

Marijuana (Cannabis)

❑ Signs of intoxication	Euphoria, relaxation, altered perception of time, increased appetite, heightened sensory perception, anxiety, paranoia

Miscellaneous Substances

❑ Substance	Examples: ▪ ecstasy (MDMA) ▪ gamma-hydroxybutyric acid (GHB) ▪ metamphetamine (crank, meth) ▪ ketamine
❑ Signs of intoxication	Euphoria, enhanced confidence, friendliness
❑ Adverse effects	Fever, circulatory collapse, dehydration, panic attacks, **arrhythmias**
❑ Interventions during drug withdrawal	Meet physical needs Ensure supervision and safety Frequent orientation Hydration, Anti-anxiety drugs
❑ What drug is used to prevent withdrawal symptoms in persons addicted to heroin or other opioids?	Methadone

Restraints

❑ What are the guidelines when using restraints?	Ask, *"Is client a danger to self or others?"* Requires an order unless emergency Assess the cause of abnormal behavior Use least restrictive alternatives first (e.g. distraction, activities, orientation) Explain risks and benefits to family Release restraint every 2 hours for hygiene, exercise and nutrition needs

Crisis Intervention

❑ Description	Failure of usual coping mechanisms → disorganization and nervous breakdown
❑ Types	Situational (bankruptcy, divorce, illness) Maturational (marriage, childbirth)
❑ Interventions in Crisis Intervention	Reduce anxiety Identify social support system Assist in problem solving Explore alternate coping mechanisms

End-of-Life Care

❑ What are the signs of impending death?	Cold or pale extremities, oliguria, bowel incontinence, hypothermia, decreased taste and smell, anorexia, reduced pain perception, Cheyne-Stokes respiration, death rattle
❑ Interventions in Comfort Measure Orders	Pain management, Elevate HOB Oxygen, Suction airway, Antiemetic, Oral care, Ice chips, Lip lubricant Continue to speak while giving care
❑ Interventions in Post-Mortem Care	Maintain respect and dignity Privacy for family and significant others Be aware of cultural practices on death Close the eyes and mouth Replace clean dentures Wash the body Determine organ donation status Remove devices (except for autopsy) Place on supine position with pillow under the head

C. Psychotropic Drugs

1. Antipsychotic Drugs

TYPICAL AND ATYPICAL ANTIPSYCHOTICS		
Blocks post-synaptic **dopamine** receptors in the brain → Decreased psychotic and bipolar symptoms Onset of effect: 7-10 days; Full effect: 3-6 weeks		
TYPICAL ANTIPSYCHOTICS (for positive symptoms) ❑ haloperidol (Haldol) ❑ loxapine (Loxitane) ❑ chlorpromazine HCl (Thorazine) ❑ pimozide (Orap) ❑ molindone HCl (Moban) ❑ thiothixene HCl (Navane) ❑ trifluoperazine (Stelazine) ❑ serentil (Mesoridazine) ❑ fluphenazine decanoate (Prolixin Decanoate) ATYPICAL ANTIPSYCHOTICS (for negative symptoms) ❑ clozapine (Clozaril) ❑ olanzapine (Zyprexa) ❑ risperidone (Risperdal) ❑ quetiapine (Seroquel) ❑ ziprasidone (Geodon) ❑ aripiprazole (Abilify)	Side Effects ❑ EXTRAPYRAMIDAL SYMPTOMS ▪ Dystonia – jerky movement ▪ Akathisia – restlessness ▪ Parkinsonian-like symptoms ▪ Tardive dyskinesia - irreversible, involuntary movements with lip smacking, tongue protrusion, facial twitching and chewing ❑ **Anticholinergic effects** ❑ Photosensitivity ❑ Orthostatic hypotension ❑ Agranulocytosis	Interventions ❑ Monitor serum glucose, lipids and CBC ❑ Give with food ❑ Contraindicated in glaucoma ❑ Use sunscreen ❑ Avoid alcohol and sedatives ❑ Change positions slowly ❑ Report sore throat and fever

NCLEX Alert! *Anticholinergic drugs are given to control the extrapyramidal side effects of antipsychotics. Examples of these drugs are benztropine (Cogentin), diphenhydramine (Benadryl), biperiden (Akineton) and trihexyphenidyl (Artane).*

Neuroleptic Malignant Syndrome

- ❑ Description — Severe, rare and fatal idiosyncratic reaction to antipsychotic drugs
- ❑ Assessment — **Fever >40°C,** muscle spasms, confusion, Parkinsonism, dysphagia, excessive drooling, oculogyric crisis, incontinence
- ❑ Interventions — Cooling measures, Seizure precautions, Stop the drug

2. Antidepressants

❑ What are the three main types of antidepressants?

(1) Selective Serotonin Reuptake Inhibitors (SSRIs)

(2) Tricyclic Antidepressants (TCAs)

(3) Monoamine Oxidase Inhibitors (MAOIs)

SELECTIVE SEROTONIN REUPTAKE INHIBITORS (SSRI)		
Increases the levels of **serotonin** in the brain → improved mood Onset of effect: 4-6 weeks		
SELECTIVE SEROTONIN REUPTAKE INHIBITORS ❑ fluoxetine (Prozac) ❑ sertraline HCl (Zoloft) ❑ citalopram (Celexa) ❑ escitalopram (Lexapro) ❑ paroxetine hydrochloride (Paxil) SEROTONIN-NOREPINEPHRINE REUPTAKE INHIBITORS ❑ duloxetine (Cymbalta) ❑ venlafaxine (Effexor) ATYPICAL ANTIDEPRESSANTS ❑ bupropion hydrochloride (Wellbutrin) ❑ trazodone (Desyrel) ❑ mirtazapine (Remeron)	Side effects ❑ Nervousness ❑ Weight loss or gain ❑ Dry mouth ❑ Nausea and vomiting ❑ CNS stimulation ❑ Decreased libido or impotence	Interventions ❑ Monitor BP ❑ Monitor weight ❑ Monitor liver and renal function ❑ Monitor WBC count ❑ Monitor for priapism ❑ Contraindicated in angle-closure glaucoma ❑ Avoid alcohol ❑ Do not abruptly stop

- ❑ What is **serotonin syndrome**?

  A fatal form of **serotonin toxicity** especially when SSRIs are used with MAOIs, cold and migraine drugs

- ❑ What are the signs and symptoms of serotonin syndrome?

  Confusion, agitation, hyperreflexia, shivering, sweating, fever, diarrhea

TRICYCLIC ANTIDEPRESSANTS (TCAs)		
Increases the levels of **norepinephrine** and **serotonin** → improved mood Onset of effect: 2-4 weeks		
Drugs ❑ doxepin hydrochloride (Sinequan) ❑ amitriptyline HCl (Elavil) ❑ protriptyline HCl (Vivactil) ❑ imipramine HCl (Tofranil) ❑ nortriptyline HCl (Aventyl) ❑ clomipramine (Anafranil) ❑ desipramine HCl (Norpramin)	Side effects ❑ **Anticholinergic effects** ❑ Photosensitivity ❑ Orthostatic hypotension ❑ Libido, ejaculation and erectile problems ❑ Weight gain	Interventions ❑ Change positions slowly ❑ Give with food or milk ❑ Avoid alcohol and driving ❑ Antidote: physostigmine (cholinesterase inhibitor)

MONOAMINE OXIDASE INHIBITORS (MAOI'S)		
Blocks the enzyme monoamine oxidase → increased norepinephrine, serotonin, and dopamine Onset of effect: 1 week		
Drugs ❑ isocarboxazid (Marplan) ❑ selegiline (Emsam) ❑ tranylcypromine sulfate (Parnate) ❑ phenelzine sulfate (Nardil)	Side effects ❑ **Anticholinergic effects** ❑ Orthostatic hypotension ❑ Lightheadedness ❑ Dry mouth ❑ Drowsiness ❑ Weight gain ❑ Delayed ejaculation	Interventions ❑ Monitor BP ❑ Change positions slowly ❑ Taper gradually ❑ Avoid alcohol and OTC meds ❑ Avoid **high tyramine** foods

❑ What will happen if the client eats foods high in **TYRAMINE**?	Hypertensive crisis
❑ What are the signs and symptoms of hypertensive crisis?	Headache, neck stiffness, nausea, vomiting, fever and chills, clammy skin, chest pain, tachycardia, photophobia
❑ What is the antidote for this type of hypertensive crisis?	phentolamine (Regitine)

NCLEX Alert! *Examples of tyramine-rich foods include* ***aged cheeses*** *like cheddar or blue cheese, avocados, bananas, chicken liver, beer, broad beans, caffeine, figs, cured or smoked meats, sausage, overripe fruit, papaya, pickled herring, raisin,* ***red wine****, miso soup, yeast extract, sour cream, soy products and yogurt.*

3. Antimanic Drugs

LITHIUM AND OTHER DRUGS		
Acts on the brain to inhibit the release of **dopamine** and **norepinephrine**→ reduced manic episode Onset of effect: 1-3 weeks		
Drugs ❑ lithium carbonate (Lithobid) Other Antimanic Drugs ❑ olanzapine (Zyprexa) ❑ carbamazepine (Tegretol) ❑ oxcarbazepine (Trileptal) ❑ risperidone (Risperdal) ❑ gabapentine (Neurontin) ❑ valproate sodium (Depakene) ❑ aripriprazole (Abilify) ❑ quetiapine (Seroquel) ❑ lamotrigine (Lamictal)	Side effects ❑ Thirst ❑ Polyuria ❑ Anorexia ❑ Dry mouth ❑ Nausea ❑ Weakness ❑ Weight gain ❑ Diarrhea ❑ Drowsiness ❑ Fine hand tremors ❑ Metallic taste	Interventions ❑ Give with meals ❑ Avoid caffeine, alcohol and diuretics ❑ Taper gradually ❑ **Maintain salt and fluid intake**

NCLEX Alert! *A client taking lithium should maintain salt and fluid intake. A sudden increase in sodium intake may result in lower serum lithium levels while a sudden decrease in sodium will increase the lithium levels resulting to lithium toxicity!*

NCLEX Alert! *Diaphoresis, dehydration, diarrhea and excessive use of diuretics can lead to hyponatremia and subsequent lithium toxicity!*

LITHIUM TOXICITY Therapeutic level: 0.6 – 1.2 mEq/L		
Mild toxicity (1.5 meq/L)	**Moderate toxicity (1.5-2.5 meq/L)**	**Severe toxicity (>2.5 meq/L)**
Diarrhea Vomiting Dry mouth Tremors Ataxia Lethargy	Nausea and vomiting Slurred speech Tinnitus Diarrhea Ataxia Muscle twitching	Nystagmus Hallucinations Oliguria Hyperreflexia Opisthotonus Seizures

NCLEX Alert! *Lithium has a narrow toxic and therapeutic range! Blood levels need to be monitored regularly to monitor toxicity.*

4. Antianxiety Drugs

BENZODIAZEPINES, BARBITURATES, SEDATIVE-HYPNOTICS		
Acts on the brain to enhance the action of the neurotransmitter, GABA (Gamma-aminobutyric acid) → decreased anxiety and muscle relaxation		
BENZODIAZEPINES ❑ clonazepam (Klonopin) ❑ diazepam (Valium) ❑ lorazepam (Ativan) ❑ midazolam (Versed) ❑ temazepam (Restoril) ❑ alprazolam (Xanax) ❑ chlordiazepoxide (Librium)	Side effects ❑ **Sedation** ❑ Dizziness ❑ Weakness ❑ Ataxia ❑ Amnesia ❑ Hypotension	Interventions ❑ Use cautiously in older adults ❑ Avoid alcohol ❑ Antidote: **flumazenil (Romazicon)**, a GABA receptor antagonist
BARBITURATES ❑ phenobarbital (Luminal) ❑ amobarbital (Amytal) SEDATIVE-HYPNOTICS ❑ meprobamate (Miltown) ❑ eszopiclone (Lunesta) ❑ zaleplon (Sonata) ❑ zolpidem (Ambien)	Side effects ❑ Drowsiness ❑ Hypersensitivity ❑ Agranulocytosis	Interventions ❑ Take 30 minutes before bedtime ❑ Avoid alcohol, driving or operating hazardous equipment

NCLEX® Assessment Test 21

The following NCLEX-style questions are for practice purposes only to test general nursing knowledge. Actual NCLEX questions will reflect practice specific contents emphasized in the NCLEX-RN and PN Test Plans. Optimal score = 60/75.

---

1. A nurse reviews the orders of a physician after a client's thyroidectomy. Which of the following orders needs to be clarified?

A. Perform coughing exercises.
B. Support head during movement.
C. Offer ice chips.
D. Bed rest until stable.

2. A pregnant female receives multivitamins as supplements. She asks the nurse why she also receives Vitamin B_9 (folic acid). The **best** nursing response is

A. "Folic acid protects the fetus from infection after delivery."
B. "Folic acid ensures that surfactant production is increased."
C. "Folic acid prevents spinal deformities."
D. "Folic acid enhances maternal production of platelets."

3. A client diagnosed with Buerger's disease is scheduled for discharge. Which of the following statements should alert the nurse for a possible non-adherence of the client to discharge plans?

A. "I have to make sure that I keep my weight within the healthy range."
B. "Sticking to a low fat diet is important for my cholesterol levels."
C. "I should cut down my cigarettes to only 2 sticks per day from now on."
D. "I have to put on extra socks to keep my feet warm during the winter season."

4. A client with a diagnosis of angina pectoris asks the nurse on how to properly take nitroglycerin sublingual tablets when experiencing chest pain. Which of the following is the **best** nursing response?

A. "Take the nitroglycerin every 5 minutes until your pain goes away."
B. "You should lie down while taking nitroglycerin for maximum effect."
C. "Take nitroglycerin every 5 minutes. If the pain is not relieved after 3 doses, you should get emergency treatment."
D. "It should take at least 15 minutes before nitroglycerin achieves its full effect, so you have to wait before taking another tablet."

5. A health care provider orders diphenhydramine (Benylin) 20 mg q 6 hours to be given to a client with asthma. The pharmacy sends a bottle of diphenhydramine (Benylin) 20 mg/5 ml. How many teaspoons should the nurse give? ______

6. A nurse is performing suctioning on a client with tracheostomy. Which of the following actions below requires further intervention?

A. Applying suction while inserting the catheter.
B. Placing the client in Fowler's position.
C. Withdrawing the catheter in a rotating motion while applying intermittent suction.
D. Lubricating the catheter with normal saline.

7. A client with laryngeal cancer is scheduled for a total laryngectomy procedure. The client should be instructed that after the surgery, he will

A. Breathe through the nose.
B. Be able to speak normally.
C. Have chest tubes to drain secretions.
D. Have a permanent tracheostomy.

8. A client with femoral fracture arrives at the emergency room after a car accident. Which of the following signs and symptoms should be reported as it indicates a complication related to this type of fracture?

A. Rales, pallor, flaring of nostrils.
B. Confusion, hypotension, fever.
C. Restlessness, dyspnea, chest pain.
D. Leg numbness, muscle twitching, tachypnea.

9. A client with osteoporosis is prescribed to take biphosphonate-alendronate sodium (Fosamax). Which of the following instructions about this medication is important to teach the client?

A. Take the medication at bedtime.
B. Remain sitting upright for 30 minutes after taking the medication.
C. Take the medication with orange juice to enhance absorption.
D. Ensure that the medication is taken with a full stomach.

10. A client is admitted to the emergency room after sustaining severe head injury in a motorcycle accident. Which of the following signs and symptoms should alert the nurse for a serious complication related to this injury?

A. Hyperglycemia.
B. Diaphoresis.
C. Polyuria.
D. Periorbital edema.

11. A nurse is providing discharge instructions to a client following Billroth 2 surgery. Which of the following is important to teach the client to prevent signs and symptoms of dumping syndrome?

A. Consume a high carbohydrate diet.
B. Lie down after eating.
C. Increase fluid intake during meals.
D. Elevate the head of bed while eating.

12. A client arrives at the emergency room due to complaints of severe abdominal pain. Upon assessment, the nurse noted severe abdominal distention, fever, absent bowel sounds and a hard abdomen. The nurse should expect which of the following interventions?

A. Insertion of a rectal tube.
B. Administration of antibiotics.
C. Application of hot water bags on the abdomen.
D. Placing the client in flat position.

13. A client takes phenytoin (Dilantin) for epilepsy. Which client teaching is important?

A. Expect change in urine color.
B. Toothache is a normal side effect.
C. Take the drug at bedtime.
D. Increase fluid intake.

14. A nurse cares for a client who had undergone total colectomy. Which of the following signs and symptoms are indications that the client is developing signs of hypovolemic shock? (Select all that apply)

❑ A. Tachycardia.
❑ B. Cold and clammy skin.
❑ C. Widened pulse pressure.
❑ D. Decreased blood pressure.
❑ E. Oliguria
❑ F. Decreased respiration.

15. A nurse is teaching the spouse of a client who developed receptive aphasia after a stroke. Which of the following outcomes is related to this condition?

A. Written communication will be helpful.
B. Speech will be slurred.
C. Verbal language will not be understood.
D. Names of objects will not be remembered.

16. After sustaining a head injury due to a traumatic accident, the nurse suspects that the client is leaking cerebrospinal fluid. Which of the following tests will confirm this observation?

A. Guthrie blood test.
B. Glucose test.
C. Barlow's test.
D. Battle's sign test.

17. A nurse observes that the client with obsessive-compulsive disorder cleans the room the entire day. Which statement explains the purpose of this behavior?

A. To gain attention from others.
B. To achieve control of the environment.
C. To avoid interaction with other clients.
D. To decrease the level of anxiety.

18. A nurse teaches a family member on how to care for the father who has advanced dementia. Which of the following is the most important instruction to provide?

A. Divide tasks into different times of the day.
B. Provide a regular, predictable schedule of activities.
C. Apply gentle restraints when the client is agitated.
D. Give detailed explanations for every activity.

19. A client takes alprazolam (Xanax) to manage his anxiety. Which of the following instructions is important to tell the client?

A. Dizziness is a temporary side effect.
B. Avoid drinking alcohol.
C. Report drowsiness immediately.
D. Drive a car only during day time.

20. A client with acute pancreatitis shows signs of alcohol withdrawal. Which of the following is the **priority** nursing action?

A. Provide cooling blankets.
B. Prepare oxygen equipment.
C. Administer antidepressant medications.
D. Initiate seizure precautions.

21. A male client is admitted to the psychiatric emergency room due to an exacerbation of a bipolar disorder. When gathering data about this client, which of the following information should the nurse expect?

A. The client went on a shopping spree.
B. The client has been eating excessively.
C. The client played video games every day.
D. The client says he cannot feel his legs.

22. A client with schizophrenia has been taking haloperidol (Haldol) for several days. Which of the following findings indicate an adverse effect to this medication?

A. Weight loss.
B. Facial twitching.
C. Tachycardia.
D. Diarrhea.

23. A nurse is teaching a client regarding his prescribed MAO inhibitor drugs. The client understands the nurse's instructions when he states that

A. "I should limit my intake of red wine."
B. "I will avoid green and leafy vegetables."
C. "I have to drink non-fat milk from now on."
D. "I cannot eat aged cheese"

24. A client with a spinal cord injury at C4 is experiencing autonomic dysreflexia. Which of the following is the **priority** nursing action?

A. Assess for bowel impaction.
B. Check the patency of the indwelling catheter.
C. Administer an antihypertensive drug.
D. Place the client in a sitting position.

25. A client is recently diagnosed as having open-angle glaucoma. When collecting information related to this condition, which client complaint would the nurse expect to hear?

A. Seeing floating spots in the visual field.
B. Occasional attacks of diplopia.
C. Hitting objects on the side when walking.
D. Gradual blurring of vision.

26. A client with full-blown AIDS is visited by a grandson who later developed chickenpox. The nurse should assess the client for signs of

A. Shingles.
B. Rubella.
C. Herpes simplex type I.
D. Impetigo.

27. A client sustained a burn injury to the entire right and left lower extremities and chest. When using the Rule of Nines to estimate the extent of body surface area burned, the total percentage would be

A. 27%.
B. 36%.
C. 45%.
D. 54%.

28. A nurse is caring for a client who recently developed diabetic ketoacidosis. Which of the following client history may have predisposed this client to develop the complication?

A. The client started taking oral hypoglycemic agents.
B. The client has a WBC count of 20,000 cells/mm3.
C. The client increased intake of salty foods.
D. The client received 2 liters of D_5NS.

29. The charge nurse of the medical-surgical unit is assigning clients to the staff. Which of the following factors is most important to consider?

A. Experience of staff.
B. Availability of supplies and equipment.
C. Care acuity of clients.
D. Number of staff present.

30. A nurse is preparing to administer insulin to a client with Type 1 diabetes mellitus. Which of the following actions below are correct steps in performing this procedure? (Select all that apply)

- ❑ A. Air is injected into the cloudy insulin first.
- ❑ B. Insulin is withdrawn from the NPH insulin vial first.
- ❑ C. The vial of insulin is rolled between the palms.
- ❑ D. Glargine is mixed with a rapid-acting insulin.
- ❑ E. Insulin is injected subcutaneously at a 45-degree angle.
- ❑ F. Insulin injection is performed using a Z-track technique.

31. The nurse has been assigned to review the clinical pathways of the unit. Which item **best** describes the purpose of clinical pathways?

A. To justify the necessity of the client's medical care.
B. To facilitate early discharge from the hospital.
C. To apply general guidelines in the care of a particular disease.
D. To ensure quality care and optimum outcomes at a lower cost.

32. A client with advanced COPD is admitted into the emergency room due to severe respiratory distress. Which of the following findings indicate the presence of the complication cor pulmonale?

A. Double vision.
B. Hypotension
C. Jugular vein distention.
D. Bloody sputum.

33. A client is taking isoniazid (INH) for treatment of tuberculosis. Which of the following signs and symptoms should the client report while taking this medication?

A. Change in urine color.
B. Drowsiness.
C. Numbness of extremities.
D. Palpitations.

34. The nurse reviews the arterial blood gas results of a client with chronic bronchitis. Which of the following items below reflects findings expected from this condition?

A. pH: 7.35, PCO_2: 22 mmHg, HCO_3:18 mEq/L.
B. pH: 7.42, PCO_2: 35 mmHg, HCO_3: 23 mEq/L.
C. pH: 7.48, PCO_2: 22 mmHg, HCO_3: 20 mEq/L.
D. pH: 7.32, PCO_2: 49 mmHg, HCO_3: 22 mEq/L.

35. A nurse is caring for a child with nephrotic syndrome. Which nursing action should be included in the plan of care for this child?

A. Assess for hypotension.
B. Measure the head circumference.
C. Restrict the intake of protein.
D. Weigh the child daily.

36. A nurse cares for several clients in the long-term care facility. Which of the following activities upholds the client's right to autonomy?

A. Teaching the client about prescribed diet and medications.
B. Allowing the client to join group trips and activities.
C. Assisting the client in completing the advance health care directive form.
D. Inviting the spouse during the quarterly care plan meeting.

37. A child with congenital heart defect receives digoxin (Lanoxin) elixir BID. The safe daily dosage is 0.08 mg/kg/day. The child's weight is 17.6 lbs. How much digoxin should the nurse administer to the child at each dose? Round off your final answer to the nearest hundred.

38. A nurse is caring for a client with chest tubes inserted for pneumothorax. Which of the following observations indicate normal functioning of the chest tube drainage system? (Select all that apply)

- ❑ A. Gentle bubbling is present in the suction control chamber.
- ❑ B. The fluid level fluctuates in the water-seal chamber.
- ❑ C. The drainage system is placed below the insertion site.
- ❑ D. Continuous bubbling occurs in the water-seal chamber.
- ❑ E. Intermittent bubbling occurs in the water-seal chamber.
- ❑ F. Vigorous bubbling is present in the suction control chamber.

39. The parent of an infant with pyloric stenosis asks the nurse about the plan of care for their child. Which of the following is the **best** nursing response?

A. Special formula will be required in the next few days.
B. A gastrostomy tube will have to be inserted.
C. Surgery is needed as soon as possible.
D. Additional diagnostic tests have to be done.

40. A mother delivers a newborn child with cleft lip and palate. She tells the nurse, "I think I did something wrong why this happened to my child." Which of the following is the **best** nursing response?

A. "There is nothing you can do in this situation."
B. "You do not have to feel this way."
C. "I understand how you feel but you did not cause this."
D. "Has this condition occurred in your family?"

41. A nurse is caring for a newborn newly-diagnosed with esophageal atresia. Which of the following interventions are appropriate for this child?

A. Full-strength milk formula and monitor urine output
B. IV fluids and NPO order.
C. Clear liquid diet and monitor bowel movements.
D. Mucolytics and oxygen via face mask.

42. A nurse is assigning clients in a skilled nursing facility. Which of the following clients can be assigned to the nursing assistant?

A. A 90-year-old client with Alzheimer's disease and has advanced liver cirrhosis.
B. A 65-year-old client recently admitted after a hip joint replacement surgery.
C. An 85-year-old client with multiple sclerosis who needs assistance with ambulation.
D. A 35-year-old client in comatose state due to a severe head injury.

43. The nurse is doing morning rounds when she noticed that a client with heart failure showed restlessness, dyspnea and pink-tinged, frothy sputum. Which of the following is the **best** nursing action?

A. Assess for the presence of pitting edema and jugular vein distention.
B. Call the physician to obtain an order for arterial blood gas procedure.
C. Administer an antidote for digoxin toxicity.
D. Place the client in High-Fowler's position.

44. A client is recently diagnosed as having pernicious anemia. Which of the following information in the medical record may have predisposed the client to develop this condition?

A. Client receives Vitamin D injections every month.
B. Client has history of total gastrectomy in the past 3 months.
C. Client has been diagnosed with hemophilia during childhood.
D. Client takes pancreatic enzymes during meals.

45. A client with myocardial infarction suddenly develops ventricular tachycardia followed by ventricular fibrillation and loss of consciousness. Which of the following is the **priority** nursing action?

A. Obtain the crash cart for immediate defibrillation procedure.
B. Count the heart rate.
C. Administer 100% oxygen via face mask.
D. Elevate the head of the bed and start CPR.

46. A client who is 34 weeks pregnant becomes lightheaded and dizzy on the examination table during a routine prenatal check-up. Which of the following is the **initial** nursing action?

A. Turn the client on the left side.
B. Check the blood pressure.
C. Assist with paper bag breathing.
D. Assess the fetal heart rate.

47. A client who is 34 weeks pregnant arrives at the emergency department and is suspected as having abruptio placenta. Which of the following assessment findings are related to this condition? (Select all that apply)

- ☐ A. Abdominal tenderness.
- ☐ B. Painless vaginal bleeding.
- ☐ C. Board-like abdominal rigidity.
- ☐ D. Presence of fetal variable decelerations.
- ☐ E. Shock.
- ☐ F. Soft abdomen.

48. When taking care of a client with psoriasis, which nursing action should be clarified?

A. Preparing a private room.
B. Ordering a full diet.
C. Managing pruritus.
D. Performing daily showers.

49. A pregnant client with pre-eclampsia complains of visual disturbances and severe epigastric pain. Which of the following is the **priority** nursing action?

A. Prepare for delivery.
B. Call the physician.
C. Initiate seizure precautions.
D. Assess the blood pressure.

50. A pregnant client undergoes a contraction stress test (CST). Which of the following information indicates a negative finding?

A. Fetal bradycardia that persists after contractions.
B. Absence of persistent late or variable decelerations.
C. Multiple fetal variable decelerations.
D. Repeated late decelerations.

51. A male client is prescribed to receive levothyroxine (Synthroid). Which of the following client statements indicate understanding of the medication therapy?

A. The client says he has to take the medication for a lifetime.
B. The client says he must take the drug at bedtime.
C. The client says the medicine will cause drowsiness.
D. The client says he should miss a dose when he feels lethargic.

52. A nurse is assigned to perform wound treatments to all of the clients in the medical-surgical floor. Which type of care delivery model is this?

A. Primary nursing.
B. Team nursing.
C. Holistic nursing.
D. Functional nursing.

53. A nurse conducts a home visit on a client recently diagnosed with hyperthyroidism. When teaching the client about adverse effects related to the use of propylthiouracil (PTU), the nurse should emphasize to the client to report which signs or symptoms?

A. Nausea and vomiting.
B. Fever and sore throat.
C. Dizziness and blurring of vision.
D. Tachycardia and insomnia.

54. Several clients are being seen in the emergency room. Which of the following clients require the most immediate attention?

A. A 30-year-old client who complains of body aches due to flu.
B. A 20-year-old client with a sprained ankle.
C. A 25-year-old client with neck rigidity, fever and sensitivity to light.
D. A 45-year-old client reporting gas pains after eating seafoods.

55. A nurse assesses a client who recently underwent a transurethral resection of the prostate (TURP) and has a triple lumen catheter for continuous bladder irrigation. Which of the following client complaints requires immediate nursing action?

A. The client says he feels thirsty.
B. The client states that he has painful bladder spasms.
C. The client reports feeling tired and weak.
C. The client complains of persistent urge to void.

56. A nurse is caring for a client who receives digoxin (Lanoxin) for right-sided heart failure. Which of the following signs and symptoms should alert the nurse for possible presence of digoxin toxicity?

A. Fatigue, headache, hypotension.
B. Bradycardia, weight gain, jugular vein distention.
C. Tachypnea, muscle weakness, chest pain.
D. Anorexia, nausea, visual changes.

57. A physician orders Schilling Test to be performed for a client suspected of having pernicious anemia. Order the steps below in completing this procedure.

1. Give oral radioactive vitamin B_{12} supplement
2. Avoid Vitamin B_{12} injections days before the test.
3. Administer IM injection of non-radioactive vitamin B_{12}
4. Measure radioactive vitamin B_{12} in urine
5. Place client on NPO for 8 hours
6. Collect urine for 24 hours

58. A client is admitted to the post-anesthesia care unit (PACU) after undergoing gastric surgery. Which of the following tasks can be safely delegated by the RN to the LPN?

A. Completing the initial assessment of the client.
B. Providing a report to the incoming charge nurse.
C. Administering oral antibiotic medications.
D. Explaining to the client the plan for pain management.

59. A nurse cares for a client after a gastroscopy procedure. Which of the following nursing actions is essential to ensure the safety of the client?

A. Auscultate for bowel sounds.
B. Assess the client's ability to speak.
C. Check the gag reflex before offering fluids.
D. Monitor the blood pressure.

60. A nurse administers a sedative to a client who is scheduled for surgery. Which of the following nursing actions should be done next?

A. Assist the client to void
B. Elevate the head of the bed.
C. Apply an identification bracelet.
D. Raise the side rails up.

61. The nurse is assigned to monitor the infection control compliance in the hospital. Which of the following observations shows a need for further staff education?

A. A nurse removes and discards the N-95 mask inside the room after caring for a client with tuberculosis.
B. A nursing assistant feeds a client with HIV without the use of gloves.
C. A nursing assistant wears a gown and gloves when caring for a client with MRSA infection.
D. A nurse initiates isolation precautions for a client with widespread rash due to shingles.

62. The nurse is doing home visits in a community. Among the following clients, which one should be seen first?

A. A client who has flu symptoms.
B. A client who needs wound care for a stage 4 pressure sore.
C. A bedridden client who has full-blown AIDS.
D. A client with multiple sclerosis who needs hygiene care.

63. The nurse is working in the emergency triage area when the following clients arrived at the same time. Which client should be seen first?

A. A client who sneezes due to colds.
B. An alert client who has small lacerations on the head.

C. An unconscious client who had a traumatic car accident.
D. A client who has diarrhea and mild stomach pain.

64. The physician orders Penicillin oral suspension 500 mg po qid for a client with pneumonia. The directions for mixing the drug reads: Add 50 mL of water and shake. Each 5 mL will contain 100 mg of Penicillin. How many teaspoons of Penicillin will you administer?

A. 3 teaspoons.
B. 4 teaspoons.
C. 5 teaspoons.
D. 6 teaspoons.

65. A 2-year-old child arrives at the emergency room after ingesting large amounts of acetaminophen pills. Which of the following interventions will be performed first?

A. Starting an intravenous line.
B. Inserting an NGT for gastric lavage.
C. Administering acetylcysteine (Mucomyst).
D. Performing a blood draw.

66. A nurse in a medical-surgical unit takes care of the following clients. Which client requires immediate nursing action?

A. A client who is complaining of pain after appendectomy.
B. A client who asks to go to the bathroom.
C. A client in wheelchair who wants to go back to bed.
D. A client with diabetes who has a blood glucose level of 40 mg/dL.

67. A nurse receives her client assignments at the start of her shift. Which of the following clients needs to be assessed first?

A. A client with hypothyroidism with a heart rate of 60 beats/minute.
B. A client with diabetes who has a fingerstick blood glucose level of 140 mg/dL..
C. A client with heart failure who has pitting edema +2 in the lower extremities.
D. A client with Addison's disease with a blood pressure of 85/60 mmHg.

68. The physician orders 2 liters of D_5 ½ NS to infuse for 6 hours. The infusion set has a drop factor of 10 gtts/mL. What flow rate (gtts/minute) will you set on the IV infusion pump? Round off your final answer to the nearest whole number.

A. 30 gtts/minute.
B. 56 gtts/minute.
C. 70 gtts/minute.
D. 110 gtts/minute.

69. A client is admitted to the hospital due to a diagnosis of Addison's disease. When providing care to this client, the nurse should

A. Limit the client's fluid intake for the first few hours.
B. Inspect the leg for swelling.
C. Assess for elevation of blood glucose.
D. Provide a stress-free environment.

70. Ranitidine (Zantac) is ordered to a client with peptic ulcer disease. Which of the following items describes the action of this medication?

A. Coats the stomach lining to protect from acid production.
B. Blocks the production of hydrochloric acid.
C. Neutralizes the acidity of the stomach.
D. Stimulates the histamine receptor sites.

71. A nurse is providing instruction to a male client who receives disulfiram (Antabuse). The client is correct when he tells that nurse that he can safely use which of the following items?

A. Mouthwash.
B. Aftershave gel.
C. Backrub lotions.
D. Adhesive bandage.

72. A male client on a psychiatric unit tells the nurse that he plans on committing suicide. Which of the following is the appropriate nursing action?

A. Search the client's room for sharp objects.
B. Administer an antidepressant drug.
C. Ask the client if he has a plan.
D. Notify the physician.

73. A client tells the nurse that she is worried about the results of her breast biopsy. Which of the following is the **best** nursing response?

A. We have the best physicians in this hospital.
B. Waiting for the result of your biopsy can really be difficult.
C. What is it about the biopsy that makes you worried?
D. Tell me how your condition started.

74. A nurse is caring for a client with Acquired Immunodeficiency Syndrome (AIDS). While reviewing the client's daily record, the nurse noted the following information: weight loss >5% in the last 2 weeks; CD_4 count – 150 cells/ul; urine output – 400 mL/24 hours; axillary temperature - 98.4° F. Based on these data, which of the following is a **priority** nursing action?

A. Obtain an order for nasogastric tube feeding.
B. Call the physician immediately.
C. Protect the client from infection.
D. Increase the client's fluid intake.

75. A unit manager of a medical-surgical unit meets with a staff nurse to discuss an annual performance appraisal. Which of the following actions below will result into a negative outcome of this session?

A. Discussing future projects related to the job role.
B. Presenting work performance based on evaluation standards.
C. Emphasizing behavior that led to negative performance.
D. Recommending opportunities for further training.

ANSWERS AND RATIONALES

1. **Answer A**. Coughing exercises should be avoided to prevent bleeding. The other choices are appropriate interventions to a client after a thyroidectomy.

2. **Answer C**. Folic acid is an important supplement during pregnancy to prevent spina bifida of the newborn. Folic acid does not provide protection against infection. It does not affect surfactant and platelet production.

3. **Answer C**. The client with Buerger's disease should stop smoking instead of cutting down on the number of cigarettes. The other choices are appropriate actions to prevent exacerbation of Buerger's disease.

4. **Answer C.** Nitroglycerin tablets should be taken every 5 minutes for 3 doses. If the chest pain is not relieved after 3 doses, the client should go to the nearest emergency room as it indicates the presence of a myocardial infarction.

5. **Answer 1 teaspoon**.
20 mg/20 mg x 5 mL = 5 mL = 1 teaspoon

6. **Answer A**. Suction should not be applied while inserting the suction catheter to prevent trauma to the mucous membranes of the airway. The other choices are appropriate nursing actions during suctioning.

7. **Answer D**. The client undergoing total laryngectomy should be told that a permanent tracheostomy will be made since the trachea is being closed after removal of the larynx. There is no longer a connection between the upper and the lower airways and a tracheostomy is necessary so the client has an opening for breathing.

8. **Answer C.** A client with a long bone fracture (femur) is at risk for developing fat embolism. This complication occurs as fat globules combine with platelets forming a clot. Signs of fat embolism include restlessness, dyspnea and chest pain.

9. **Answer B**. The client should remain sitting upright after taking the medication to prevent esophageal irritation. Biphosphonate-alendronate sodium should be taken in the morning upon awakening on an empty stomach.

10. **Answer C**. A head injury can cause dysfunction of the pituitary gland and can lead to diabetes insipidus. Increased urination (polyuria) is the hallmark manifestation of diabetes insipidus due to decreased secretion of antidiuretic hormone (ADH).

11. **Answer B**. Dumping syndrome occurs due to the rapid entrance of hypertonic chyme in the small intestines resulting to fluid shifting. This can be prevented by encouraging the client to lie down after eating. A low carbohydrate diet and restriction of fluid intake with meals are also recommended.

12. **Answer B**. The client is showing signs and symptoms typical of peritonitis. This is a fatal infection and antibiotics should be administered immediately. The other choices are not appropriate actions.

13. **Answer A**. A common side effect of phenytoin (Dilantin) is a change in urine color (pink-red or red-brown) and is considered to be harmless. Another side effect is gingival hyperplasia. Toothache is not a side effect of phenytoin.

14. **Answer A, B, D, E**. Signs of shock include tachycardia, cold and clammy skin, decreased blood pressure, decreased urine output, increased respiration and narrowing of pulse pressure.

15. **Answer C**. Receptive (Wernicke's aphasia) is characterized by the client's inability to understand spoken and written words. Slurred, effortful speech is associated with expressive aphasia. The other choices are not related to this condition.

16. **Answer B**. The cerebrospinal fluid (CSF) normally contains glucose. The glucose test will confirm the presence of a CSF leak which indicates the presence of severe brain injury or increased intracranial pressure. Guthrie blood test is a test to diagnose phenylketonuria. Barlow's test is an assessment test for congenital hip dysplasia. Battle's sign is the ecchymosis of the mastoid area due to a head injury.

17. **Answer D**. A client with obsessive-compulsive disorder performs repetitive rituals as a method to reduce the levels of anxiety. If attempts to perform the rituals are interrupted, the client's anxiety level will increase.

18. **Answer B**. Care for a client with dementia requires the provision of a structured, predictable environment to minimize confusion. Use of restraints for agitated behavior is not recommended. Short and simple instructions should be used when communicating with the client.

19. **Answer B**. Alprazolam can cause drowsiness and alcohol intake will potentiate this effect. The client should also avoid operating dangerous machinery such as driving a car while taking the medication. Dizziness is not a temporary side effect of alprazolam.

20. **Answer D**. A client with alcohol withdrawal can develop seizure episodes. Initiating seizure precautions is important to prevent injury. The other choices are not priority nursing actions.

21. **Answer A**. The manic phase of a bipolar disorder is characterized by excessive spending. Inability to feel the legs is found in patients with conversion disorder. Eating excessively is not a sign of bipolar disorder.

22. **Answer B**. Haloperidol is an antipsychotic medication that can cause tardive dyskinesia, a condition characterized by involuntary muscle spasms and facial twitching. The other choices are not adverse effects directly related to the use of haloperidol.

23. **Answer D**. A client taking a MAO inhibitor drug should avoid consuming foods and drinks that are rich in tyramine such as red wine, strong or aged cheeses like cheddar, soy products like miso soup or tofu and cured or smoked meats or fish, such as salami or sausage. Avoiding, not limiting, red wine is advised.

24. **Answer D**. Autonomic dysreflexia is characterized by severe hypertension. The immediate goal is to reduce the blood pressure to prevent a stroke. Placing the client in sitting or High-Fowler's position will lower the blood pressure. The other interventions are important but not the first priority in this condition.

25. **Answer C.** Tunnel vision is common among clients with open-angle glaucoma. Hitting objects on the side occurs due to the loss of peripheral vision. Floating spots in vision occurs in retinal detachment. Blurring of vision occurs in cataract. Attacks of diplopia is not related to open-angle glaucoma.

26. **Answer A**. Shingles is caused bv the reactivation of chickenpox infection. A person with negative titer can develop chickenpox when exposed to a client with shingles. The other choices do not relate to chickenpox.

27. **Answer C**. The entire right and left lower extremities (36%) and chest (9%) has a total of 45%.

28. **Answer B**. One of the most common causes of diabetic ketoacidosis (DKA) is infection manifested by an increased WBC count. Infection causes the body to produce cortisol and adrenaline hormones that elevate the blood glucose levels. This increases the body's demand for insulin.

29. **Answer C**. The most important consideration when assigning tasks to the staff is to assess the care needs of clients. The other choices have to be considered but are not the most essential.

30. **Answer A, C, E**. When preparing insulin, insulin should be injected first into the cloudy insulin. Insulin is withdrawn from the clear vial. Insulin should be rolled between the palms to maintain clarity of the solution. Glargine is a long-acting insulin that should not be mixed with any type of insulin. Insulin is injected at a 45-degree angle. Z-track technique is not necessary for a subcutaneous injection of insulin.

31. **Answer D**. The purpose of clinical pathways is to standardize care interventions and timeframes using evidence-based research to achieve quality care at a lower cost. Clinical pathway guidelines are specific to the disease condition. The other choices describe outcomes related to clinical pathways but are not the primary purposes.

32. **Answer C.** Cor pulmonale is right ventricular hypertrophy (heart failure) secondary to a pulmonary disorder that causes pulmonary artery hypertension. Signs of right-sided heart failure include hepatomegaly, jugular vein distention and lower extremity edema.

33. **Answer C**. A common side effect of isoniazid (INH) is peripheral neuropathy. Signs of this condition include tingling and numbness of the extremity, muscle weakness and cramping. Change in urine color, drowsiness and palpitations are not expected side effects.

34. **Answer D**. Respiratory acidosis is the primary acid-base imbalance among clients with chronic obstructive pulmonary disease (COPD) and is reflected in this choice. Choice B is a normal ABG reading. The other choices do not show respiratory acidosis.

35. **Answer D**. Nephrotic syndrome is a condition characterized by the loss of protein in the urine. Hypoalbuminemia causes weight gain due to fluid retention. Protein should not be restricted. Hypertension, not hypotension, is a common finding. There is no need to measure the head circumference.

36. **Answer C.** Autonomy refers to the client's right to make informed decisions regarding their care. Completing the advance health care directive is one way to ensure that the client's wishes are followed when receiving care. The other choices are not activities that address the client's autonomy.

37. **Answer 0.32 mg per dose.**
Step 1. Convert 17.6 lbs. to kg. = 8 kg
Step 2. Calculate the daily safe dose:
0.08 mg x 8 = 0.64 mg daily
Step 3. Divide by frequency ordered:
0.64 divided by 2 (BID) = 0.32 mg per dose

38. **Answer A, B, C, E**. Gentle bubbling in the suction control chamber indicates that the suction is working properly. Fluctuation (tidaling) of the fluid level and intermittent bubbling in the water-seal chamber are expected as fluid and air are drained. The drainage system should always be placed below the insertion site to prevent backflow of drainage. Continuous bubbling in the water-seal chamber indicates an air leak is present. Vigorous bubbling in the suction control chamber indicates an air leak is present.

39. **Answer C**. An infant with pyloric stenosis requires immediate surgery to prevent life-threatening dehydration and electrolyte imbalance due to projectile vomiting. The surgery, called

pyloromyotomy, is usually well-tolerated and has a high success rate. There is no need for a gastrostomy.

40. **Answer C**. This response shows empathy by acknowledging the client's feelings. It is important to point out that the condition is not the client's fault. The other responses are not therapeutic and does not address the client's concerns.

41. **Answer B**. Esophageal atresia is characterized by coughing, choking and cyanosis. The newborn should be placed on NPO with IV fluid administration to correct nutritional deficits. Feeding with a full-strength formula, a clear liquid diet and mucolytics are not part of the interventions.

42. **Answer C.** A nursing assistant can be assigned to a stable client who needs assistance with ambulation. The other choices represent conditions that require critical nursing judgment and monitoring and should not be delegated.

43. **Answer D**. Placing the client in a High-Fowler's position is the priority action during an episode of acute pulmonary edema to facilitate breathing. The client is not manifesting digoxin toxicity. Assessing for pitting edema and jugular vein distention and calling the physician are not priority nursing actions.

44. **Answer B.** Pernicious anemia is caused by the lack of intrinsic factor that is needed for the absorption of Vitamin B_{12}. The removal of the stomach leads to the absence of the intrinsic factor that leads to this condition. The other choices do not relate to the risk factors for pernicious anemia.

45. **Answer A**. The priority nursing action for ventricular fibrillation is to defibrillate immediately. There is no need to count the heart rate as the situation already implied that the client is having ventricular fibrillation. Giving oxygen and elevating the head of the bed are important but not the priorities.

46. **Answer A**. The client should be turned to the left side to improve maternal and fetal perfusion. Supine hypotension syndrome occurs when the mother lies on a supine position while being examined. Checking the blood pressure, paper bag breathing and assessing the fetal heart rate are not the first nursing actions.

47. **Answer A, C, D, E**. A client having abruptio placenta will show abdominal tenderness, board-like abdominal rigidity and signs of shock due to hemorrhage. Presence of fetal variable decelerations indicate fetal distress related to the condition. The other choices describe findings present in placenta previa.

48. **Answer A.** Psoriasis is not infectious and there is no need to prepare a private room for the client. A full diet, managing pruritus and daily showers are appropriate nursing interventions.

49. **Answer C**. Visual disturbances and severe epigastric pain are warning signs of eclampsia which is characterized by seizures. The nurse should promote client safety by initiating seizure precautions. Preparing for delivery, calling the physician and assessing the blood pressure are not priority nursing actions.

50. **Answer B**. A negative contraction stress test (CST) means a "normal" result which is characterized by absence of late or variable decelerations. The other choices describe abnormal findings during a CST.

51. **Answer A**. Medications for hypothyroidism should be taken consistently for life. The drug must be taken during day time as it can cause insomnia. Skipping a dose is not recommended.

52. **Answer D**. Functional nursing is a task-oriented model of care delivery. An example of this would be a nurse who is assigned to specific responsibilities

such as wound care and administration of medications.

53. **Answer B**. Propylthiouracil (PTU) is an anti-thyroid drug that can cause agranulocytosis. To monitor this effect, the client should be told to report signs of infection such as fever and sore throat. The other choices do not describe the symptoms of agranulocytosis.

54. **Answer C**. The client is manifesting signs and symptoms indicative of meningitis. Isolation precautions must be implemented and antibiotic medications must be given to prevent worsening of infection.

55. **Answer B**. Painful bladder spasms indicate that there is blockage in the irrigation system and must be addressed immediately to prevent bleeding. Feeling thirsty and weak and a persistent urge to void are important to address but not the first priority.

56. **Answer D**. Signs of digoxin toxicity include anorexia, nausea and vomiting, bradycardia, diarrhea and visual changes. The other choices are not signs of digoxin toxicity.

57. **Answer 2, 5, 1, 3, 6, 4**. This is the correct sequence when performing a Schilling Test. Avoid Vitamin B_{12} injections days before the test; Place client on NPO for 8 hours; Give oral radioactive Vitamin B_{12} supplement; Administer IM injection of non-radioactive Vitamin B_{12}; Collect urine for 24 hours; Measure radioactive B_{12} in urine.

58. **Answer C**. Administering oral antibiotic medications is within the scope of practice of the LPN and can be safely delegated. Completing the initial assessment, providing a report to the incoming nurse and explaining the plan for pain management require critical assessment, evaluation and teaching skills that can be performed only by the RN.

59. **Answer C**. The nurse should ensure that the gag reflex is present before allowing the client to consume fluids to prevent aspiration. Assessing the bowel sounds, ability to speak and blood pressure are not priority nursing actions.

60. **Answer D**. Sedatives can cause drowsiness and falls. Safety should be ensured after the client takes a sedative prior to surgery. Assisting the client to void and applying the ID bracelet are not the next nursing actions.

61. **Answer A**. The N-95 mask should be removed outside the room. Tuberculosis is an airborne infection and can be transmitted while inside the room. Use of gloves is not needed when feeding a client with HIV. A gown and gloves must be worn for contact precautions such as MRSA. A client with disseminated shingles requires airborne and contact isolation precautions.

62. **Answer C**. The client with AIDS is immunosuppressed and should be seen first to prevent the likelihood of transmitting infection from other clients who have ongoing infections or wounds.

63. **Answer C**. A client who is unconscious after an accident should be assessed first to identify signs of internal trauma such as bleeding. Clients with colds, small lacerations on the head, diarrhea and mild stomach pain need attention but are not priorities.

64. **Answer C**. 500 mg/100 mg x 5 = 25 mL; 1 teaspoon is equal to 5 mL. Hence, 25 mL divided by 5 = 5 teaspoons.

65. **Answer B**. The immediate goal is to remove the drug to prevent further absorption and poisoning. Starting an IV line, administering acetylcysteine and blood draw are important but not the first intervention.

66. **Answer D**. A blood glucose level of 40 mg/dL indicates severe hypoglycemia. Severe hypoglycemia is a serious condition that can lead to irreversible brain damage.

67. **Answer D**. Addison's disease is characterized by low blood pressure. However, a blood pressure of 85/60 mmHg requires immediate attention and may need evaluation of the client's cortisol levels. Severe lack of adrenal hormones can lead to a fatal Addisonian crisis.

68. **Answer B**. 2000 mL x 10 divided by 6 hours x 60 minutes = 55.5 gtts/minute = 56 gtts/minute.

69. **Answer D**. Stress can increase the demand for cortisol. A client with Addison's disease has a shortage of the cortisol hormones and will be unable to adapt to a stressful environment. If cortisol levels drop severely, this can lead to a life-threatening adrenal crisis. Hypoglycemia, not hyperglycemia, is common in Addison's disease.

70. **Answer B**. Ranitidine is a histamine 2 antagonist and works by suppressing the production of hydrochloric acid. Antacids neutralize the acidity of the stomach. Sucralfate coats the stomach lining to protect from acid production.

71. **Answer D**. A client taking disulfiram should avoid products containing alcohol such as mouthwashes, aftershave gel and backrub lotions. Adhesive bandage does not contain alcohol and can be safely used.

72. **Answer C**. The nurse should directly ask the client if there is any plan of actually carrying out the suicide attempt. The possibility of a suicide is higher if the client has thought of a way on how to perform the act.

73. **Answer B.** This response shows empathy and understanding of the client's concerns. Choice A is a defensive response that is not helpful. Choice C is not correct as the client already stated about being worried of the results of the biopsy. Asking the client how the condition started does not address the client's feelings.

74. **Answer C.** The client's CD_4 cell count is very low and is diagnostic of AIDS. Immunosuppression can lead to serious infections in a client with AIDS. The client's weight loss needs to be addressed but the risk for infection is the first priority.

75. **Answer C**. Performance appraisal should create an atmosphere of respect and constructive feedback. Behavior that led to poor performance is not the focus. When managers look forward to future plans and actions, the appraisal process turns into a productive session for the staff.

Index

Made in the USA
Middletown, DE
14 July 2019